Bone Regulatory Factors
Morphology, Biochemistry,
Physiology, and Pharmacology

NATO ASI Series

Advanced Science Institutes Series

A series presenting the results of activities sponsored by the NATO Science Committee, which aims at the dissemination of advanced scientific and technological knowledge, with a view to strengthening links between scientific communities.

The series is published by an international board of publishers in conjunction with the NATO Scientific Affairs Division

A	**Life Sciences**	Plenum Publishing Corporation
B	**Physics**	New York and London
C	**Mathematical and Physical Sciences**	Kluwer Academic Publishers
		Dordrecht, Boston, and London
D	**Behavioral and Social Sciences**	
E	**Applied Sciences**	
F	**Computer and Systems Sciences**	Springer-Verlag
G	**Ecological Sciences**	Berlin, Heidelberg, New York, London,
H	**Cell Biology**	Paris, and Tokyo

Recent Volumes in this Series

Series A: Life Sciences

Bone Regulatory Factors
Morphology, Biochemistry, Physiology, and Pharmacology

Edited by

Antonio Pecile

University of Milan
Milan, Italy

and

Benedetto de Bernard

University of Trieste
Trieste, Italy

Plenum Press
New York and London
Published in cooperation with NATO Scientific Affairs Division

Proceedings of a NATO Advanced Study Institute on
Advances in Bone Regulatory Factors:
Morphology, Biochemistry, Physiology, and Pharmacology,
held May 2–12, 1989,
in Erice, Sicily, Italy

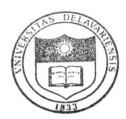

QP
88
.2
, N37
1989

Library of Congress Cataloging in Publication Data

NATO Advanced Study Institute on Advances in Bone Regulatory Factors: Morphology, Biochemistry, Physiology, and Pharmacology (1989: Erice, Italy)
  Bone regulatory factors: morphology, biochemistry, physiology, and pharmacology / edited by Antonio Pecile and Benedetto de Bernard.
     p.   cm.—(NATO ASI series. Series A, Life sciences; v. 184)
  "Proceedings of a NATO Advanced Study Institute on Advances in Bone Regulatory Factors: Morphology, Biochemistry, Physiology, and Pharmacology, held May 2–12, 1989, in Erice, Sicily, Italy."—T.p. verso.
  "Published in cooperation with NATO Scientific Affairs Division."
  Includes bibliographical references.
  ISBN 0-306-43500-4
  1. Bones—Growth—Regulation—Congresses. 2. Growth factors—Congresses. 3. Bones—Pathophysiology—Congresses. 4. Biomineralization—Regulation—Congresses. I. Pecile, A. (Antonio) II. De Bernard, Benedetto. III. North Atlantic Treaty Organization. Scientific Affairs Division. IV. Title. V. Series.
  [DNLM: 1. Bone and Bones—physiology—congresses. WE 200 N279b 1989]
QP88.2.N37   1989
612.7'5—dc20
DNLM/DLC   90-6777
for Library of Congress   CIP

© 1990 Plenum Press, New York
A Division of Plenum Publishing Corporation
233 Spring Street, New York, N.Y. 10013

PREFACE

This book includes all lectures presented at Erice during the NATO
ASI Course on Advances in Bone Regulatory Factors. It covers morphological, chemical, biochemical, physiological and pathophysiological aspects of bone formation and resorption, focusing on
regulatory factors and indicating the new directions that are opening
up.

The physicochemical principles of biomineralization are reviewed,
with particular attention to the crystal nucleation and growth. The
studies on embryology of calcified tissues confirm that embryonic
cartilage and bone involve differently competent ectomesenchyme cells
and that a sequential endogenous developmental program for regulatory
factors may be critical in the autocrine and/or paracrine regulation
of cartilage and bone formation. The morphological and quantitative
aspects of bone formation and mineralization concern bone cells, bone
calcification and bone matrix formation and resorption, with emphasis
on osteoblast maturation into osteocytes or lining cells, structure-
function relationships in osteocytes and osteoclasts, alkaline
phosphatase and tartrate-resistant acid phosphatase activities; the
role of collagen fibrils, non-collageneous proteins and matrix
vesicles in bone calcification; the relationship between inorganic
substance and crystal ghosts and osteoclast-osteoblast coupling.
Three points of the osteogenetic process are illustrated in most
detail: 1) osteoblast dynamics; 2) the osteoblast-osteocyte transformation; 3) osteoblast control of collagen orientation.

The biochemistry of the intercellular matrix is presented to indicate
modifications of cells and matrix components before mineralization.
The properties of membrane proteins and glycoproteins, matrix proteoglycans and alkaline phosphatase are considered in depth. The role of
bone morphogenic proteins and especially of osteogenin in the induction of bone is treated exhaustively. Classical bone regulatory
factors are examined and particularly: the vitamin D endocrine system
as regulator of calcium absorption and bone cell metabolism; PTH as
modulator of osteoblasts and osteoclasts activities; calcitonin as
responsible for the maintenance of bone mass, mainly by inhibiting
osteoclasts activity. The critical review of methods to evaluate the
biological activities of bone regulatory factors is intended to serve
as a basis for new research proposals, to improve the results and to
consider the entire spectrum of factors or drugs active on bone and
mineral metabolism. The emerging data on calcium regulating hormone-

like peptides, which are suggested to be neuromodulators in brain behavioural control, are also discussed.

The pathophysiology of bone formation and resorption is illustrated through the characteristic features of primary hyperparathyroidism, hypoparathyroidism, Paget's bone disease, marble bone disease and the various kinds of osteoporosis and osteomalacia. The treatment of bone diseases with bone regulatory factors is discussed, giving due space also to the therapeutic use of estrogens for postmenopausal osteoporosis and of fluoride or diphosphonates for different bone pathologic conditions.

The book is an essential up-to-date reference for future research, urgently needed in the area of hard tissue physiology and pathology.

We take this opportunity to thank the NATO Scientific Affairs Committee for its support. The contribution of the Centro Nazionale delle Ricerche (C.N.R.) of Italy is also acknowledged. Warm thanks are also due to Sclavo S.p.A. for their financial contribution.
We wish to thank each of the lecturers and ASI participants for their efforts in making the Course a success.
We thank the International School of Pharmacology for housing the Course at the "Ettore Majorana Centre for Scientific Culture" at Erice, admirably directed. In a very real sense, the unique organizational skills of Dr. Maria Luisa Pecile have been crucial to the success of the Course.

A. Pecile
B. de Bernard

ACKNOWLEDGEMENTS

DIRECTORS

A. Pecile, Head of the Dept. of Pharmacology, Chemotherapy and Medical Toxicology, University of Milan, Italy

B. De Bernard, Head of the Dept. of Biochemistry, Biophysics and Chemistry of Macromolecules, University of Trieste, Italy

ORGANIZING COMMITTEE

A. Pecile, Professor of Pharmacology, University of Milan, Italy

B. De Bernard, Professor of Biochemistry, University of Trieste, Italy

D.H. Copp, Professor of Physiology, University of British Columbia, Vancouver, Canada

J.M. Zanelli, Ph.D., National Institute for Biological Standards & Control, Potters Bar, Herts, U.K.

SECRETARY

Maria Luisa Pecile, International Congresses & Courses Secretariat, Department of Pharmacology, Chemotherapy and Medical Toxicology, University of Milan, Italy

CONTENTS

PHYSICO-CHEMICAL PRINCIPLES OF BIOMINERALIZATION

Edward D. Eanes

National Institute of Dental Research
Bone Research Branch Research Associate Program
National Institute of Standards and Technology
Gaithersburg, Maryland

INTRODUCTION

Fundamental physico-chemical knowledge of the mineral components in skeletal tissues has increased substantially during the 3 decades since the publication of Neuman and Neuman's (1958) pioneering treatise on this subject. In particular, the dominant apatitic phase has become especially well characterized in terms of its chemical, structural, and morphological features. Substantial progress has also been made in our understanding of the dynamics of calcium phosphate precipitation in aqueous synthetic and in vitro systems. Less complete, however, is our knowledge of the actual deposition processes by which the bony extracellular matrix is invested with these mineral salts in vivo. Even though early notions of biomineral formation as merely a mass action effect has been supplanted by more sophisticated appreciation of the multistep complexities of the process, a fully proper understanding of biomineral deposition still eludes our grasp. Principally for this reason, the more dynamic aspects of biomineralization have received increased research emphasis in recent years. Moreover, much of this research has been directed toward better elucidating the physical and chemical bases for the subtle interplay between the bone cells, the extracellular matrix components, and the tissue fluid environment which initiate and regulate mineral formation in vivo. This paper reviews our current knowledge in this area as well as discusses deficiencies in this knowledge that could profitably be the foci for future research. Particular emphasis is placed on the physico-chemical principles of nucleation and growth and how the application of these principles, together with our present knowledge on the ultrastructural properties of bone mineral, has provided valuable insight into the bioorganic control of the calcification process.

MINERAL NUCLEATION -- GENERAL CONSIDERATIONS

The first step in mineral formation whether in vivo or in synthetic solutions, is the formation of a stable nucleus, which can be defined as the smallest cluster of ions of the precipitated phase capable of survival and growth as a crystal. A necessary thermodynamic condition for nuclei formation is that the reactant ions in solution exceed the equilibrium free

energy (i.e. solubility) of the precipitated phase (Walton, 1967).
Otherwise, such clusters, if they form at all, would rapidly dissolve.
However, supersaturation alone is no guarantee that nucleation will occur.
An additional barrier to nucleation is imposed by the fact that during the
initial sub-nucleus stage of cluster formation the energy expended in
creating the cluster surface (i.e., the interfacial energy) exceeds the
energy released by ion bonding within the cluster (i.e., the volume free
energy) (Nielsen, 1964; Walton, 1967). For a sparingly soluble salt such
as apatite, relatively high surface energies can make this barrier quite
large. This excess energy requirement must be lowered substantially if
nucleation is to take place in a timely manner. One way this can be
accomplished is by raising the cluster volume free energy through
increasing the supersaturation. Classical nucleation theory (Nielsen,
1964; Walton, 1967) predicts that when the energy barrier is lowered in
this manner a critical supersaturation is reached below which the solutions
are quite stable but above which the onset of precipitation is very rapid.
Precipitation initiated in this way is said to be homogeneously nucleated.

However, the initial precipitate formed by homogeneous nucleation is
not always the most thermodynamically stable phase possible. This is
strikingly illustrated in synthetic preparations of apatite. Although
apatite would normally be the expected phase under basic pH conditions, the
first solids to form by homogeneous precipitation are often amorphous in
nature (Eanes et al., 1965; Eanes and Posner, 1965). These amorphous
calcium phosphates (ACP) are considerably more soluble than apatite , and
in time will transform into the latter. At pH 9 and above, this
transformation is direct, but below this pH the reaction becomes even more
complicated with an octacalcium phosphate (OCP)-like crystalline
intermediate developing before the apatite phase appears (Eanes and Meyer,
1977; Meyer and Eanes, 1978). These highly hydrated phases occur in
preference to apatite because, although less stable thermodynamically, they
apparently have much lower surface energies which reduces the net energy
required for their _de novo_ formation to below that for anhydrous apatite.

The critical supersaturation value marks the upper limit of stability
for supersaturated solutions. However, the presence of foreign solids in
these solutions often have a strong destabilizing influence, lowering the
nucleation threshold to values considerably below that required for
homogeneous precipitation (Walton, 1967). In almost every case, the solids
act to reduce interfacial energy requirements by providing advantageous
sites for nucleation on their surfaces. The most effective heterogeneous
nucleators have two surface properties in common: a strong affinity for
the ions being precipitated, and a topology closely matching that of the
precipitated surface. Both of the properties are of equal importance. If
ion/substrate affinity is high but the positions of the adsorbed ions on
the surface of the substrate do not closely match their normal lattice
arrangement, then the surface activation energy needed to shift them into
this arrangement will be too great for local ordering into a stable nuclei
to occur. This is the major reason why many high affinity biomolecules
such as Ca-binding proteins make poor nucleators. Although strongly
adsorbed, the reactant ions are incorrectly positioned on these
biomolecules for nucleus formation. On the other hand, the lattice match
between the precipitating phase and the substrate may be favorable for
nucleation but the adsorptive forces are too weak to hold the ions on the
surface long enough for them to desolvate and bind together into stable
clusters capable of crystal growth. Collagen fibers may possibly be an
example of this latter situation. Although collagen can adsorb relatively
large amounts of PO_4 (150 moles P/mole collagen) with some becoming
possibly covalently bonded, Ca^{2+} binding to collagen is relatively weak and
easily dissociable (Glimcher, 1976).

The dimensions of an apatite nucleus, being dependent upon such factors as supersaturation and substrate properties, are difficult to determine exactly, but are probably of the order of 1-2 nm (Eanes and Posner, 1970), considerably smaller than the smallest known apatite crystals such as those found in bone ($\approx$10-50 nm). Therefore, the subsequent growth of the initial nucleus accounts for the bulk of the crystal's mass. Crystal growth, in general, occurs by two primary mechanisms : screw dislocation propagation and two-dimensional (2D) surface nucleation (Walton, 1967). Very small crystals such as bone apatite probably grow via the second mechanism as they don't possess the proper type of dislocations required for the first (Nielsen, 1964). In 2D nucleation, the crystal grows by successive layering of the reactant ions, with each layer initiated by a nucleation event on the surface of the previously deposited layer. The initial nucleation step for each layer can be looked upon as a special form of heterogenous nucleation. But since the substrate is identical, both in structure and composition, to the forming surface cluster, the supersaturation required for growth, although non-zero because of the edge energy of the growing cluster, is generally much lower than that required to form the primary crystal nucleus. The expectation, therefore, is for growth to dominate the precipitation reaction once a few primary nuclei are formed. However, this situation is generally not observed in synthetic preparations of apatite. Instead, what occurs more frequently is a proliferation of numerous, uniformly small crystals similar to those seen in bone, rather than the development of a few large ones (Eanes and Posner, 1970).

The exact reason for polycrystalline apatite growth is not known. One possibility is that it arises from an aberration of the surface-nucleated growth process sometimes known as secondary nucleation (Garside, 1982). A characteristic feature of this type of nucleation is that the growing crystal upon reaching a certain initial size becomes shape unstable and branches into satellite or daughter crystals (Cahn, 1967). One condition under which this type of dendritic instability can develop is moderate to high supersaturation where growth occurs so rapidly that it becomes diffusion limited, i.e. the rate of ion accretion at surface growth sites becomes controlled by the ion transport capacity of the growth medium. Because of the nature of the diffusion fields and concentration gradients surrounding small crystals at these supersaturations, as the crystal faces enlarge with growth, regions near edges and corners become more accessible to solute ions than the center of the faces. The result is more frequent layering at these locations promoting growth in new directions.

One weakness in the above explanation is that diffusion limited polycrystalline growth should be insensitive to surface controlling factors, which is contrary to observation. As an example, many substances present even in very small amounts in the growth medium (e.g. $P_2O_7^{4-}$) can slow appreciably the growth process (Meyer, 1984). These substances, however, act not by controlling diffusion but by interfering with the incorporation of the reactant ions into the surface layer.

An alternative explanation, but one which would be operative only in solutions supersaturated with respect to OCP as well as apatite, is that proliferative, polycrystalline apatite growth is the consequence of two opposing solution factors (Eanes, 1985) : solution supersaturation which, as described earlier, favors OCP formation, and solution pH which facilitates in situ hydrolysis of OCP into apatite. Since OCP can readily form on apatite crystal surfaces (Nelson et al., 1986), 2D surface nucleation and growth becomes a two-phase, three step process of epitaxial OCP nucleation, growth, and hydrolytic transformation to a double-thick

3

apatite layer. However, x-ray diffraction evidence (Eanes and Meyer, 1977; Brown et al., 1979) that interlayers of the two phases occur in OCP-hydrolyzed apatite indicates that this last step is not always completed before the next overgrowth takes place. Because the structural arrangements of the two phases, although close, are not exact, such interlayering could result in internal lattice stresses which, in turn, would lead to fracturing and separation into smaller crystals. One should bear in mind, however, that this two-phase explanation as well as the diffusion-controlled one discussed earlier are still largely speculative, and that a more complete understanding of polycrystalline apatite formation awaits further experimental details.

MINERAL FORMATION IN VIVO -- GENERAL COMMENTS

All extracellular fluids in equilibrium with serum are supersaturated with respect to apatite, and possibly to OCP as well (Eidelman et al., 1987). Although not sufficiently supersaturated for homogeneous nucleation, these fluids bathe a variety of bioorganic structures whose surfaces could potentially serve as substrates for heterogeneous nucleation. It is remarkable, then, that the body has the ability to restrict mineralization to skeletal and other selected tissues under such potentially unstable systemic supersaturated conditions. Indeed, the latency for soft-tissue calcification is amply illustrated by many pathophysiological examples.

One commonly advanced hypothesis to account for the ability of soft-tissue fluids to remain metastable is that they are normally prevented from mineralizing by the local production and/or systemic circulation of potent nucleation inhibitors, e.g. $P_2O_7^{4-}$, (Meyer, 1984). To effect mineralization, these inhibitors must first be enzymatically broken down and removed. Furthermore, in skeletal tissues such inhibitor inactivation would have to be very selective, both temporally and spatially, to account for the orderly fashion in which mineral deposition occurs in these tissues.

However, once inhibitors are deactivated and/or removed, one of two additional events must occur before precipitation can commence : either local solute concentrations must be raised to homogeneous nucleation levels or suitable substrates must be present or provided for heterogeneous nucleation at humoral solute concentrations. Each of these two factors appear to have a role in skeletal tissue calcification.

HOMOGENEOUS NUCLEATION IN VIVO

The local tissue elevation of supersaturation needed for homogeneous nucleation requires substantial increases in the free solute concentrations of the reactant ions. Passive processes such as ion-binding to extracellular biomolecules, although capable of appreciably increasing total ion levels in some tissues, cannot of themselves bring about such supersaturation changes. When matrix fluids are in equilibrium with the serum compartment, ion complexing often will not measurably affect free solute levels at all. Even in cartilage, where proteoglycan binding can increase total Ca^{2+} up to 9 times the levels in synovial fluid, and Donnan equilibrium effects correspondingly increase free solute Ca^{2+} twofold, offsetting decreases in solute PO_4 leaves the supersaturation essentially unchanged (Maroudas, 1979). Similarly, Ca^{2+}-releasing enzymatic processes such as degradation of high Ca^{2+} affinity biomolecules into less ion selective fragments, are probably equally ineffective in raising the supersaturation. Diffusion coefficients in calcifiable matrices like those

4

found in cartilage, although less than one-half their free solution values (Maroudas, 1979), are still sufficiently large that diffusion would dissipate local ion accumulations from sites of such metabolic activity as rapidly as they occur.

However, there is good experimental evidence for active membrane transport processes locally raising free Ca^{2+} and PO_4 concentrations to precipitable levels in vivo. The best documented example of such facilitated precipitation occurs in mitochondria where mineral deposition within the interior spaces of these intracellular organelles have been clearly linked to countergradient ion transport across their outer membranes (Lehninger, 1970). That these transmembrane ion movements were sufficient to achieve critical supersaturation is evidenced by the ACP-like nature of the deposits. Although such intramitochondrial precipitation frequently occurs in cells of mineralizing tissues (e.g. growth-plate chondrocytes (Sutfin et al., 1971)) and possibly provides a ready store of Ca^{2+} and PO_4 for extracellular calcification, there is no compelling experimental evidence that intact particles from these deposits find their way directly into the extracellular matrix. Such active, membrane-driven mineralization appears to be primarily associated with cytosolic Ca^{2+} regulation.

MATRIX VESICLE CALCIFICATION

An even more intensively studied example of biomineral formation where membranes and their associate transport processes possibly play a key role is matrix vesicle calcification. The reason for such intense interest is that these cell-derived, membrane-bound vesicular structures appear to be the extracellular loci for initial mineral deposition in many skeletal tissues (Bonucci, 1967; Anderson, 1969; Katchburian, 1973; Yamada, 1976; Bab et al., 1979), with the first identifiable crystals in these tissues appearing in the aqueous interiors of the vesicles. By providing such protected enclosures for initial nucleation and growth, matrix vesicles appear to give hard tissue cells the means to directly control the mineralization process and integrate it with other cellular functions such as extracellular matrix production and organization.

Matrix vesicles can accumulate appreciable Ca^{2+} and PO_4 in their interior spaces before the first mineral crystals are observed (Wuthier, 1977). Although a large fraction of the PO_4 may come from cytosolic sources at the time the vesicles are formed from the plasma membrane, most of the accumulation, especially that of Ca^{2+}, appear to occur after the vesicles are released into the extracellular matrix. Such Ca^{2+} and PO_4 accumulations (50-100 and 30-50 mM, respectively, (Wuthier, 1977)) would have had to gain entry, then, by passage across the vesicular membrane from extracellular sources. However, the exact manner and extent of involvement of the various vesicular membrane transport processes in sequestering these ions is still not fully elucidated. Even though the reactants far exceed in total concentrations their corresponding extracellular fluid levels, it is unlikely that energy-dependent enzymatic pumps of the type that are responsible for mitochondrial ion uptake are involved in vesicle transport. One mitigating factor is that ATP energy sources for driving such pumps become scarce once the vesicles detach themselves from the cell. Another factor is that the Ca^{2+} pumps in the vesicle membrane are derived from the plasma membrane without inversion (Wuthier, 1982). Thus, if operative, they would remove Ca^{2+} from the vesicle interior, rather than add Ca^{2+} to it. On the other hand, the finding that Ca^{2+} uptake is accompanied by intravesicular Na^+ and K^+ exchanges (Wuthier, 1977) suggest that membrane proteins or proteolipids may passively transport and release Ca^{2+} into the vesicle interior by ionophore-like, cation exchange mechanisms.

5

It is not clear what level of supersaturation is established by the passage of extracellular Ca^{2+} and PO_4 ions across the vesicular membrane. This assessment is complicated by the uncertainty in the fraction of these ions that are complexed with proteins in the vesicle interior and with membrane lipid. Also, the apparent lack of energy-dependent pumping mechanisms poses problems as to how the detached vesicle is able to sustain whatever free Ca^{2+} and PO_4 levels that may have existed at the time of separation from the cell. Particularly important in this regard is the fate of the free PO_4 that may have initially been provided by the cytosol. Studies with model membrane and liposome systems (Eanes and Costa, 1983; Eanes et al., 1984) suggest that with the level of PO_4 present in the interior at the time the vesicle is released from the cell membrane (≈ 25 mM), extracellular Ca^{2+} entry by passive ion exchange may be sufficient to establish a state of critical supersaturation if this initial PO_4 level does not decrease by leakage from the vesicle. Unfortunately, the presence of ACP-like precursor phases prior to the appearance of the first crystals, evidence that would support this conjecture, has not been conclusively demonstrated.

The option, therefore, must be kept open that the first crystals formed inside the vesicles were heterogeneously nucleated. The TEM observation (Anderson, 1976; Morris et al., 1983) that these crystals are often closely associated with the vesicle membrane in vivo suggest that sites favorable for nucleation may be present on the inner membrane surface. The membrane constituent most often suggested as best suited for establishing the proper substrate for nucleation is phosphatidylserine (PS) (Boskey, 1981; Wuthier, 1982). There is marked enrichment of this lipid in the vesicle membrane compared to the plasma membrane, and most of this extra PS appears to localize in the inside lipid layer as a complex with both Ca^{2+} and PO_4. However, such complexes alone do not appear to be sufficient to establish a nucleation site. In in vitro systems, free-standing PS-Ca-PO_4 complexes are very slow nucleators of metastable solutions (Boskey and Posner, 1977; Wuthier, 1982). Although efficient Ca^{2+} and PO_4 binders, they appear not to have the correct spatial geometry inducive for forming stable nuclei. Studies with the calcifying microorganism Bacterionema matruchotii (Boyan-Salyers et al., 1978) show that it is possible that PS-Ca-PO_4 complexes can only become actively involved in nucleation when they become tightly bound with small hydrophobic membrane proteins to form larger proteo-lipid complexes whose surface topology may better match the lattice geometry of the nucleus.

In addition to the uncertainty as to the exact manner by which the first mineral in matrix vesicles is formed, i.e. whether it is by homo- or heterogeneous nucleation, there is also some question as to the nature of the initial crystalline phase seen. Although the first observable crystals are commonly assumed to be stable apatite, recent infrared evidence (Sauer and Wuthier, 1988) suggest that OCP may possibly form preferentially. The formation of OCP does not necessarily imply that intravesicular supersaturation is higher than that for the extracellular fluids surrounding the vesicles. The slight supersaturation that is observed in serum ultrafiltrate (Eidelman et al., 1987) may be adequate for intravesicular OCP formation if the internal substrates are particularly effective in reducing the interfacial energy barrier to nucleation. Another factor favoring OCP nucleation is that it has a much lower intrinsic surface free energy to begin with than apatite (Brown, 1966).

The first-formed crystals seen in the vesicle interior represent only a very small fraction of the total crystalline mass associated with matrix vesicle calcification. The bulk of the crystals occur subsequently outside the vesicles. The observation (Anderson, 1980) that the first of these extravesicular crystals cluster in the fluid space immediately adjacent to the vesicle surface suggest that the interior crystals played a role in their formation. Although enzymatic disruption of the vesicle membrane is a possibility, liposome model studies (Eanes et al., 1984; Eanes and Hailer, 1985) suggest that the interior crystals can gain access to the extravesicular space simply by physically breaching the bilayer structure. The exposed crystals then either continue growing or, as the TEM appearance of the clusters would suggest (Akisaka et al., 1988; Arsenault et al., 1988), seed directly new crystals, possibly by one of the polycrystalline nucleation mechanisms described earlier. Polycrystalline growth would also account for the observed proliferative, spherulitic expansion of the crystalline mass away from the vesicle surface into the body of the extracellular matrix.

An interesting feature of extravesicular mineral formation is that the crystals progressively expand within an extracellular fluid environment presumably protected from extraneous precipitation by inhibitors of apatite nucleation and growth. Either the inhibitors are non-functional in this case because they provide protection only from primary de novo crystal nucleation and do not protect against secondary nucleation or they are cleared away from the path of growth. Alkaline phosphatase (AP), an enzyme markedly enriched in matrix vesicle-containing tissues, may be a vital element in this latter process by destroying inhibitors such as $P_2O_7^{4-}$ which can continuously diffuse into areas of active mineralization (Wuthier and Register, 1985). Another possible barrier to proliferative crystal expansion are macromolecular matrix species such as proteoglycans and anionic proteins which are capable of impeding apatite growth in vitro (Blumental et al., 1979; Termine et al., 1980). Whether they totally inhibit growth in vivo and, therefore, must be modified or removed for mineral expansion to occur, or simply act to modulate the kinetics of the expansion remains to be clarified.

COLLAGEN CALCIFICATION -- FIRST STAGE

Mineral deposition in a few hard tissues such as calcified growth plate cartilage appears to be controlled almost entirely by the matrix vesicle mechanism just described. Little, if any, of the mineral in these tissues is observed associated with non-vesicular components such as collagen. In other tissues such as intramembranous bone, mantle dentin and calcified turkey leg tendon both collagenous as well as vesicular mineral deposits occur. Moreover, the two types of deposits in the turkey tendon frequently exist in close association, sometimes with no clear demarcation between them (Landis, 1985). This latter observation suggests that in these instances the vesicular deposits, which usually formed first, may have triggered the mineralization of the collagen fibers. However, the unique periodic pattern of axial and lateral mineralization seen in the turkey collagen fibers is evidence that the fibers were not simply invaded by a relentless multiplicative expansion of vesicular-spawned crystals. Instead the crystals, upon contacting the fiber surface, most likely stimulated a separate, secondary chain of nucleation and growth events as discussed more fully in the next section.

In bone tissues, however, such a connection between matrix vesicles, even when present, and collagen calcification has not been established. This raises the possibility that the first crystals associated with the collagen phase in these tissues are formed de novo. Since the fluid phase surrounding the collagen fibers is not sufficiently supersaturated for homogeneous nucleation, the inference is that these first crystals are heterogeneously nucleated on substrates in the collagenous matrix. Considerable evidence suggest, however, that collagen fibers alone are not responsible for this primary nucleation. They bind Ca^{2+} weakly (Glimcher, 1976), their crystallographic parameters do not match those of apatite

(Schiffmann et al., 1970), and when highly purified, they have proven to be poor catalysts for apatite growth in vitro (Eanes, 1985).

The most plausible hypothesis for de novo collagen mineralization is that one or more non-collagenous matrix macromolecules, either by themselves or in association with the collagen fibers, define the localized surface necessary for the initial heterogeneous nucleation step. A number of anionic non-collagenous proteins (NCPs), e.g., osteonectin (Termine et al., 1981), phosphoproteins (Veis, 1985), and γ-carboxyglutamate-containing proteins (Price et al., 1976; Hauschka, 1985), have been proposed to fill this role. These various NCPs appear to have been suggested, in part, because they are all good Ca^{2+} binders, an essential although apparently not a very exclusive criterion for heterogeneous nucleation. But to be effective nucleators, NCPs must also satisfy the second criterion for heterogeneous nucleation : that their active surface conformation closely match structurally, and complement electrically, the contiguous surface of the overlying crystal nucleus. Fulfilling these latter conditions apparently requires that the molecules in turn be securely anchored to the surface of the collagen fiber. When freely suspended in solution, NCPs behave as inhibitors rather than as promoters of apatite crystal growth in vitro, presumably by binding to and thereby blocking access of solution ions to surface growth sites (Diamond and Neuman, 1979; Termine et al., 1980; Doi et al., 1989). On the other hand, preadsorption onto the surfaces of solid biopolymeric substrates such as agarose enables NCPs to adopt a molecular conformation capable of inducing mineral formation in metastable calcium phosphate solutions (Linde et al., 1989). At least two of the above listed NCPs, osteonectin (Termine et al., 1981) and dentin phosphoprotein (Veis, 1985), appear to have the high affinity for collagen consonant with the second nucleation requirement.

It is not known whether the adsorbed NCPs function alone and the collagen is merely a supporting phase or whether the two phases together in some way define the nucleating site. If this second possibility occurs, the most probable location would be the region of solution-exposed collagen surface at the boundary with an adsorbed NCP molecule. At this location, the Ca^{2+} ions bound to the edge of the NCP molecule would lie on the same surface as collagen-adsorbed PO_4 ions. If these edge sites are correctly positioned in relation to the surface PO_4 locations, then the close juxtaposition of the two reactants could possibly result in the formation of a critical cluster on the collagen surface. In fact, Ca^{2+} and PO_4 ions probably come into closer surface contact with each other at the NCP-collagen boundary than they would on the anionic, PO_4-repelling surface of the NCP itself. For nucleation to occur on this latter surface, the PO_4 would have to be complexed as a second layer to the substrate-bound Ca^{2+} ions, a kinetically more complicated and possibly less favorable route to crystal formation than edge nucleation.

Little specifically is known about where on the collagen fibers the NCPs are situated. The finding that the first mineral crystals in collagen appear in the hole zones would indicate that those NCPs involved in the primary nucleation process would be located in this region. Also unknown is the exact molecular conformation of the adsorbed NCP molecules. Traub et al. (1985) have postulated that the compact surface regularity of proteins in antiparallel ß-pleated sheet conformations is well suited as a substrate for crystal nucleation. The lack of direct evidence for ß-sheet structures in collagenous matrices does not exclude this possibility. Even NCPs with low intrinsic ß-structure could possibly convert into this conformation upon interaction with the collagen surface. Another question that is not fully answered is whether the nucleation sites on the collagen fibers are formed at the time the fibers are assembled and later are uncovered by removal of inhibitors or protective substances, or whether site preparation and nucleation are concurrent events. The observation (Weinstock and Leblond, 1973) that certain NCPs, e.g. dentin phosphoproteins, are directly transported to and concentrate in newly mineralized areas suggest that substrate activation and crystal nucleation, if not concurrent, are closely coordinated in some hard tissue.

COLLAGEN CALCIFICATION -- SECOND STAGE

Once collagenous mineralization is initiated, whether de novo or by matrix vesicles, the mineral spreads throughout the fibers in an orderly, progressive manner by the multiplicative proliferation of many small plate-like crystals, all of which are of nearly the same size. This spread occurs initially in and around the hole zone, where the first crystals are usually observed, then extends into the overlap regions until the entire aqueous space of the fiber is filled with crystals.

Although the spatial pattern of this spread has been known for some time (Glimcher, 1959; Nylen et al., 1960), the underlying mineralization mechanism is still not well understood. The proliferative invasion of the crystalline mass from primary foci suggest that the crystals at the leading edge of this expansion are propagated by the crystals immediately preceding them. It is not known, however, whether this occurs directly by secondary nucleation or indirectly by heterogeneous nucleation at sites in the matrix which are activated by the advancing crystal front. A possible mechanism for accomplishing this latter activation has not been established but presumably would involve surface configurational changes at the nucleating site induced by neighboring crystal/matrix interactions.

Another interesting but poorly understood feature of this proliferative pattern of mineralization is the high frequency in which the collagen-deposited crystals are aligned with their crystallographic c-axes parallel to the fiber axis (Engstrom and Zetterstrom, 1951). It is unlikely that these preferred alignments result from the crystals simply conforming to the spatial dimensions of the aqueous compartments within which they grow. More probably, the co-orientation is the consequence of direction-specific crystallochemical interactions between the crystals and the collagen surface. Less certain is the point in the growth process in which these interactions come into play. Orientation could occur as early as the nucleation stage. For instance, crystallochemical interactions may be too weak for oriented overgrowth except at sites of crystal nucleation such as NCP-collagen boundaries. However, c-axis growth would continue in the direction established by the orientation of the nuclei if the ion binding at these boundaries is sufficiently strong to keep the growing crystals from detaching from the collagen surface and rotating into other orientations. Another possibility is that the NCP-collagen surfaces control orientation during the entire nucleation and growth process, with c-axis growth continually constrained to the direction originally established at the nucleating site.

Alternatively, nucleation and orientation could be separate events dictated by different regions of the collagen surface. In this regards, a possibly important non-nucleating role of adsorbed NCPs would be to provide direction-specific anionic surfaces for constraining c-axis orientations to principally along the fiber axis. Growing crystals not already properly positioned would be brought into alignment by electrostatic interactions with these surfaces. Such realignments, however, would require that the interactions be strong enough to break any attachments holding the crystals in their original positions. Similar direction-constraining forces may also be operative in secondary-nucleated growth, if substrate interactions favor growth only of daughter nuclei with c-axes parallel to the fiber axis.

However, regardless of which of these factors, if any, control axial crystal orientation, the interactions responsible for them is less evident in directions normal to the fiber axis. Apatite crystals appear to be more randomly oriented in these lateral directions within the fiber than along its length.

As with many of its other features, the factors establishing the rate of collagen fiber mineralization are obscure. However, the sharp division between fully and sparsely mineralized fibers that marks the boundary with the osteoid zone suggests that, once started, mineralization of individual fibers in bone tissue occurs relatively rapidly compared to the overall advancement of the mineralization front. This discrepancy in rates can be taken as evidence that cellularly-controlled events such as matrix elaboration and maturation are the primary rate limiting factors in bone tissue mineralization.

CONCLUSION

In conclusion, the physico-chemical principles governing nucleation and growth of crystalline salts from aqueous solutions have provided a theoretical framework for understanding mineral deposition in skeletal tissues. Additionally, the ultrastructural features of the mineral crystals and of mineral/matrix relationships have offered important clues as to the physiological constraints on these physico-chemical processes. But as we have seen, many fundamental questions remain, especially those regarding crystallochemical interactions at the mineral/matrix interface which form the molecular-level basis for the regulation of bone mineral formation. Hopefully, by bringing into clearer focus some these ambiguities in this paper, we will be better able to address them experimentally in future research.

REFERENCES

Akisaka, T., Kawaguchi, H., Subita, G. P., Shigenaga, Y., and Gay,C. V., 1988, Ultrastructure of matrix vesicles in chick growth plate as revealed by quick freezing and freeze substitution., Calcif. Tissue Int., 42:383

Anderson, H. C., 1976, Matrix vesicles of cartilage and bone, in: "The Biochemistry and Physiology of Bone," G. H. Bourne, ed., Academic Press, New York.

Anderson, H. C., 1980, Calcification processes, Pathol. Annu., 15:45

Anderson, H. C., 1969, Vesicles associated with calcification in the matrix of epiphyseal cartilage., J. Cell Biol., 41:59

Arsenault, A. L., Ottensmeyer, F. P., and Heath, I. B., 1988, An electron microscopic and spectroscopic study of murine epiphyseal cartilage: analysis of fine structure and matrix vesicles preserved by slam freezing and freeze substitution., J. Ultrastruct. Mol. Struct. Res., 98:32

Bab, I. A., Muhlrad, A., and Sela, J., 1979, Ultrastructural and biochemical study of extracellular matrix vesicles in normal alveolar bones of rats., Cell Tiss. Res., 202:1

Blumenthal, N. C., Posner, A. S., Silverman, L. C., and Rosenberg, L. C., 1979, The effect of proteoglycans on in vitro hydroxyapatite formation., Calcif. Tissue Int., 27:75

Bonucci, E., 1967, Fine structure of early cartilage
     calcification, J. Ultrastruct. Res., 20:33
Boskey, A. L., 1981, Current concepts of the physiology and
     biochemistry of calcification., Clin. Orthop. Rel. Res.,
     157:225
Boskey, A. L., and Posner, A. S., 1977, The role of synthetic
     and bone extracted Ca-Phospholipid-PO$_4$ complexes in
     hydroxyapatite formation., Calcif. Tiss. Res., 23:251
Boyan-Salyers, B. D., Vogel, J. J., Riggan, L. J., Summers, F., and Howell,
     R. E., 1978, Application of a microbial model to biologic
     calcification, Metab. Bone Dis., 1:143
Brown, W. E., 1966, Crystal growth of bone mineral., Clin.
     Orthop. Rel. Res., 44:205
Brown, W. E., Schroeder, L. W., and Ferris, J. S., 1979,
     Interlayering of crystalline octacalcium phosphate and
     hydroxyapatite., J. Phys. Chem., 83:1385
Cahn, J. W., 1967, On the morphological stability of growing
     crystals, in: "Crystal Growth," H. S. Peiser, ed.,
     Pergamon Press Ltd., Oxford.
Diamond, A. G., and Neuman, W. F., 1979, Macromolecular
     inhibitors of calcium phosphate precipitation in bone.,
     in: "Vitamin K Metabolism and Vitamin K Dependent
     Proteins," J. W. Suttie, ed., University Park Press,
     Baltimore.
Doi, Y., Okuda, R., Takezawa, Y., Shibata, S., Moriwaki, Y.,
     Wakamatsu, N., Shimizu, N., Moriyama, K., and Shimokawa, H., 1989,
     Osteonectin inhibiting de novo formation of apatite in the presence
     of collagen., Calcif. Tissue Int., 44:200
Eanes, E. D., 1985, Dynamic aspects of apatite phases of
     mineralized tissues-model studies., in: "The Chemistry and
     Biology of Mineralized Tissues," W. T. Butler, ed.,
     EBSCO Media, Birmingham.
Eanes, E. D., and Costa, J. L., 1983, X-537A ionophore-mediated
     calcium transport and calcium phosphate formation in
     Pressman cells., Calcif. Tissue Int., 35:250
Eanes, E. D., Gillessen, I. H., and Posner, A. S., 1965,
     Intermediate states in the precipitation of
     hydroxyapatite., Nature, 208:365
Eanes, E. D., and Hailer, A. W., 1985, Liposome-mediated calcium
     phosphate formation in metastable solutions., Calcif.
     Tissue Int., 37:390
Eanes, E. D., Hailer, A. W., and Costa, J. L., 1984, Calcium
     phosphate formation in aqueous suspensions of
     multilamellar liposomes., Calcif. Tissue Int., 36:421
Eanes, E. D., and Meyer, J. L., 1977, The maturation of
     crystalline calcium phosphates in aqueous suspension at
     physiologic pH., Calcif. Tissue Res., 23:259
Eanes, E. D., and Posner, A. S., 1965, Kinetics and mechanism of
     conversion of noncrystalline calcium phosphate to
     crystalline hydroxyapatite., Trans. NY Acad. Sci., 28:233
Eanes, E. D., and Posner, A. S., 1970, A note on the crystal
     growth of hydroxyapatite precipitated from aqueous
     solutions., Mat. Res. Bull., 5:377
Eidelman, N., Chow, L. C., and Brown, W. E., 1987, Calcium
     phosphate saturation levels in ultrafiltered serum.,
     Calcif. Tissue Int., 40:71
Engstrom, A., and Zetterstrom, R., 1951, Studies on the
     ultrastructure of bone, Exp. Cell Res., 2:268
Garside, J., 1982, Nucleation, in: "Biological Mineralization
     and Demineralization.," G. H. Nancollas, ed., Springer-
     Verlag, Berlin.

Glimcher, M. J., 1959, Molecular biology of mineralized tissues with particular reference to bone., Rev. Mod. Phys., 31: 359

Glimcher, M. J., 1976, Composition, structure, and organization of bone and other mineralized tissues and the mechanism of calcification., in: "Handbook of Physiology-Endocrinology VII.," Williams and Wilkins Co., Baltimore.

Hauschka, P. V., 1985, Osteocalcin and its functional domains., in: "The Chemistry and Biology of Mineralized Tissues.," W. T. Butler, ed., EBSCO Media, Inc., Birmingham.

Katchburian, E., 1973, Membrane-bound bodies as initiators of mineralization of dentine., J. Anat., 116:285

Landis, W. J., 1985, Temporal sequence of mineralization in calcifying turkey leg tendon., in: "The Chemistry and Biology of Mineralized Tissues.," W. T. Butler, ed., EBSCO Media Inc., Birmingham.

Lehninger, A. L., 1970, Mitochondria and calcium ion transport., Biochem. J., 119:129

Linde, A., Lussi, A., and Crenshaw, M. A., 1989, Mineral induction by immobilized polyanionic proteins., Calcif. Tissue Int., 44:286

Maroudas, A., 1979, Physicochemical properties of articular cartilage., in: "Adult Articular Cartilage," M. A. R. Freeman, ed., Pitman Medical, Tunbridge Wells.

Meyer, J. L., 1984, Can biological calcification occur in the presence of pyrophosphate?, Arch. Biochem. Biophys., 231:1

Meyer, J. L., and Eanes, E. D., 1978, A thermodynamic analysis of the amorphous to crystalline calcium phosphate transformation., Calcif. Tissue Res., 25:59

Morris, D. C., Vaananen, H. K., and Anderson, H. C., 1983, Matrix vesicle calcification in rat epiphyseal growth plate cartilage prepared anhydrously for electron microscopy., Metab. Bone Dis., 5:131

Nelson, D. G. A., Salimi, H., and Nancollas, G. H., 1986, Octacalcium phosphate and apatite overgrowths: A crystallographic and kinetic study., J. Colloid Interface Sci., 110:32

Neuman, W. F., and Neuman, M. W., 1958, "The Chemical Dynamics of Bone Mineral," University of Chicago Press, Chicago.

Nielsen, A. E., 1964, "Kinetics of Precipitation," Pergamon Press, Oxford.

Nylen, M. U., Scott, D. B., and Mosley, V. M., 1960, Mineralization of turkey leg tendon. II. Collagen-mineral relations revealed by electron and x-ray microscopy, in: "Calcification in Biological Systems.," R. F. Sognnaes, ed., AAAS, Washington.

Price, P. A., Otsuka, A. S., Poser, J. W., Kristaponis, J., and Raman, N., 1976, Characterization of a γ-Carboxyglutamic acid-containing protein from bone., Proc. Natl. Acad. Sci. USA, 73:1447

Sauer, G. R., and Wuthier, R. E., 1988, Fourier transform infrared characterization of mineral phases formed during induction of mineralization by collagenase-released matrix vesicles in vitro., J. Biol. Chem., 263:13718

Schiffmann, E., Martin, G. R., and Miller, E. J., 1970, Matrices that calcify, in: "Biological Calcification: Cellular and Molecular Aspects," H. Schraer, ed., Appleton-Century-Crofts, New York.

Sutfin, L. V., Holtrop, M. E., and Ogilvie, R. E., 1971, Microanalysis of individual mitochondrial granules with diameters less than 1000 A., Science, 174:947

12

Termine, J. D., Kleinman, H. K., Whitson, S. W., Conn, K. M., McGarvey, M. L., and Martin, G. R., 1981, Osteonectin, a bone-specific protein linking mineral to collagen., Cell, 26:99

Termine, J. D., Eanes, E. D., and Conn, K. M., 1980, Phosphoprotein modulation of apatite crystallization., Calcif. Tissue Int., 31:247

Traub, W., Jodaikin, A., and Weiner, S., 1985, Diffraction studies of enamel protein-mineral structural relations., in: "The Chemistry and Biology of Mineralized Tissues," W. T. Butler, ed., EBSCO Media, Inc., Birmingham.

Veis, A., 1985, Phosphoproteins of dentin and bone., in: "The Chemistry and Biology of Mineralized Tissues.," W. T. Butler, ed., EBSCO Media, Inc., Birmingham.

Walton, A. G., 1967, "The Formation and Properties of Precipitates," Interscience, New York.

Weinstock, M., and Leblond, C. P., 1973, Radioautographic visualization of the deposition of a phosphoprotein at the mineralization front in the dentin of the rat incisor., J. Cell Biol., 56:838

Wuthier, R. E., 1977, Electrolytes of isolated epiphyseal chondrocytes, matrix vesicles, and extracellular fluid., Calcif. Tissue Res., 23:125

Wuthier, R. E., 1982, A review of the primary mechanism of endochondral calcification with special emphasis on the role of cells, mitrochondria and matrix vesicles., Clin. Orthop., 169:219

Wuthier, R. E., 1982, The role of phospholipid-calcium-phosphate complexes in biological mineralization., in: "The Role of Calcium in Biological Systems.," L. J. Anghileri, and A. M. Tuffet-Anghileri, eds., CRC Press, Boca Raton.

Wuthier, R. E., and Register, T. C., 1985, Role of alkaline phosphatase, a polyfunctional enzyme, in mineralizing tissues., in: "The Chemistry and Biology of Mineralized Tissues," W. T. Butler, ed., EBSCO Media, Inc., Birmingham.

Yamada, M., 1976, Ultrastructural and cytochemical studies on the calcification of the tendon bone joint., Histol. Jap., 39:347

THE HISTOLOGY, HISTOCHEMISTRY, AND ULTRASTRUCTURE OF BONE

Ermanno Bonucci

Department of Human Biopathology, Section of Pathological Anatomy, La Sapienza University, Rome

INTRODUCTION

Bone is a composite tissue whose properties (mechanical and meta-bolic) closely depend on its structure and composition. Although its complexity is accentuated by the existence of different types and levels of tissue organization, knowledge of the histological, histochemical and ultrastructural characteristics of its individual components is funda-mental for understanding its physiological activities (modality of for-mation and resorption, mechanism of calcification, metabolic turnover) and pathological changes. Because the bone tissue consists of cells and intercellular matrix, these constituents will be considered separately.

THE CELLS OF THE BONE TISSUE

When the cells of the bone tissue are considered, it is necessary to differentiate the elements strictly pertaining to bone from those pertaining to bone marrow. Although these different cells are corre-lated, only the bone cells are considered in this chapter. Because of its function, also the osteoclast is considered a bone cell, although the presence of its progenitors in hematopoietic tissues (cfr. Vaes[1]) can rise doubts on the opportunity of this choice. Consequently, osteo-blasts, osteocytes, lining cells, and osteoclasts are considered in this chapter as the cellular elements of bone. The subject has been recently reviewed by Peck and Woods .

The osteoblast

The osteoblast is responsible for the synthesis and secretion of the organic constituents of the bone matrix and, to some extent, of their calcification. Moreover, they might release local factor(s) which probably mediate bone resorption (see below).

Osteoblasts are cuboidal or low columnar cells which either form a continuous layer on the growing osseous surfaces (Fig. 1, inset) or in

15

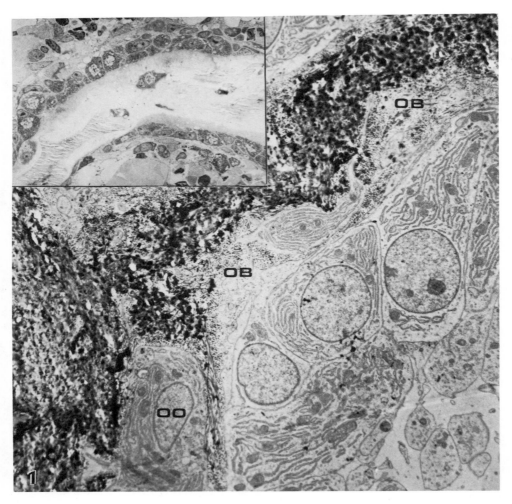

Fig. 1 - Border of an area of ossification: active osteoblasts with abundant granular endoplasmic reticulum, osteoid border (OB), and an osteoid osteocyte (OO) are visible; calcified matrix black. Uranyl acetate and lead citrate, x 7,000. Inset: osteoblasts along borders of a trabecula; note apparently empty cytoplasmic area corresponding to Golgi apparatus. Azure II - Methylene blue, x 250.

particular cases, such as in intramembranous ossification, encircle roundish bone areas. Part of its peripheral membrane is in contact with the osteoid border, that is, the not yet calcified matrix, and is in relationship with the calcification front, that is, the area of the osteoid border where mineralization occurs. These connections are favoured by many cytoplasmic processes which penetrate the uncalcified and calcifying matrix. The roundish nucleus is often polarized, that is, it is placed at the end of the cell farthest from the osteoid surface; the nucleolus is prominent. Because of the high RNA content, the wide cytoplasm is basophilic, excepting the wide Golgi area which is eosino-phylic or apparently empty and is frequently placed between the nucleus and that part of the cell which is in contact with the osteoid border (Fig. 1, inset).

Since the early studies of Cameron[3] and Dudley and Spiro[4], the ultrastructure of the osteoblast is well known (Fig. 1). As other cells actively engaged in protein synthesis, the osteoblast is chiefly charac- terized by the aboundant rough endoplasmic reticulum, and the developed Golgi area. The former consists of elongated cisternae which contain a loose fibrillar material and whose ribosomes are often arranged in polyribosomes; the latter is formed by small smooth vesicles whose content is of variable electron density. Several mitochondria, lysosomes, and occasional multivesicular bodies are present in the cytoplasm, which contains also irregular bundles of filaments[5], at least part of which are actin-like[6]. Pinocytosis vesicles are recognizable along the peripheral membrane. Adjacent osteoblasts are connected by gap and tight junctions[7,8].

Histochemistry confirms that the osteoblast cytoplasm has a high content of RNA and sometimes contains glycogen and lipid droplets[9]. Moreover, enzymatic histochemistry has shown that osteoblasts have a strong alkaline phosphatase activity (see review by Bourne[10]). Recent histochemical investigations, carried out by the azo-dye method of Burstone[11] on semithin (1 μ thick) sections (which allow to obtain a high microscopic resolution) of undecalcified bone (to avoid solubili- zation and/or inactivation of the enzyme during decalcification), have shown that the enzyme is mainly located on the peripheral membrane of osteoblasts and osteoblast processes facing and penetrating the osteoid border. Immunoperoxidase and immunogold-silver procedures[12] and electron microscopy[13] confirm this localization, which is the same as that of adenosine triphosphatase activity[14,15]. Alkaline phosphatase activity is present also in matrix vesicles of the osteoid border, as discussed below. Moreover, osteoblasts have acid phosphatase activity which is associated with single membrane bound lysosomal bodies[13] and Golgi saccules[16]. This is in agreement with the recent observation that osteo- blasts of growing rat bone have tartrate-resistant acid phosphatase activity[17], an enzyme generally known as a distinctive cytochemical feature of osteoclasts (see below).

The principal product of osteoblast activity is type I collagen, as shown by autoradiographic[18] and immunohistochemical[19,20] methods. Bone matrix contains a number of non-collagenous proteins (different types of proteoglycans and glycoproteins, phosphoproteins, phospholipids, osteocalcin, osteonectin, osteopontin; recently reviewed by Marks and Popoff.[21]). Most of them are secreted by the osteoblast, as shown by their presence in the osteoblast cytoplasm. These include glycoproteins and sulfated glycoconiugates[16], 44kDa phosphoprotein[22], osteocalcin[22-24], osteonectin[25,26]. Of particular interest is the immunohistochemical demonstration that osteoblasts produce a neutral collagenase[27,28] which could be sequestered in the calcified matrix and could be active during bone resorption.

A number of substances and factors, present in bone organ cultures but not yet demonstrated by morphological methods, are worth of consideration because of their possible role in bone formation and resorption. They will be considered in the paragraph concerning the coupling between osteoblast and osteoclast activity.

The osteocyte

Although its activity is fundamental for the survival of the bone tissue, the osteocyte is probably the least known of the bone cells. This is due to its localization within the calcified matrix, which makes its study extremely difficult, especially in undecalcified specimens.

Histological investigations carried out in different types of bone have shown that the osteocyte is placed in enclosed lacunae, the wall of which is completely calcified. However, the cell is not completely reclused, because many canaliculi, containing cytoplasmic processes, extend from the lacunae into the surrounding matrix and establish several contacts with canaliculi of other osteocytes. Their volume and shape change with the type of bone[29], woven bone containing relatively large, roundish osteocytes, lamellar bone relatively small osteocytes of elongated, ovoidal shape, whose greater diameter is parallel to the direction of the adjacent lamellae[30].

Most of our knowledge on the morphology of the osteocyte has been obtained by electron microscopy[6,31-35]. As recently reviewed[35], this shows that most of the osteocyte lacuna (Fig. 2) is occupied by a roundish or elongated nucleus with a small nucleolus; the scanty cytoplasm contains a reduced amount of organelles consisting of a few cisternae of endoplasmic reticulum, isolated mitochondria, inconspicuous Golgi apparatus, and very few lysosome-like bodies. Microtubules and actin-like filaments[8,36] and the occasional presence of cilia[37], have been reported. The plasma membrane is not in direct contact with the calcified bone matrix: in some cases, especially in osteocytes of woven bone, it is separated by the wall of the lacuna by interposition of uncalcified collagen fibrils and amorphous material; in other cases, probably corresponding to osteocytes which have completed the formation of their lacuna, filament-like apatite crystallites (so-called coastal crystals[38]), not connected to collagen fibrils, protrude side by side from the lacunar wall toward the cell membrane forming a "lacunar brush border"[39]. It is possible that these crystals correspond to and mask the osmiophilic lamina which can be seen on the inner border of the lacunae in specimens decalcified before embedding[32,34,38,40-42]. The cytoplasmic processes which are contained in the osteocyte canaliculi have very few organelles; however, they contain microtubules and actin-like filaments similar to those of the cytoplasm[36]. The membrane of the processes is not in direct contact with the calcified matrix because of the interposition of a thin sheath of amorphous material. Tight junctions between cytoplasmic processes of adjacent osteocytes, and between processes of an osteocyte and the cytoplasm of another osteocyte have been described both in normal and pathological conditions[4,36-39].

The above reported findings concern the "mature" osteocyte, that

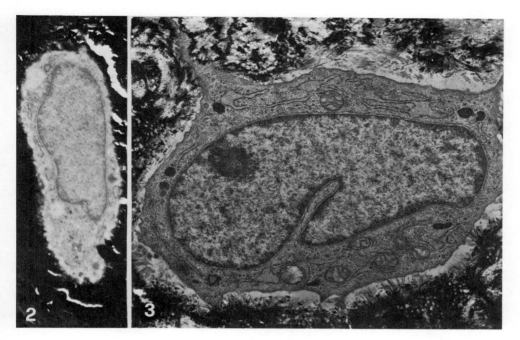

Fig. 2 - "Mature" osteocyte; note reduced amount of cytoplasm and cytoplasmic organelles, and close contact between osteocytic cytoplasm and bone matrix. Uranyl acetate and lead citrate, x 13,000.

Fig. 3 - Osteoid osteocyte: persistence of osteoblastic morphology. The lacunar wall is incompletely calcified. Uranyl acetate and lead citrate, x 13,000.

is, the osteocyte which is placed in the fully calcified matrix and is in an apparent "resting" or "inactive" functional state. However, the morphological results suggest that other "active" functional phases are possible, that is, formative, resorptive, and degenerative phases, which could represent successive different steps of the osteocyte life[35].

The formative phase derives its name from the fact that, in this period, the cells maintain their osteoblastic activity and synthesize the bone matrix necessary to form their definitive lacunae. As a consequence, the osteoblast is first entrapped into a partially calcified osteoid tissue (osteoid osteocyte;[6] Figs. 1, 3), then is gradually buried in calcified matrix and transformed into a definitive osteocyte. During this period, the osteoblastic characteristics of the cytoplasm are gradually lost, chiefly by reduction of the rough endoplasmic reticulum[6,43-45], so that at the stage of "mature" osteocyte the volume of the osteoblast has fallen by about 70% of the initial value[46].

The resorptive phase corresponds to a period of the osteocyte life during which the cell is considered capable of resorbing the bone matrix which forms the border of its lacuna. This process, called osteocytic or periosteocytic osteolysis[47] and supported by a number of investigators (see Bélanger[48] for review) has not received a general consensus[49-51].

The theory that the osteocyte has a resorptive phase is chiefly based on the histological observation that in cases of increased bone resorption many osteocyte lacunae are enlarged and irregularly shaped[39,43,52-56], on the histochemical finding that the osteocytes of these lacunae can have proteolytic activity[57], and on the ultrastructural evidence that the enlarged lacunae not only have irregular borders[31], but show a pericellular space containing fragmented and flocculent material which is supposed to derive from the resorption of the calcified matrix; moreover, the osteocytic cytoplasm shows numbers of mitochondria (which are sometimes calcified), lysosomes, and granular endoplasmic reticulum greater than those of resting osteocytes[32,39,41-43,56,58-63]. However, these data, which should demonstrate the existence of an osteocytic resorptive phase, can be interpreted in another way. First, the shape and size of the lacunae vary with, and depend on the type of bone, size of osteoblasts, and orientation of specimens[30,46,64]; second, the enlarged pericellular space could be due to cytoplasm shrinkage during fixation and dehydration; third, the increased size of the lacunae could be due to defective calcification of the perilacunar matrix[41,65]. Moreover, the SEM has never shown evidence of perilacunar matrix resorption[50].

All these problems call for further investigations. In this connection, it is worth considering that the osteocytes, especially those placed near active osteoclasts, contain acid phosphatase and, above all, tartrate-resistant acid phosphatase[17] (see Fig. 5 B) which is considered a marker of osteoclasts and their precursors[66,67]. These findings, and the observation that osteocytes have other proteolytic enzymes[68], although at the present not conclusive, might support the theory of osteocytic osteolysis.

The osteocyte might regulate its intracellular calcium concentration by resorption or deposition of the coastal crystals described above. Because these crystals are not connected to collagen fibrils, their dissolution might occur without changes of the lacunar spaces. Although ultrastructural findings support this possibility[35], it must be verified by further investigation.

The degenerative phase, which probably ends with the death of the osteocyte, is characterized by pyknosis and fragmentation of the nucleus, vacuolation or condensation of the cytoplasm, derangement of the coastal crystals, and/or complete fragmentation and disappearance of the cell (Fig. 4), a series of event which, after the first description by Recklinghausen[69], has been reported several times[32,34,41,62]. The reason of the osteocyte degeneration is not known. It might be simply the final stage of the normal evolution of the osteocyte, or might be due to condition of hypoxia and/or aging[34,31].

The lining cells

The inactive surfaces of bone are covered by a layer of very flat, endothelial-like cells, which are called lining cells. It is very difficult to study these cells under the light microscope because their

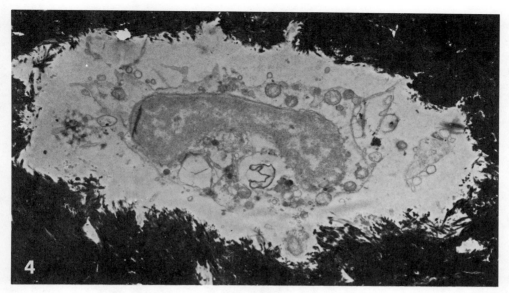

Fig. 4 – Degenerated osteocyte contained in irregular lacuna. Uranyl acetate and lead citrate, x 8,000.

cytoplasm is excessively thin to be recognized. The nucleus is elongated and thin and is the only structure which is visible in usual histological preparations. However, the cytoplasm of most of them can be visualized by its alkaline phosphatase activity. In this case, the lining cells appear in close relationships with the reticular cells of the bone marrow. It has been shown that they are connected also with the osteocytes through the canalicular system[70]. Under the electron microscope, the lining cells appear as elements with thin, elongated nucleus and very thin cytoplasm which separates the bone marrow cells from the bone matrix and contains very few organelles (scanty cisternae of the endoplasmic reticulum, few mitochondria, microfilaments), and small clusters of glycogen[70-72]. Adjacent lining cells are connected by gap junctions[70].

The function of these cells is practically unknown, although they may have the principal role of separating the interstitial from the bone fluids[73], may contribute to maintain plasma calcium concentration[74], and may retain osteonic potentiality[72]. The possibility that they have a role in mediating osteoclast activity is discussed below.

The osteoclast

Numerous findings are available on the osteoclast, its origin and fate, and the way it resorbs bone. They have been reviewed several times[1,2,21,75-84]. Histologically, the osteoclast appears as a giant, multinucleated cell attached to the bone surface, in connection with a resorption lacuna of variable depth, along the surface of which a developed brush or ruffled border is usually present (Fig. 5 A). This well known cytological pattern is probably not unique, because in case of

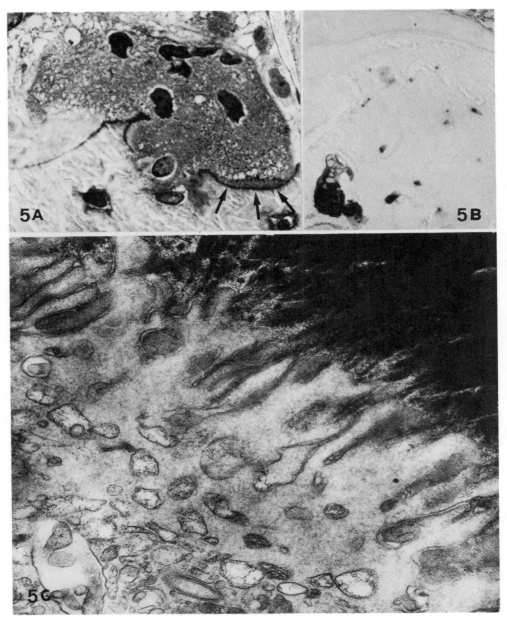

Fig. 5 - A. Histological appearance of an osteoclast: note vacuolation of cytoplasm, brush border (arrows), and a partially phagocytosed osteocyte; Azure II – Methylene blue, x 300. B. TRAP activity in osteoclast (lower left) and adjacent osteocytes; x 120. C. Part of an osteoclast and its ruffled border: note numerous cytoplasmic vacuoles containing needle-shaped crystals; the bone matrix undergoing resorption does not appear decalcified. Uranyl acetate and lead citrate, x 30,000.

increased bone resorption, such as in severe hyperparathyroidism, small mononucleate cells have osteoclastic characteristics and properties.

Under the electron microscope (Fig. 5 C), the osteoclast is chiefly characterized by its developed ruffled border, which is formed by a number of membrane infoldings, the development of which is proportional to the degree of resorption activity[80]. The ruffled border is surrounded by the clear zone, that is the zone, containing actin-like filaments , which allows cellular attachment to bone surface. The cytoplasm contains numerous mitochondria, a few cisternae of the granular endoplasmic reticulum, one or more, small Golgi areas, and several vacuoles, part of which seem to be empty and part contain free crystallites deriving from the disaggregation of the calcified matrix (Fig. 5 C). At the level of the ruffled border, the osteoclast-bone interface is characterized by the presence of dissociated collagen fibrils and free crystals, which are present also in the thin channels formed by the membrane infoldings (Figs. 5 C, 6). Only the former, however, are gradually introduced and completely solubilized in cytoplasmic vacuoles, whereas the digestion of the fibrils completely occurs in the extracellular space[85]. The presence in this space of "denuded" collagen fibrils has been reported by Hancox and Boothroyd[86]. These fibrils are more frequently found in some types of bone than in others and probably correspond to collagen fibrils which had never been calcified[85].

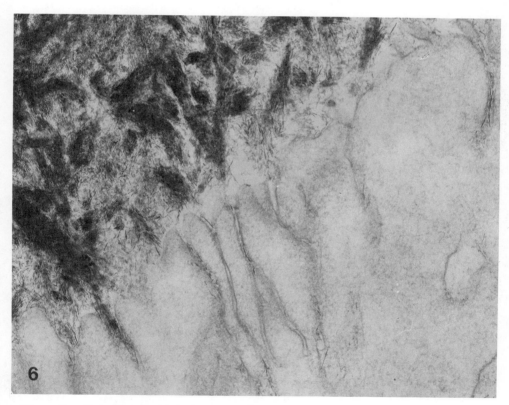

6

Fig. 6 - Detail of osteoclast ruffled border and adjacent disaggregated bone matrix; note lack of decalcification, dissociated collagen fibrils, and free crystals in the channels of the ruffled border. Uranyl acetate and lead citrate, x 92,000.

The presence of intense acid phosphatase activity in the cytoplasm of the osteoclast has long been known and this activity represents the main histochemical feature distinguishing osteoclasts from other bone cells, although it can be found also in osteoblasts and osteocytes. The osteoclast contains the isoenzyme resistant to tartrate inhibition (TRAP; tartrate resistant acid phosphatase), which can be considered a marker of osteoclasts and preosteoclasts[66,67], although it is present also in osteoblasts and osteocytes[17] (Fig. 5 B). Acid phosphatase, and other hydrolytic enzymes, are present not only in phagocytic vacuoles of the cytoplasm, but also in the channels of the ruffled border, in the osteoclast-bone interspace, and even in the bone matrix undergoing resorption[2,87-89].

The current ideas on the mechanism of bone resorption have been recently reviewed by Vaes[1], who underlines that at present most of the findings support an extracellular dissolution of the bone mineral followed by digestion of the organic components. According to this view (see Marks and Popoff[21] and Vaes[1] for review), the osteoclast decalcifies bone matrix by a mechanism similar to that which occurs in gastric parietal cells[90]. The CO_2 produced by cell metabolism is converted into bicarbonate and hydrogen ions by the enzyme carbonic anhydrase (isoenzyme II), which has been described to be present in the cytosol, Golgi apparatus, cytoplasmic vesicles of the osteoclast, and on the plasma membrane of its ruffled border[91-93]. An ATP-mediated proton pump, active on the membrane of the ruffled border, transfers H+ ions in the osteoclast-bone interspace delimited at the periphery by the clear zone, thus creating in this segregated space an acidified environment[94]. This on one hand induces decalcification of bone matrix, on the other facilitates the digestion of organic components by acid hydrolases secreted by the osteoclast[1]. The digestion products are then taken up in cytoplasmic vacuoles and secondary lysosomes, and further degraded.

This mechanism is supported by a number of histochemical and biochemical findings, but not by the results of morphological investigations. Electron microscopy of normal osteoclasts and adjacent bone matrix does not show, in fact, any evidence of matrix decalcification. On the contrary, as reported above, the area of resorption is characterized by the presence of free crystals dissociated and freed from the disrupted calcified matrix, oriented at random, and partly contained within the channels of the ruffled border; they are contained also in cytoplasmic vacuoles[85]. The resorption zone contains also undecalcified collagen fibrils, their fragments, and only in some type of bone (chick embryo tibia, for instance) a few "denuded" collagen fibrils which probably had been never calcified. Thus, the electron microscope findings suggest that bone resorption begins with fragmentation and dissociation of bone matrix, which is responsible of release of crystals; these are then phagocytosed and dissolved in cytoplasmic vacuoles, while digestion of organic material continues in the extracellular space[85].

To explain the discrepancy between these results and those obtained by histochemical and biochemical methods, and to support the theory that the first step of bone resorption is decalcification of the matrix, Vaes[1] suggests that the presence of free crystals in the space supposed to be acidified might be due to the fact either that they represent a late stage in the resorption of bone matrix, i.e., are crystals which are not yet solubilized, or that they are formed by re-precipitation of calcium and phosphate during preparation of the specimens. However, free crystals are often more abundant in areas of initial resorption than in fully developed Howship's lacunae; moreover, their presence and concentration in the osteoclast–bone interspace is not dependent on the procedures used to prepare the bone specimens for electron microscopy; finally, they are completly similar to the crystals present in the matrix which is not undergoing resorption. It seems necessary to conclude that further investigation is needed to fully understand the mechanism of bone mineral resorption (see also Sakamoto and Sakamoto[28]).

The bone remodeling unit (BRU)

The normal bone metabolism implies a continuous bone remodeling, which occurs at the level of the so called bone remodeling unit (BRU)[95] in such a way that the bone volume is maintained costant by a coupling between osteoclast and osteoblast activity[96]. A BRU consists of the different phases of a dynamic process which begins with activation of osteoclasts on the bone surface (activation phase) and continues with resorption of bone matrix and formation of Howship's lacuna (resorption phase), disappearance of osteoclasts which are substituted by mononuclear cells (reversion phase), disappearance of these cells and reappearance of osteoblasts with reparation of the resorption lacuna (formation phase). All of these phases can be documented morphologically[97]. However, morphological investigations are static and cannot easily elucidate a dynamic process which involves a complex series of cellular stimulation and inhibition by systemic (PTH, vitamin D, calcitonin, glucocorticoids, sex steroid, thyroid hormone, vitamin A) and local factors (cytokines, growth factors, prostaglandins). On the other hand, most of the results on this subject have been obtained by biochemical analysis, especially of in vitro cultures, and for their detailed discussion reference may be made to recent excellent reviews[2,82–84,98,99]. The main finding emerging from the bulk of these investigations is that osteoblasts and lining cells have a primary role in inducing the activation phase. Although research on this field is still in progress, several results indicate that osteoblasts, and not osteoclasts, have receptors for PTH, $1,25(OH)_2D_3$, prostaglandins, and other factors stimulating bone resorption, and that in response to stimulation by these substances osteoblasts, or osteoblast–like cells, can retract and secrete collagenase and chemotactic factors; in this way, the osteoid tissue which covers the calcified matrix is exposed and digested, thus allowing a direct contact between calcified matrix and osteoclasts, which are attracted in the exposed area by the osteoblast chemotactic factors[70,100–106].

Much remains to be done on the local mechanisms which regulate the coupling between osteoblast and osteoclast activity. Although a number of factors (cytokines, including osteoclast activating factor(s), or

OAF, and tumour necrosis factor alpha; interferon gamma; colony stimulating factors; transforming growth factors) are probably involved in this
regulation, demonstration of their presence in the BRU by morphological
investigations is lacking. These, however, have shown that during the
reversion phase the Howship's lacuna is occupied by mononuclear cells
which have TRAP-activity, thus resembling active osteoclasts, from which
they might derive ("post-osteoclasts")[98]. These cells might have the
main function of resorbing the last bone particles left behind by the
osteoclast, and synthesizing the cement line[98]. Moreover, these cells
might release a coupling factor. It is interesting that acid phosphatase
activity can be demonstrated in the cement lines, even at distance from
the active BRU.

THE INTERCELLULAR MATRIX OF BONE

Bone is a heterogeneous, highly anysotropic tissue, so that its
intercellular matrix shows different structure and properties in different types of bone. However, its basic constituents are always the same
and can be considered as if their composition and distribution was
uniform. Bone intercellular matrix consists of two main components,
organic and inorganic, which will be considered separately.

The organic matrix of bone

The main constituent of the organic matrix of bone is collagen type
I, which accounts for 90-95% of the organic matrix. Its fibrils are
similar to those of collagen type I present in other tissues and are
essentially characterized by a periodic banding of about 640 Å. Both the
polarizing[107] and the transmission[34] and scanning[49,51] electron microscopy show that these fibrils are randomly arranged in the so-called
woven bone, whereas have preferential orientations and are aggregated in
laminar layers or lamellae in other types of bone. The physical and
mechanical properties of bone largely depend on this preferential disposition of the collagen fibrils[108].

Besides collagen fibrils, the organic matrix of bone consists of
other organic, non-collagenous material[21,109-111], the main component of
which is osteonectin[110-112]. Although not exclusive of bone matrix, this
phosphoprotein could interact at the same time with collagen and inorganic substance. Ultrastructural immunohistochemical investigation using
the protein A-gold method has shown that bone matrix is strongly reac-
tive with antiosteonectin antiserum, especially in areas with the
highest degree of calcification[113]. Osteocalcin, or Gla-protein, an
acidic molecule characterized by the presence of three residues of
gamma-carboxyglutamic acid, and the "matrix Gla-protein"[114], have a
similar localization[24,113].

A number of other non-collagenous molecules are present in bone
matrix. They include sialoprotein I (osteopontin) and II, phosphoproteins, bone morphogenetic proteins, lipids, proteoglycans. Morphological
investigation on these molecules is scanty, although at least part of
them can have a fundamental role in calcification. As far as acid pro-

teoglycans are concerned, the available results show that their concentration is greater in osteoid tissue than in calcified matrix[16]. This subject will be considered again in the paragraph on the mechanism of calcification.

The inorganic substance of bone

Although it has long known that the mineral substance of bone is principally hydroxyapatite, there are still many doubts about its structure, composition and phisico-chemical properties (see Posner[115] for review). In 1968, in their review on the organization and structure of bone, Glimcher and Krane[116] reported that although the mineral phase consists of hydroxyapatite, or of crystals whose structure is similar to hydroxyapatite, its exact nature is unknown. Since then, knowledge on the inorganic substance of bone has not greatly improved and many doubts still remain. This seems to depend on one hand on the difficulty which is intrinsic to the study of hydroxyapatites, on the other on the fact that the mineral phase is intimately mixed with the organic substance which can change its properties.

Under the electron microscope, the mineral phase of bone shows two principal aspects[116-118] (Fig. 7): a) an electron-dense, finely granular or amorphous mineral substance which forms dense bands about 400 Å thick, separated by clear interbands about 300 Å thick, oriented transversally to the axes of the collagen fibrils and apparently reinforcing or "staining" their period; b) thin (from 25 to 50 Å thick), needle- and filament-like crystalline structures which in areas of inital calcification form roundish aggregates called calcification nodules and in fully calcified areas are collected in bundles which have the same orientation as that of the collagen fibrils.

Much has been debated about the true shape and dimensions of the components of the mineral phase (see Posner[115] and Bonucci[119] for review). However, the two types of organization reported above – thin elongated crystalline structures and transversally oriented bands of apparently amorphous inorganic substance – seem to represent the true organization of the mineral phase in bone. Their presence and distribution vary with the different types of bone, the frequence of the latter decreasing proportionally with the density of the collagen fibrils.

The calcification process

The close relationship which links the mineral phase in bands with the periodic banding of the collagen fibrils (Fig. 7) has led to the suggestion that the early stage of the calcification process occurs by heterogeneous nucleation of the mineral substance in the holes or hole regions of the collagen fibrils[116,120,121]. This attractive hypothesis is principally supported by electron microscope findings of calcifying tissues with dense collagen organization, as compact bone (osteonic and lamellar) and turkey leg tendons[117,122-124]. In these tissues, in fact, the morphological evidence of the relationship between the mineral phase and the periodic banding of the collagen fibrils is always prominent.

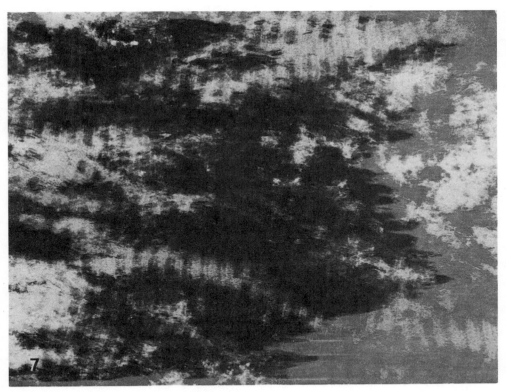

Fig. 7 – Area of calcification in osteonic bone: electron–dense bands reinforcing the collagen periodic banding, and needle-shaped crystals, are visible. Unstained, x 90,000.

However, ultrastructural investigations show that other organic components can have a role in induction and regulation of bone calcification. These are probably components of the interfibrillar ground substance, as suggested by the presence of crystals in the interfibrillar spaces[119,125]. It is not known at present which component(s) could be active in promoting the formation of these interfibrillar crystallites. However, chiefly on the basis of the calcification process which occurs in cartilage (see Ali[126] for review), it is possible to suggest that at least two of them have a principal role: acid proteoglycans and matrix vesicles.

The amount of acid proteoglycans in bone matrix is low, although it is greater in osteoid matrix undergoing calcification than in calcified matrix (see above). Their role in calcification is debated, and there is still disagreement if calcification is promoted or inhibited by, and is associated to a rise or decrease of, these substances[127]. The bulk of evidence shows that they increase before calcification starts and decrease afterwards.

Recent investigations on early stages of cartilage and osteoid tissue calcification suggest that they could be primarily controlled by acid proteoglycans[128]. It is known that, when decalcification is carried out after embedding (post embedding decalcification and staining method, or PEDS)[129] the organic structures are not extracted by the decalcifying solution so that those present in calcified areas are preserved and can be studied under the electron microscope[130]. In this way, it has been possible to show that the calcification nodules of cartilage and bone contain organic structures (<u>crystal ghosts</u>) which have the same needle- and filament-like shape as that of the untreated crystallites and are closely associated with the inorganic substance[119,125,129-133]. These results have been confirmed with the same or other techniques in a number of calcified tissues (for review see Bonucci)[119,125,132]. Without examining thoroughly this topic, which on the other hand needs further investigation, it is important to underline that the crystal ghosts have strongly acidic, sulphate groups and consequently seem to correspond to acid proteoglycans[128]. They could have a close relationships with other crystal-bound organic molecules[125] such as osteonectin[26] and alkaline phosphatase[134]; their relationship with lipids (see Boskey[135]) is uncertian.

<u>Matrix vesicles</u> (Fig. 8) represent the locus of initial calcification in cartilage, bone, predentin, and other tissues (for review see Anderson[136,137] and Bonucci[138]). They are roundish structures of cellular origin which, however, have no direct connection with the cells, being located in the intercellular matrix (longitudinal septa of epiphyseal cartilage, osteoid borders of bone, predentine), probably because most of them derive from budding of the tip of cytoplasmic processes[139-141]. They are of variable size (from 250 to 2500 Å) and consist of an amorphous substance surrounded by a trilaminar membrane which has the same structure and characteristics as those of the

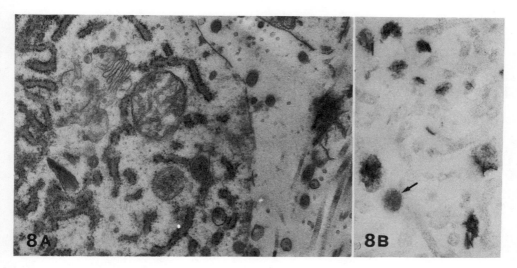

Fig. 8 – Periosteal bone of chick embryo. A. Detail of the cytoplasm of an osteoblast and of the adjacent osteoid border, in which collagen fibrils, calcification nodule, and matrix vesicles are visible. B. Uncalcified (arrow) and calcifying matrix vesicles. Uranyl acetate and lead citrate, A x 60,000, B x 90,000.

cellular plasma membrane. Early aggregates of crystals are found within them and on their membrane. As these aggregates increase in size, the whole vesicle is calcified and transformed into a roundish "calcification nodule" from which the crystals successively spread into the surrounding matrix.

Matrix vesicles have been found in areas of osteogenesis in a wide variety of bone tissues. However, they are less frequent in bone than in epiphyseal cartilage. Moreover, different types of bone have different concentration of matrix vesicles, their frequence being roughly proportional to the amount of interfibrillar ground substance.

The mechanism by which matrix vesicles mediate the early stage of the calcification process is not known. Matrix vesicles of epiphyseal cartilage can be studied more easily, and consequently are better known, than matrix vesicles of bone. Thus, numerous morphological and biochemical investigations have shown that cartilage vesicles contain glycoproteins and phospholipids, are surrounded by acid proteoglycans, and have alkaline phosphatase, ATPase, and pyrophosphatase activities. These components and enzymatic activities could be involved in the mechanism of matrix vesicle calcification (see Ali[126]): the hypothesis has been suggested that calcium ions, probably accumulated in matrix vesicles by a calcium pump at the vesicle membrane, are sequestered by phospholipids and react with phosphate ions produced by alkaline phosphatase activity, pyrophosphatase probably inactivating local inhibitors of the process[136]. In this connection, the observation that the alkaline phosphatase of matrix vesicles is a calcium-binding glycoprotein[135], and that it is inactivated with the onset of calcification[135,142], suggests that the enzyme could bind at the same time calcium and phosphate ions, in so doing promoting calcification and remaining incorporated into, and inactivated by, the mineral phase[135].

Assuming that there are no differences between matrix vesicles of cartilage and bone, it may be supposed that the mechanism of calcification is the same. However, in epiphyseal cartilage the early phase of the calcification process is mediated by matrix vesicles alone, and only the successive phases occur in, and involve the components of, the intercellular matrix, whereas in bone calcification occurs at the same time in matrix vesicles and in relationship with collagen fibrils and interfibrillar ground substance. It is obvious that further investigation is needed to fully understand the role of matrix vesicles in bone.

REFERENCES

1. G. Vaes, Cellular biology and biochemical mechanism of bone resorption, Clin. Orthop. 231: 239-271 (1988).
2. W.A. Peck, and W.L. Woods, The cells of bone, in: "Osteoporosis: Etiology, Diagnosis, and management", B.L. Riggs and L.J. Melton, eds., Raven Press, New York (1988).
3. D.A. Cameron, The fine structure of osteoblasts in the metaphysis of the tibia of the young rat, J. Biophys. Biochem. Cytol. 9: 583-595 (1961).

4. R.H. Dudley, and D. Spiro, The fine structure of bone cells, J. Biophys. Biochem. Cytol. 11: 627–649 (1961).

5. G. Göthlin, and J.L.E. Ericsson, Electron microscopic studies of cytoplasmic filaments and fibers in different cell types of fracture callus in the rat. Virchows Arch. Abt. B Zellpath. 6: 24–37 (1970).

6. G.J. King, and M.E. Holtrop, Actine–like filaments in bone cells of cultured mouse calvaria as demonstrated by binding to heavy meromyosin, J. Cell Biol. 66: 445–451 (1975).

7. S.B. Doty, Morphological evidence of gap junctions between bone cells, Calcif. Tiss. Int. 33: 509–512 (1981).

8. S.W. Whitson, Tight junction formation in osteon, Clin. Orthop. 86: 206–213 (1972).

9. R.L. Cabrini, Histochemistry of ossification, Int. Rev. Cytol. 11: 283–306 (1961).

10. G.H. Bourne, Phosphatase and calcification, in: "The biochemistry and physiology of bone", G.H. Bourne, ed., Academic Press, New York and London (1972).

11. M.S. Burstone, Histochemical observations on enzymatic processes in bone and teeth, Ann. N. Y. Acad. Sci. 85: 431–444 (1960).

12. D.C. Morris, J.C. Randall, and H.C. Anderson, Light microscopic localization of alkaline phosphatase in fetal bovine bone using immunoperoxidase and immunogold–silver staining procedures, J. Histochem. Cytochem. 36: 323–327 (1988).

13. S.B. Doty, and B.H. Schofield, Enzyme histochemistry of bone and cartilage cells, Progr. Histochem. Cytochem. 8: 1–38 (1976).

14. G. Göthlin, and J.L.E. Ericsson, Studies on the ultrastructural localization of adenosine triphosphatase activity in fracture callus, Histochemie 35: 111–126 (1973).

15. O. Fukushima, and N. Goshi, Neutral ATP–hydrolyzing enzyme activity on the plasma membrane of osteoblasts, Acta Histochem. Cytochem. 16: 216–222 (1983).

16. M. Takagi, R.T. Parmley, Y. Toda, and F.R. Denys, Ultrastructural cytochemistry of complex carbohydrates in osteoblasts, osteoid, and bone matrix, Calcif. Tiss. Int. 35: 309–319 (1983).

17. P. Bianco, P. Ballanti, and E. Bonucci E., Tartrate–resistant acid phosphatase activity in rat osteoblasts and osteocytes. Calcif. Tiss. Int. 43: 167–171 (1988).

18. M. Weinstock, Elaboration of precursor collagen by osteoblasts as visualized by radioautography after ^{3}H–proline administration, in: "Extracellular matrix influence on gene expression", H.C. Slavkin and R.C. Greulich, eds., Academic Press, New York (1975).

19. K. Von der Mark, H. Von der Mark, and S. Gay, Study of differential collagen synthesis during development of the chick embryo by immuno–fluorescence. II. Localization of type I and type II collagen during long bone development, Dev. Biol. 53: 153–170 (1976).

20. G.M. Wright, and C.P. Leblond, Immunohistochemical localization of procollagens. III. Type I procollagen antigenicity in osteoblasts and prebone (osteoid), J. Histochem. Cytochem. 29: 791–804 (1981).

21. S.C.Jr. Marks, and S.N. Popoff, Bone cell biology: the regulation of development, structure, and function in the skeleton, Am. J. Anat. 183: 1–44 (1988).

22. M.P. Mark, C.W. Prince, S. Gay, R.L. Austin, M. Bhown, R.D.

Finkelman, and W.T. Butler, A comparative immunocytochemical study on the subcellular distribution of 44kDa bone phosphoprotein and bone –carboxyglutamic acid (Gla)–containing protein in osteoblasts. J. Bone Min. Res. 2: 337–346 (1987).

23. A.L.J.J. Bronckers, S. Gay, M.T. Dimuzio, and W.T. Butler, Immunolocalization of –carboxyglutamic acid–containing proteins in developing molar tooth germs of the rat, Collag. Rel. Res. 5: 17–22 (1985).

24. A.J. Camarda, W.T. Butler, R.D. Finkelman, and A. Nanci Immunocytochemical localization of –carboxyglutamic acid–containing protein (Osteocalcin) in rat bone and dentin, Calcif. Tiss. Int. 40: 349–355 (1987).

25. G. Jundt, K.-H. Berghauser, J.D. Termine, and A. Schulz, Osteonectin – a differentiation marker of bone cells, Cell Tiss. Res. 248: 409–415 (1987).

26. P. Bianco, G. Silvestrini, J.D. Termine, and E. Bonucci, Immunohistochemical localization of osteonectin in developing human and calf bone using monoclonal antibodies, Calcif. Tiss. Int. 43: 155–161 (1988).

27. S. Sakamoto, and M. Sakamoto, Biochemical and immunohistochemical studies on collagenase in resorbing bone in tissue culture, J. Periodont. Res. 17: 523–526 (1982).

28. S. Sakamoto, and M. Sakamoto, Bone collagenase, osteoblasts and cell-mediated bone resorption, in: "Bone and mineral research/4", W.A. Peck, ed., Elsevier, Amsterdam, New York, Oxford (1986).

29. G. Marotti, Three dimensional study of the osteocyte lacunae, in: "Bone histomorphometry", W.S.S. Jee, A.M. Parfitt, eds., Armour Montagu, Paris (1981).

30. G. Marotti, Osteocyte orientation in human lamellar bone and its relevance to the morphometry of periosteocytic lacunae, Metab. Bone Dis. Rel. Res. 1: 325–333 (1979).

31. A. Baud, Morphologie et structure inframicroscopique des ostéocytes, Acta anat., 51: 209–225 (1962).

32. S.S. Jande, Fine structural study of osteocytes and their surrounding bone matrix with respect to their age in young chicks, J. Ultrastruct. Res. 37: 279–300 (1971)

33. S.S. Jande, and L.F. Bélanger, Electron microscopy of osteocytes and the pericellular matrix in rat trabecular bone, Calcif. Tiss. Res. 6: 280–289 (1971).

34. S.C. Luk, C. Nopajaroonsri, and G.T. Simon, The ultrastructure of cortical bone in young adult rabbits, J. Ultrastruct. Res. 46: 184–205 (1974).

35. E. Bonucci, The ultrastructure of the osteocyte, in: "Ultrastructure of skeletal tissues – Bone and cartilage in normalcy and pathology", E. Bonucci and P.M. Motta, eds., CRC Press, Boca Raton (1989; in press).

36. J.M. Weinger, and M.E. Holtrop, An ultrastructural study of bone cells: the occurrence of microtubules, microfilaments and tight junctions. Calcif. Tiss. Res. 14: 15–29 (1973).

37. M. Federman, and G.Jr. Nichols, Bone cell cilia: vestigial or functional organelles? Calcif. Tiss. Res. 17: 81–85 (1974).

38. F. Wassermann, and J.A. Yaeger, Fine structure of the osteocyte

capsule and of the wall of the lacunae in bone, Z. Zellforsch. 67: 636–652 (1965).

39. E. Bonucci, and G. Gherardi, 1977, Osteocyte ultrastructure in renal osteodystrophy, Virchows Arch. A Path. Anat. Histol. 373, 213–231 (1977).

40. K. Donath, and G. Delling, Elektronenmikroskopische Darstellung der periosteocytaren Matrix durch Ultradunnschnitt–EDTA–entkalkung, Virchows Arch. 354 A: 305–311 (1971).

41. S.S. Jande, and L.F. Bélanger, The life cycle of the osteocyte, Clin. Orthop. 94: 281–305 (1973).

42. E.A. Tonna, Electron microscopic evidence of alternating osteocytic-osteoclastic and osteoplastic activity in the perilacunar walls of aging mice, Connect. Tiss. Res. 1: 221–230 (1972).

43. V.L. Yeager, S. Chiemchanya, and P. Chaiseri, Changes in size of lacunae during the life of osteocytes in osteons of compact bone, J. Gerontol. 30: 9–14 (1975).

44. A. Zambonin Zallone, A. Teti, B. Nico, M.V. Primavera, Osteoplastic activity of mature osteocytes evaluated by ^{3}H-proline incorporation, Basic Appl, Histochem. 26: 65–67 (1982).

45. C. Palumbo, A three-dimensional ultrastructural study of osteoid-osteocytes in the tibia of chick embryos, Cell Tiss. Res. 246: 125–131 (1986).

46. G. Marotti, Decrement in volume of osteoblasts during osteon formation and its effect on the size of the corresponding osteocytes, in: "Bone histomorphometry", P.J. Meunier, ed., Armour Montagu, Paris (1977).

47. L.F. Bélanger, Osteocytic osteolysis, Calcif. Tiss. Int. 4: 1–12 (1969).

48. L.F. Bélanger, Osteocytic resorption, In: "The biochemistry and physiology of bone", 2nd ed., v. 3, G.H. Bourne, ed., Academic Press, New York (1971).

49. A. Boyde, Scanning electron microscope studies of bone, in: "The biochemistry and physiology of bone", 2nd ed., v. 1, G.H. Bourne, ed., Academic Press, New York (1972).

50. A. Boyde, S.J. Jones, and J. Ashford, Scanning electron microscope observations and the question of possible osteocytic bone mini-(re)-modelling, in: "Current advances in skeletogenesis", M. Silbermann, H.C. Slavkin, eds., Excerpta Medica, Amsterdam (1982).

51. G. Marotti, The original contribution of the SEM to the knowledge of bone structure, in: "Ultrastructure of skeletal tissues – Bone and cartilage in normalcy and pathology", E. Bonucci and P.M. Motta, eds., CRC Press, Boca Raton (1989, in press).

52. L.F. Bélanger, and J. Robichon, Parathormone-induced osteolysis in dogs, J. Bone Joint Surg. 46A: 1008–1012 (1964).

53. P. Meunier, J. Bernard, and G. Vignon, La mesure de l'élargissement périostéocytaire appliquée au diagnostic des hyperparathyroidies, Path. Biol. 19: 371–378 (1971).

54. B. Krempien, G. Geiger, E. Ritz, and S. Buttner, Osteocytes in chronic uremia. Differential count of osteocytes in human femoral bone, Virchows Arch. Abt. A Path. Anat. 360: 1–9 (1973).

55. J. Duriez, Les modifications calciques péri-ostéocytaires. Etude microradiographique à l'analyseur automatique d'images, Nouv. Presse Méd. 3: 2007–2010 (1974).

56. E, Bonucci, V. Lo Cascio, S. Adami, L. Cominacini, G. Galvanini, and A. Scuro, The ultrastructure of bone cells and bone matrix in human primary hyperparathyroidism, Virchows Arch. Abt. A Path. Anat. 379: 11-23 (1978).

57. L.F. Bélanger and B.B. Migicovsky, Histochemical avidence of proteolysis in bone: the influence of parathormone, J. Histochem. Cytochem. 11: 735-737 (1963).

58. D.A. Cameron, H.A. Paschall, and R.A. Robinson, Changes in the fine structure of bone cells after the administration of parathyroid extract, J. Cell Biol. 33: 1-14 (1967).

59. W. Remagen, H.J. Höhling, T.T. Hall, and R. Caesar, Electron microscopical and microprobe observations on the cell sheath of stimulated osteocytes, Calcif. Tiss. Res. 4: 60-68 (1969).

60. A. Schulz, K. Donat, and G. Delling, Ultrastruktur und Entwicklung des Corticalisosteocyten. Tiereexperimentelle Untersuchungen an der Rattentibia, Virchows Arch. A Path. Anat. Histol. 364: 347-356 (1974).

61. S.E. Weisbrode, C.C. Capen, and L.A. Nagode, Effects of parathyroid hormone on bone of thyroparathyroidectomized rats, Am. J. Path. 75: 529-542 (1974).

62. M.P. Anderson, and C.C. Capen, Fine structural changes of bone cells in experimental nutritional osteodystrophy of green iguanas, Virchows Arch. B Cell Path. 20, 169-184 (1976).

63. B. Krempien, and E. Ritz, Effects of parathyroid hormone on osteocytes. Ultrastructural evidence for anisotropic osteolysis and involvement of the cytoskeleton, Metab. Bone Dis. Rel. Res. 1: 55-65 (1978).

64. V. Canè, G. Marotti, G. Volpi, D. Zaffe, S. Palazzini, F. Remaggi, and M.A. Muglia, Size and density of osteocyte lacunae in different regions of long bones, Calcif. Tiss. Int. 34: 558-563 (1982).

65. R. Steendijk, and A. Boyde, Scanning electron microscopic observations on bone from patients with hypophosphatemic (vitamin D resistant) rickets, Calcif. Tiss. Res. 11: 242-250 (1973).

66. C. Minkin, Bone acid phosphatase: tartrate-resistant acid phosphatase as a marker of osteoclast function, Calcif. Tiss. Int. 34: 285-290 (1982).

67. F.P. Van de Wijngaert, and E.H. Burger, Demonstration of tartrate-resistant acid phosphatase in undecalcified, glycolmetacrylate-embedded mouse bone: a possible marker of (pre)osteoclast identification, J. Histochem. Cytochem 34: 1317-1323 (1986).

68. P.L. Sannes, B.H. Schofield, and D.F. McDonald, Histochemical evidence of cathepsin B, dipeptidyl peptidase I, and dipeptidyl peptidase II in rat bone, J. Histochem. Cytochem. 34: 983-988 (1986).

69. Recklinghausen, F.v., "Untersuchungen über Rachitis und Osteomalacia", Gustav Fischer, Jena (1910).

70. Miller, S.C., and Jee, W.S.S., The bone lining cell: a distinct phenotype? Calcif. Tiss. Int. 41: 1-5 (1987).

71. C.J. Vander Wiel, S.A. Grubb, and R.V. Talmage, The presence of lining cells on surfaces of human trabecular bone, Clin. Orthop. 134: 350-355 (1978).

72. B.M. Bowman, and S.C. Miller, The proliferation and differentiation

of the bone-lining cell in estrogen-induced osteogenesis, <u>Bone</u> 7: 351-357 (1986).

73. F. Canas, A.R. Terepka, and W.F. Neuman, Potassium and milieu interior of bone, <u>Am. J. Physiol.</u> 217: 117-120 (1969).

74. H. Norimatsu, C.J. Vander Wiel, and R.V. Talmage, Morphological support of a role for cells lining bone surfaces in maintenance of plasma calcium concentration, <u>Clin. Orthop.</u> 138: 254-262 (1979).

75. D.A. Cameron, The ultrastructure of bone, in: "The biochemistry and physiology of bone", G.H. Bourne, ed., 2nd ed., v. 1, Academic Press, New York, San Francisco, London (1972).

76. N.M. Hancox, "Biology of bone", University Press, Cambridge (1972).

77. U. Lucht, The ultrastructure of osteoclasts under normal and experimental conditions, Thesis, University of Aarhus (1974).

78. B.K. Hall, The origin and fate of osteoclasts, <u>Anat. Record</u> 183: 1-12 (1975).

79. G. Göthlin, and J.L.E. Ericsson, The osteoclast. Review of ultrastructure, origin, and structure-function relationship, <u>Clin. Orthop.</u> 120: 201-231 (1976).

80. M.E. Holtrop, and G.J. King, The ultrastructure of the osteoclast and its functional implications, <u>Clin. Orthop.</u> 123: 177-196 (1977).

81. E. Bonucci, New knowledge on the origin, function and fate of osteoclasts, <u>Clin. Orthop.</u>, 158: 252-269 (1981).

82. G.R. Mundy, and G.D. Roodman, Osteoclast ontogeny and function, in: "Bone and mineral research/V", W.A. Peck, ed., Elsevier, Amsterdam, New York, Oxford (1987).

83. W.E. Huffer, Biology of disease. Morphology and biochemistry of bone remodeling: possible control by vitamin D, parathyroid hormone, and other substances, <u>Lab. Invest.</u> 59: 418-442 (1988).

84. S.C.Jr. Marks, and S.N. Popoff, Ultrastructural biology and pathology of the osteoclast, in: "Ultrastructure of skeletal tissues - Bone and cartilage in normalcy and pathology", E. Bonucci and P.M. Motta, eds., CRC Press, Boca Raton (1989, in press).

85. E. Bonucci, The organic-inorganic relationships in bone matrix undergoing osteoclastic resorption, <u>Calcif. Tiss. Res.</u> 16: 13-36 (1974).

86. N.M. Hancox, and B. Boothroyd, Structure-function relationships in the osteoclast, in: "Mechanisms of hard tissue destruction", R.F. Sognnaes, ed., Amer. Ass. for the Advancement of Science, Washington (1963).

87. G. Göthlin, and J.L.E. Ericsson, Fine structural localization of acid phosphomonoesterase in the brush border region of the osteoclasts, <u>Histochemie</u> 28: 337-344 (1971).

88. S.B. Doty, and B.H. Schofield, Electron microscopic localization of hydrolytic enzymes in osteoclasts, <u>Histochem. J.</u> 4: 245-258 (1972).

89. U. Lucht, Acid phosphatase of osteoclasts demonstrated by electron microscopic histochemistry, <u>Histochemie</u> 28: 103-117 (1971).

90. R.E. Anderson, D.M. Woodbury, and W.S.S. Jee, Humoral and ionic regulation of osteoclast acidity, <u>Calcif. Tiss. Int.</u> 39: 252-258 (1986).

91. C.V. Gay, and W.J. Mueller, Carbonic anhydrase and osteoclasts:

localization by labelled inhibitor autoradiography, Science 183: 432–434 (1974).

92. R.E. Anderson, H. Schraer, and C.V. Gay, Ultrastructural immunocytochemical localization of carbonic anhydrase in normal and calcitonin-treated chick osteoclasts, Anat. Record 204: 9–20 (1982).

93. H.K. Väänänen, and E.-K. Parvinen, High active isoenzyme of carbonic anhydrase in rat calvaria osteoclasts. Immunohistochemical study, Histochemistry 78: 481–485 (1983).

94. R. Baron, L. Neff, C. Roy, A. Boisvert, and M. Caplan, Cell-mediated extracellular acidification and bone resorption: evidence for a low pH in resorbing lacunae and localization of a 100-kD lysosomal membrane protein at the osteoclast ruffled border, J. Cell Biol. 101: 2210–2222 (1986).

95. H. Rasmussen, and P. Bordier, "The physiological and cellular basis of metabolic bone disease", Williams and Wilkins, Baltimore (1974).

96. H.M. Frost, Dynamics of bone remodelling, in: "Bone biodynamics", H.M. Frost, ed., Little, Brown, and Co., Boston (1964).

97. P. Tran Van, A. Vignery, and R. Baron, An electron-microscopic study of the bone-remodeling sequence in the rat, Cell Tiss. Res. 225: 283–292 (1982).

98. R. Baron, A. Vignery, and M. Horowitz, Lymphocytes, macrophages and the regulation of bone remodeling, in: "Bone and Mineral Research Annual 2", W.A. Peck, ed., Elsevier, Amsterdam, New York, Oxford (1984).

99. G.A. Rodan, and S.B. Rodan, Expression of the osteoblastic phenotype, in: "Bone and mineral research annual 2", W.A. Peck, ed., Elsevier, Amsterdam, New York, Oxford (1984).

100. G.A. Rodan, T.J. Martin, Role of osteoblasts in hormonal control of bone resorption – a hypothesis. Calcif. Tiss. Int. 33: 349–351 (1981).

101. E.G. Burger, J.W.M. Van der Meer, and P.J. Nijweide, Osteoclast formation from mononuclear phagocytes: role of bone-forming cells, J. Cell Biol. 99: 1901–1906 (1984).

102. J.K. Heath, S.J. Atkinson, M.C. Meikle, and J.J. Reynolds, Mouse osteoblasts synthesize collagenase in response to bone resorbing agents, Biochim. Biophys. Acta 802: 151–154 (1984).

103. G.L. Wong, Paracrine interactions in bone-secreted products of osteoblasts permit osteoclasts to respond to parathyroid hormone, J. Biol. Chem. 259: 4019–4022 (1984).

104. T.J. Chambers, and K. Fuller, Bone cells predispose bone surface to resorption by exposure of mineral to osteoclastic contact, J. Cell Sci. 76: 155–165 (1985).

105. R.L. Jilka, Are osteoblastic cells required for the control of osteoclast activity by parathyroid hormone?, Bone and Miner. 1: 261–266 (1986).

106. P.M.J. McSheehy, and T.J. Chambers, 1,25-dihydroxyvitamin D stimulates rat osteoblastic cells to release a soluble factor that increases osteoclastic bone resorption, J. Clin. Invest. 80: 425–429 (1987).

107. A. Ascenzi, and E. Bonucci, A quantitative investigation of the birefringence of the osteon, Acta anat. 44:236–262 (1961).

108. A. Ascenzi, The micromechanics versus the macromechanics of corti-

cal bone – A comprehensive presentation, J. Biomechan. Engineer. 110: 357–363 (1988).

109. J.D. Termine, Phenotypic proteins of calf lamellar bone, in: "Current advances in skeletogenesis", M. Silbermann, and H.C. Slavkin, eds., Excerpta Medica, Amsterdam, Oxford, Princeton (1982).

110. J.D. Termine, Osteonectin and other newly described proteins of developing bone, in: "Bone and mineral research, annual 1", W.A. Peck, ed., Excerpta Medica, Amsterdam, Oxford, Princeton (1983).

111. W.T. Butler, Matrix macromolecules of bone and dentin, Collagen Rel. Res. 4: 297–307 (1984).

112. J.D. Termine, A.B. Belcourt, K.M. Conn, and H.K. Kleinman, Mineral and collagen-binding proteins of fetal calf bone, J. Biol. Chem. 256: 10403–10408 (1981).

113. P. Bianco, Y. Hayashi, G. Silvestrini, J.D. Termine, and E. Bonucci, Osteonectin and GLA-protein in calf bone: ultrastructural immunohistochemical localization using the protein A-gold method, Calcif. Tiss. Int. 37: 684–686 (1984).

114. P.A. Price, M.R. Urist, and Y. Otawara, Matrix Gla protein, a new -carboxyglutamic acid-containing protein which is associated with the organic matrix of bone, Biochem. Biophys. Res. Comm. 117: 765–771 (1983).

115. A.S. Posner, Bone mineral and the mineralization process, in: "Bone and mineral research/5", W.A. Peck, ed., Elsevier, Amsterdam, New York, Oxford (1987).

116. M.J. Glimcher, and S.M. Krane, The organization and structure of bone, and the mechanism of calcification, in: "Treatise on collagen; v. 2, Biology of collagen", B.S. Gould, ed., Academic Press, London and New York (1968).

117. A. Ascenzi, E. Bonucci, and D. Steve Bocciarelli, An electron microscope study of osteon calcification, J. Ultrastruct. Res. 12: 287–303 (1965).

118. A. Ascenzi, E. Bonucci, and D. Steve Bocciarelli, An electron microscope study on primary periosteal bone, J. Ultrastruct. Res. 18: 605–618 (1967).

119. E. Bonucci, The structural basis of calcification, in: "Ultrastructure of the connective tissue matrix", A. Ruggeri and P.M. Motta, eds., Martinus Nijhoff Publ., Boston, The Hague, Dordrecht, Lancaster (1984).

120. M.J. Glimcher, Molecular biology of mineralized tissues with particular reference to bone, Rev. Mod. Phys. 31: 359–393 (1959).

121. M.J. Glimcher, Composition, structure, and organization of bone and other mineralized tissues and the mechanism of calcification, in: "Handbook of physiology: Endocrinology", v. 7, R.O. Greep, E.B. Astwood, eds., Am. Physiol. Soc., Washington (1976).

122. M.U. Nylen, D.B. Scott, and V.M. Mosley, Mineralization of turkey leg tendon. II. Collagen-mineral relations revealed by electron and X-ray microscopy, in: "Calcification in biological systems", R.F. Sognnaes, ed., Am. Ass. Adv. Sci., Washington (1960).

123. W.J. Landis, A study of calcification in the leg tendons from the domestic turkey, J. Ultrastruct. Molec. Struct. Res. 94: 217–238 (1986).

124. A.L. Arsenault, Crystal-collagen relationships in calcified turkey

leg tendons visualized by selected-area dark field electron microscopy, Calcif. Tiss. Int. 43: 202-212 (1988).

125. E. Bonucci, Is there a calcification factor common to all calcifying matrices?, Scann. Microsc. 1: 1089-1102 (1987).

126. S.Y. Ali, Calcification of cartilage, in: "Cartilage", v. 1, B.K.
Hall, ed., Academic Press, New York, London (1983).

127. B. De Bernard, N. Stagni, I. Colautti, F. Vittur, and E. Bonucci,
Glycosaminoglycans and endochondral calcification, Clin. Orthop.
126: 285-291 (1977).

128. E. Bonucci, G. Silvestrini, R. Di Grezia, The ultrastructure of the
organic phase associated with the inorganic substance in calcified
tissues, Clin. Orthop. 233: 243-261 (1988).

129. E. Bonucci, and J. Reurink, The fine structure of decalcified
cartilage and bone: a comparison between decalcification procedures
performed before and after embedding, Calcif. Tiss. Res. 25: 179-190
(1978).

130. E. Bonucci, Fine structure of early cartilage calcification, J.
Ultrastruct. Res. 20: 33-50 (1967).

131. E. Bonucci, Further investigation on the organic-inorganic relationships in calcifying cartilage, Calcif. Tiss. Res. 3: 38-54
(1969).

132. E. Bonucci, The locus of initial calcification in cartilage and
bone, Clin. Orthop. 78: 108-139 (1971).

133. E. Bonucci, The organic-inorganic relationships in calcified
organic matrices, In: "Physico-chimie et crystallographie des apa-
tites d'intéret biologique", Coll. Int. CRNS n. 230, Paris (1975).

134. B. De Bernard, P. Bianco, E. Bonucci, M. Costantini, G.C. Lunazzi,
P. Martinuzzi, C. Modricky, L. Moro, E. Panfili, P. Pollesello, N.
Stagni, and F. Vittur, Biochemical and immunohistochemical evidence
that in cartilage an alkaline phosphatase is a Ca^{2+}-binding glycoprotein, J. Cell Biol. 103: 1615-1623 (1986).

135. A.L. Boskey, The role of calcium-phospholipids, phosphate complexes in tissue mineralization, Metab. Bone Dis. Rel. Res. 1: 137-
142 (1978).

136. H.C. Anderson, Matrix vesicles of cartilage and bone, in: "The
biochemistry and physiology of bone", 2nd ed., v. 4, G.H. Bourne,
ed., Academic Press, New York, San Francisco, London (1976).

137. H.C. Anderson, Mineralization by matrix vesicles, Scann. Electr.
Micr. 2: 953-964 (1984).

138. E. Bonucci, Matrix vesicles: their role in calcification, in:
"Dentin and dentinogenesis", A. Linde, ed., CRC Press, Boca Raton
(1984).

139. E. Bonucci, Fine structure and histochemistry of "calcifying globules" in epiphyseal cartilage, Z. Zellfor. 103: 192-217 (1978)

140. E. Bonucci, Matrix vesicles formation in cartilage of scorbutic
guinea pigs: electron microscope study of serial sections, Metab.
Bone Dis. Rel. Res. 1: 205-212 (1978).

141. J.E. Hale, and R.E. Wuthier, The mechanism of matrix vesicle formation, J. Biol. Chem. 262: 1916-1925 (1987).

142. F.M. McLean, P.J. Keller, B.R. Genge, S.A. Walters, and R.E.
Wuthier, Disposition of preformed mineral in matrix vesicles.
Internal localization and association with alkaline phosphatase, J.
Biol. Chem. 262: 10481-10488 (1987).

MORPHOLOGICAL AND QUANTITATIVE ASPECTS
OF BONE FORMATION AND MINERALIZATION

Gastone Marotti

Istituto di Anatomia umana normale, Università di Modena

Policlinico, Via Del Pozzo 71, Modena (Italy)

INTRODUCTION

Bone formation is a biphasic process. During the first phase, the osteoblasts secrete an organic matrix, called preosseous matrix or osteoid, made up of type I collagen and ground substance (proteoglycans, glycoproteins, non-collagenous proteins). During the second phase, mineralization occurs, transforming the osteoid into bone tissue. Analyzed from the morphological viewpoint, three main aspects must be taken into account in osteogenesis of cellular bone: **osteoblast dynamics**, namely the mechanism by which the osteoblasts modulate the bone appositional growth rate; **osteoblast-osteocyte transformation**; **osteoblast control of collagen orientation.**

OSTEOBLAST DYNAMICS

Since the preosseous matrix does not mineralize as soon as it is elaborated, the osteoblastic laminae appear to be separated from the already mineralized pre-existing bone by a layer of unmineralized organic matrix, named osteoid seam. Unlike the mineralized bone matrix, the preosseous matrix is highly acidophilic, PAS-positive and orthochromatic. The boundary between the two matrices is given by a thin granular line, called mineralizing surface (or front), for it corresponds to the site of nucleation of hydroxyapatite crystals; while the boundary between the osteoblastic lamina and the osteoid seam is called osteoidogenetic surface (or front). Briefly the following formations appear to be stratified onto the osteogenetic surfaces: 1) mineralizing surface, 2) osteoid seam 3) osteoidogenetic surface, 4) osteoblastic lamina (fig. 1).

In normal conditions, the mineralizing surface and the osteoidogenetic surface grow at the same rate; the thickness of the osteoid seam ranges between 2 and 14 μm, and in general the greater its thickness the higher the rate of accretion of an osteogenetic surface. It must be noted, however, that the thickness of the osteoid seam does not

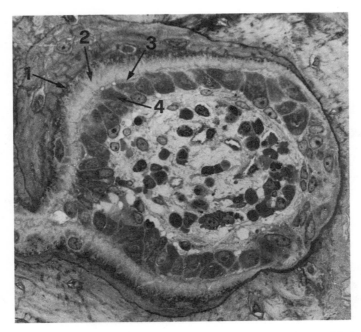

Figure 1. Microphotograph under transmitted ordinary light (x 790) of a cross-sectioned growing osteon. 1-mineralizing surface, 2-osteoid seam, 3-osteoidogenetic surface, 4-osteoblastic lamina.

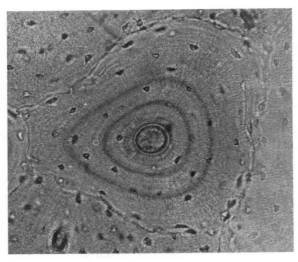

Figure 2. Microphotograph under transmitted ordinary light (x 400) of a growing osteon in compact bone of a 4-month-old dog, treated with a single intravenous injection of alizarin (ARS 20mg/Kg) every 20 days for 3 times. Note that the distance between the outer and the intermediate ARS bands, which are also visible under ordinary light, is greater than the distance between the intermediate and the inner bands, even though the time interval between the intravenous injections was kept constant at 20 days. This indicates that the appositional growth rate decreases during osteon formation.

always represent a good index of osteoblast secreting activity. For instance under certain pathological conditions (osteomalacia and rachitism), that are characterized by defects of bone calcification, the thickness of the osteoid seams may reach values higher than 30-40 μm without any increase of osteoblast activity; osteoblasts may even be absent in these situations (osteoid without osteoblasts).

The mineralizing surface can be precisely labeled with fluorochromes (tetracyclines, alizarin, uroporphyrine, ematoporphyrine, lumomagneson, etc.), for the molecules of these fluorescent substances adsorb on the surface of hydroxyapatite crystals during the initial phase of their accretion. Thus by means of the multiple or double fluorochrome-labeling technique, it is possible to measure, under U.V. light, the "linear rate of mineralization" that corresponds, in normal conditions, to the "linear rate of bone apposition", i.e. the so-called "appositional growth rate". With the use of this technique, it has been shown that the appositional growth rate differs considerably not only in various skeletal regions, but even in adjacent areas of a given osteogenetic surface, on both trabecular bone[1,2] and the wall of Haversian canals. On the latter, moreover, the rate decreases exponentially during osteon formation[3,4,5] (fig. 2).

The problem concerning the mechanisms by means of which the osteoblasts modulate the rate of bone apposition is rather complicated; it has been solved only in recent years thanks to precise histomorphometric evaluations carried out on osteoblastic laminae carpeting osteogenetic surfaces having different rates of accretion[6,7,8]. It has been observed that where the rate is very high, as for instance in large canals of osteons at the initial stage of formation, the osteoblastic laminae are made up of tightly packed cells of large size and columnar shape, i.e. with a narrow surface in contact with the osteoid seam (secretory territory = S.T.). On the contrary, in progressively smaller canals, parallel with the diminution of the radial growth rate, the osteoblasts become smaller, separated from one another by larger intercellular spaces and flattened so as to adhere to the osteoid seam with a relatively broad S.T.. Typical situations are given in Table 1, and figs. 3 and 4.

Table 1. Data recorded from serial semithin sections of growing Haversian systems in a 4 month-old dog (from Marotti[6]).

Haversian canal μm^2	Linear rate μm/day	Osteoblast volume μm^3	Osteoblast S.T. μm^2
13,000	1.8	910	100
3,000	0.9	675	114
900	0.4	500	224

In growing shafts of chick embryo, it has been shown that between the columnar osteoblasts and the flat ones, up to the bone lining cells which are no longer active, there is an infinite number of intermediate

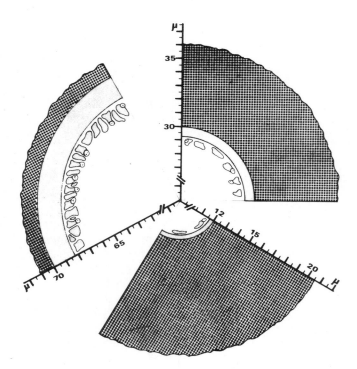

Figure 3. Diagram showing 3 sectors of a growing osteon, each
depicting a stage of formation. Left sector shows the initial stage: the
appositional growth rate, indicated by the thickness of the grey band, is
very high (1.8 µm/day), and correspondingly the osteoblasts are columnar
and tightly packed. Right sector shows the intermediate stage: the rate
is decreased (0.9 µm/day) and the osteoblasts have a cuboidal shape.
Lower sector shows the final stage: the rate is very low (0.4 µm/day) and
the osteoblasts are small and flattened.

stages which seem likely to depend on gradual modifications undergone in
time by the same osteoblasts rather than from differentiation of new
osteoblasts of progressively smaller size[8]. The lining bone cells appear
therefore to derive mainly from flat osteoblasts. It has also been
observed that all the osteoblasts, independently of their shape and size
show the cytoplasm completely filled with granular endoplasmic reticulum
and Golgi apparatus. As a consequence of this, the big columnar
osteoblasts, compared with the small flat ones, secrete a thicker osteoid
seam, and thus induce the osteoidogenetic surface to grow at a higher
rate, for two reasons: first because they secrete a greater amount of
organic matrix, for they have a higher content in cytoplasmic organelles;
second because they have a smaller secretory territory (S.T.) and thus
they arrange their secreted material ove a smaller surface. Briefly, the
bone appositional growth rate before the S.T. of each osteoblast seems to
depend on the ratio V/S.T., which expresses the volume (V) of
osteoblastic protoplasm engaged in organic matrix secretion on a given

osteoidogenetic area (S.T.). In other words, the bigger the osteoblast relative to the surface at which it is active the more columnar the cell, and the higher the linear rate of its osteoid deposition.

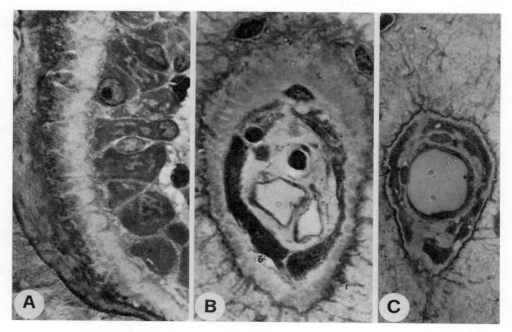

Figure 4. Osteogenetic surfaces growing, from A to C, at progressively lower rate. Microphotographs under transmitted ordinary light all taken at the same magnification (x 2,000). Note the different shape and size of the osteoblasts.

OSTEOBLAST-OSTEOCYTE TRANSFORMATION

According to the previous description, it is evident that during the deposition of the preosseous matrix the osteoblastic laminae move away from the pre-existing bone and, in normal conditions, at the same rate as the mineralizing surface. Obviously this does not occur for the osteoblasts committed to transforming into osteocytes. In response to signals which, as we shall presently show, are very probably emitted by the osteocytes, these osteoblasts transform into dendritic cells and reduce the rate at which they move away from the bone, so that the mineralizing surface catches up with them and overtakes them to the point where they are included into the bone matrix.

The sequence of events occurring in the osteoblastic protoplasm during the radiation of cytoplasmic processes and the mechanism of its incorporation into the bone have recently been studied in our laboratory by means of computerized three-dimensional reconstruction of the cells from transmission electron micrographs of serial ultrathin sections[9,10].

Going from the osteoblast to the mature osteocyte, we distinguished in growing bone surfaces of rabbits three types of preosteocytes on the basis of cell position, shape and ultrastructure.

Type 1-preosteocyte is still located in the osteogenetic lamina and like the osteoblasts its cytoplasm is rich in organelles. It may be distinguished from the non-committed osteoblasts since it shows the vascular facing side completely covered by the adjacent osteoblasts, a wide secretory territory (2-3 times broader than those of the adjacent osteoblasts), and a well defined outline of the plasma membrane facing the osteoidogenetic surface. Type 1-preosteocyte additionally radiates inside the osteoid seam short and thick cytoplasmic processes that are surrounded by matrix vesicles originating from them (fig. 5A).

Type 2-preosteocyte is located inside the osteoid seam (osteoid-osteocyte); however its vascular-facing plasma membrane remains in contact with the osteoblastic lamina. Compared with type 1-preosteocyte, type 2 shows a cellular body flattened against the mineralizing surface, an increased nucleus-to-cytoplasm ratio, and longer but structurally similar cytoplasmic processes radiating only into the mineralizing surface. Owing to its high content of cytoplasm organelles, type 2-preosteocyte still appears to be an osteoid-forming cell polarized towards the mineralizing surface (fig. 5B).

Type 3-preosteocyte is detached from the osteoblastic lamina and partly surrounded by calcified matrix. Compared with type 2-preosteocyte, type 3 has a smaller cell body with more definite ellipsoidal shape, central nucleus, higher nucleus-to-cytoplasm ratio, and a markedly decreased content of cytoplasmic organelles. The main feature of type 3-preosteocyte is the presence of cytoplasmic processes on both the mineral- and the vascular-facing sides. The processes radiating towards the minerals are short and thick, like the corresponding processes in type 1- and type 2-preosteocytes. The processes radiating towards the vessels, compared with those of the opposite side, are longer, more slender and have a regular outline since they never appear associated with globular structures (fig.5C). Some processes were found to contact the osteoblastic lamina.

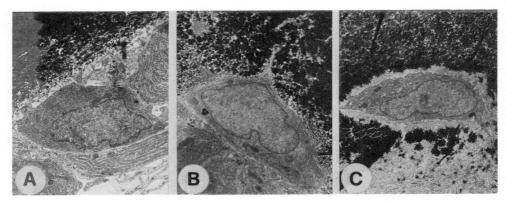

Figure 5. Transmission electron micrographs (x 5,000) showing osteoblast-osteocyte transformation: A) type 1-preosteocyte, B) type 2-preosteocyte, C) type 3-preosteocyte.

To summarize, according to our findings, the formation of osteocyte cytoplasmic processes appears to be an asynchronous and asymmetrical phenomenon that seems to precede the mineralization of the organic matrix; in other words, osteocyte cytoplasmic processes do not seem to be able to grow inside the mineralized bone matrix. We also collected preliminary data showing that mature osteocytes too are asymmetrical cells as regards their cytoplasmic arborization. According to classical histology, this finding would appear to be unexpected. However, if one considers that all bone cells live in an asymmetrical environment as regards their vascular nutrition, it appears logical that not only the osteoblasts but also the preosteocytes and the osteocytes are morphofunctional asymmetrical cells.

We suggest that the short and thick cytoplasmmic processes, that the preosteocytes first radiate towards the mineralizing matrix, mainly have an osteoformative function. This may be true at the beginning of the formation of these precesses; later it seems likely that they are involved in canaliculi formation together with the vascular processes of more mature cells. On the contrary, the long cytoplasmic processes, that the preosteocytes later radiate from their vascular-facing side, seem not to be involved in matrix secretion and calcification. They certainly have a nutritional function, namely in the formation of canaliculi, and probably also a modulatory effect on the metabolic activity of adjacent osteoblasts, for some of them were found to contact the osteoblastic lamina.

What is the mechanism by which the osteoblast "enters" the bone matrix to become an osteocyte? There are two possibilities: (1) the osteoblast participates in its incorporation into the bone or (2) it is buried inside the calcified matrix by the adjacent osteoblasts. In the first instance the cell would invert its functional polarization and lay down bone matrix from its vascular facing side. In the second case, the bone appositional growth rate before the secretory territory (S.T.) of the committed osteoblast must necessarily reduce, compared with the adjacent osteoblasts. Our findings strongly support the latter possibility. In fact, both type 1- and type 2-preosteocytes always appear to be polarized towards the mineralizing surface, as may be inferred from both the reciprocal position of their nucleus and cytoplasmic organelles, and the presence of cytoplasmic processes and matrix vesicles on their mineral-facing side only. Type 3-preosteocyte seems to lose the morphofunctional polarization, but it also shows a marked reduction of cytoplasmic organelles. Thus the loss of the morphofunctional polarization seems to occur at the same time as the diminution of the bone secreting activity. At the stage of type 3, the preosteocyte seems to be mainly engaged in radiating the processes directed towards the vessels, i.e. the osteoblastic lamina.

How does the appositional growth rate manage to diminish before the secretory territory (S.T.) of the osteoblast committed to transforming into osteocyte? It should be recalled in this connection that the appositional growth rate before the S.T. of each osteoblast has been shown to depend on the ratio V/S.T. (see previous section). On the basis of this fact, and considering that type 1-preosteocytes were found to have much larger S.T. than the adjacent osteoblasts, we believe that the enlargement of S.T. represents the first phenomenon occurring in the

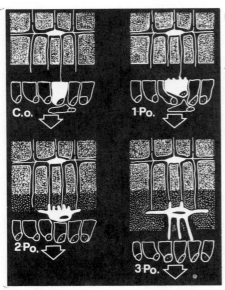

Figure 6. Schematic drawing of the morphological events we suggested as occurring during the differentiation of the osteoblast into osteocyte. Committed osteoblast (C.o.) in contact with the cytoplasmic process of a mature osteocyte. Type 1-preosteocyte (1-Po.) enlarges its secretory territory, thus reducing its appositional growth rate, and starts to radiate processes towards the osteoid. Type 2-preosteocyte (2-Po.) located inside the osteoid seam, but still in contact with the osteoblasts, continues to radiate short and thick cytoplasmic processes only from the mineral-facing side. Type 3-preosteocyte (3 Po.), before being completely buried by minerals, radiates from the vascular-facing side long and slender processes that touch the osteoblastic lamina.

committed osteoblast that reduces the appositional growth rate before its S.T.. In fact, even though the committed osteoblast should continue to secrete the same amount of bone matrix as before, when it had a columnar shape, it produces a thinner osteoid seam than the adjacent osteoblasts, owing to the fact that it has to arrange its secreted material over a wider surface. As a consequence, the committed osteoblast "enters" the bone fluid compartment, i.e. an ionic enviroment different from the perivascular extracellular fluid[11]. It is possible that the successive morphofunctional changes undergone by the preosteocyte also depend on the new environment as well as on its increasing distance from the vascular source. The sequence of events we postulated as occuring during the process of osteocyte differentiation is schematically drawn in fig. 6.

OSTEOBLAST CONTROL OF COLLAGEN ORIENTATION

Before taking into account the problem of cellular control of fiber orientation, one must mention in advance that recent SEM investigations, carried out in our laboratory, while substantiating the existence of the 3 classical types of bone tissue (woven-fibred bone, parallel-fibred bone, lamellar bone), have also pointed out that lamellar bone is a variety of woven bone and not of parallel-fibred bone as previously believed[12,13].

It should be recalled in this connection, that according to the classic model of bone lamellation, the so-called Gebhardt's model[14], which is currently by far the most widely accepted - and in fact it is given in all the textbooks of histology as an established datum - the lamellae basically have the same structure, all being dense fibrous layers in which collagen fibers lie parallel. The lamellar appearance depends solely on the orientation of the fibrils that may change through an angle of 0°-90° in successive lamellae. For this reason, the lamellar bone was rightly regarded, until now, as a variety of parallel-fibred bone.

Gebhardt and the several authors supporting his interpretation on bone lamellation based their opinion on the fact that bony lamellae, viewed under polarized light, alternately appear to be birifringent and extiguished. They believed that birifringent, anisotropic lamellae (transverse or horizontal lamellae) were made up of collagen fibers lying **only** in the plane of the section; and that extinguished, isotropic lamellae (longitudinal or vertical lamellae) were made up of fibers running **only** perpendicular to the plane of the section. But these are two blunders: first, because if birifringent lamellae also contain fibers running in planes other than that of the section, they cannot be seen under polarized light because they are extinguished; second, because the extinguished isotropic lamellae are not necessarily made up of perpendicular fibers; on the contrary, it would, if anything, be more correct to suppose that they are afibrillar. It must be noticed, moreover, that in none of the investigations so far reported in literature was the same bony lamella observed in both cross and longitudinal section. In other words, evidence has never been given that a transverse (birifringent) lamella takes on the aspect of a longitudinal (extinguished) lamella when orthogonally sectioned, and vice versa.

We approach the problem by analysing under the scanning electron microscope (SEM) solid samples of human compact bone with edges having angles of 90°. Fig. 7 shows the cross and the longitudinal sectional

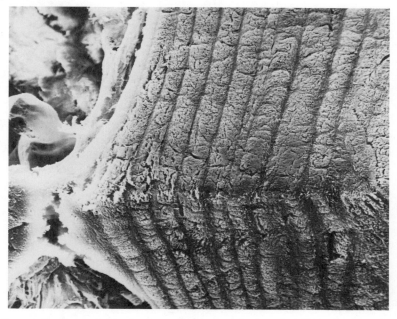

Figure 7. Scanning electron micrograph (x 1,200) of the edge of a lamellar human osteon. Note that each single lamella shows the same structural aspect in both the cross and the longitudinal sectional surfaces of the osteon.

surfaces of a lamellar osteon, and it reveals that Gebhardt's model is wrong. For, according to this model, the longitudinal lamellae, which appear stippled in the cross-sectional surface of the osteon, should show a striped aspect in the longitudinal surface, and vice versa the transverse lamellae. But this is not the case; in fact, it clearly appears that the lamellae showing a striped or a stippled aspect in the cross surface, respectively appear striped and stippled in the longitudinal surface as well. We recently substantiated this observation by analysing the edges of ground sections of lamellar bone also under polarized light (fig. 8). This unexpected finding was observed in all the samples of human lamellar bone examined, without any exception as regards the age of the subjects.

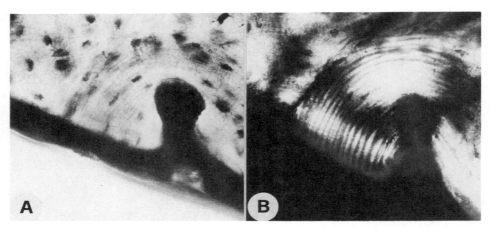

Figure 8. Edge of an undecalcified ground section of human compact bone under ordinary light (A) and polarized light (B): x 180. Note in B that each single lamella appears birifringent (bright) or extinguished (dark) both in the cross and in the longitudinal surfaces of the section.

To explain why any single lamella always shows the same appearance whatever the plane of the section, one must necessarily postulate that within each lamella the collagen fibers follow different orientations and not a preferential one. Indeed, at higher magnification it appears that bone lamellation is largely due to a different density of fibrillar matrix rather than to a different orientation of collagen fibers in adjacent lamellae (fig. 9). The collagen-rich layers (dense lamellae) are in general thinner than the collagen-poor layers (loose lamellae), and show compact and interwoven bundles of longitudinally-, cross- and variously obliquely-sectioned fibers. The loose lamellae are bands of interwoven delicate fibers; most of these fibers seem to arise, according to various angles, from the peripheral part of an adjacent dense lamella and, after an oblique or transverse course, they penetrate into the dense lamella of the opposite side. The interwoven texture of the lamellae with collagen bundles running in various directions is also visible on the surface of the lamellae lining the endosteum (fig. 10). It must be noted, however, that the interlacement of fibers within the lamellae does not

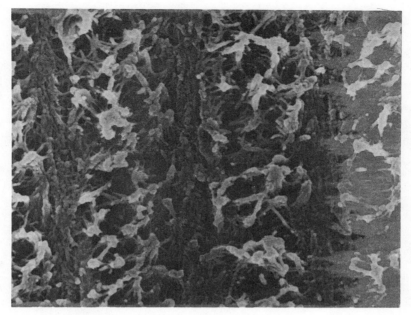

Figure 9. Scanning electron micrograph (x 6,300) showing the interwoven texture of <u>dense</u> and <u>loose lamellae</u> in a cross-sectioned human osteon.

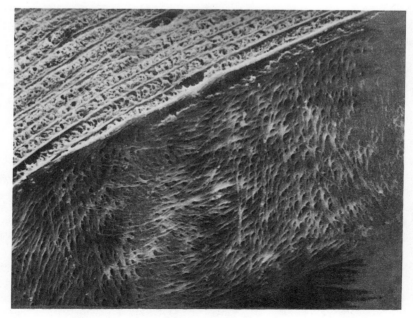

Figure 10. Scanning electron micrograph (x 800) of the surface of a lamella lining the endosteum in a human tibial shaft. Note the criss-cross texture of collagen fibers.

appear to be completely haphazard. Small patches of preferred fiber orientation similar to Boyde's[15] domains were observed. Moreover, the bundles conjoining adjacent dense lamellae sometimes form, while crossing in loose lamellae, ogival arches recalling Gothic vaults. This artistic microarchitecture may explain why TEM analysis, being restricted to small microscopic fields in ultrathin sections, gives the impression of a lamellar collagen pattern more orderly arranged than it really is[16,17,18].

The result of the comparative analysis with polarized light and the SEM shows that the dense lamellae are anisotropic and the loose lamellae are isotropic. The birifringence of the dense lamellae seem to be due to the compact bundles of fibres lying in the plane of the section, while the anisotropy of the loose lamellae is not evidenced by polarized light probably because the delicate fibres lying in the plane of the section are not aligned in dense bundles. By means of X-ray microprobe analysis we recently found that Calcium and Phosphorus content in loose lamellae is 10-15% higher than in dense lamellae (unpublished data). Thus bone minerals really seem mostly associated with the components of the amorphous ground substance, as suggested in literature[19,20].

A lamellar bone made up of layers all having an interwoven fibrous texture, and only differing in collagen and ground substance density, enables the interpretation of many findings that do not fit in with Gebhardt's model (see Marotti[13]); in particular, as far as cellular control of collagen fibers orientation is concerned.

It has been shown, in this connection, that the orientation of collagen tends to be the same as the osteoblast that formed it[21]. It has also been suggested that the alignment of collagen fibers occurs only if the osteoblasts are able to move, with respect to the matrix they produce, according to the direction of the main axis of the fibers[15,21]. If orientation and movement of osteoblasts are the main factors in collagen orientation, Gebhardt's model and a fortiori, by virtue of its complexity, the twisted plywood model too, recently proposed by Giraud-Guille[18], appear impossible to explain in terms of osteoblastic activity. For, in order to build such models, one must assume not only that all the osteoblasts of an osteogenetic lamina should shift in the same direction and presumably for a certain distance to orient the collagen fibers of a single lamella (or plywood) but also, after having completed a lamella (or a plywood) and before the deposition of the successive one, they should also rotate all together by about 90° (by a small but constant angle in the case of plywoods) and then move again according to the direction of the collagen in the new lamella (or plywood). A complicated process like this cannot occur, since the space for mass shifting of the osteoblastic laminae is materially lacking. Where do the cells situated on the periphery of the osteoblastic laminae end up?

On the contrary, cell movement and rotation do not need to occur during the deposition of dense and loose lamellae, because the osteoblasts continue to lay down an interwoven fibrillar matrix.

The problem is now to explain the formation of successive collagen-rich and collagen-poor layers. Obviously this might depend on waves in fibrillogenetic activity by osteoblasts. But this phenomenon too is not simple to explain from the viewpoint of osteoblast metabolism.

From a careful examination of our material, especially as regards distribution of the osteocyte lacunae and their relationship with collagen, it emerges that: a) in all types of bone tissues, osteocyte lacunae appear to be surrounded by a rather thick layer (osteocyte perilacunar matrix) of loosely arranged collagen fibers whose structure looks like that of loose lamellae; b) osteocytes in lamellar bone are found to be almost exclusively located inside loose lamellae. On the basis of these two findings, I have come to the provisional conclusion that the difference in the collagen textures between woven-fibred bone and lamellar bone mainly depends on the manner of recruitment of osteoblasts that transform into osteocytes - a phenomenon that, in turn, is probably connected with the rate at which bone matrix is laid down.

In woven-fibred bone, which is generally laid down very rapidly, the osteoblasts are recruited haphazardly and "enter" the bone confusedly; with the result that woven bone consists of an irregular distribution of osteocyte-rich areas, where the collagen is loosely arranged because it corresponds to that of the perilacunar matrices, interposed with osteocyte-poor or acellular areas, recalling the structure of dense lamellae (fig. 11A).

In lamellar bone, osteoblast recruitment seems to occur in an orderly manner, probably because the matrix is laid down at a lower rate than in woven bone. Since cellular lamellae are only the loose ones, one may logically suppose that the osteoblasts committed to transforming into osteocytes are recruited in successive groups, i.e. when the formation of a loose lamella is required. Given that the osteoblasts of each individual group are distributed in a single plane, i.e. corresponding to that of a loose lamella, it follows that the latter could simply form by the fusion of the loosely arranged fibers pertaining to the osteocyte perilacunar matrices (fig. 11B) It is likely that the low collagen content of the loose lamellae also depends on the reduction in fibrillogenetic activity of the osteoblasts that occurs as they transform into osteocytes[9,10].

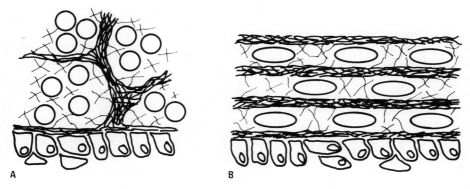

A   B

Figure 11. Schematic drawings of the deposition of woven-fibred bone (A) and lamellar bone (B). Osteocyte lacunae are indicated as open circles in the former and as open ellipses in the latter. Below the osteoblastic laminae. See text for explanation.

To summarize, according to our hypothesis, the osteoblasts always secrete the same type of dense fibrillar matrix in both woven and lamellar bone; the loose fibrillar matrix is laid down only during the trasformation of osteoblasts into osteocytes, and this leads to the formation of the osteocyte perilacunar matrices. In woven bone, the irregular arrangement of collagen-rich areas and collagen-poor areas depends on the random distribution of the osteocytes, the latter resulting from the haphazard recruitment of osteoblasts. In lamellar bone, the alternation of collagen-rich layers (dense lamellae) with collagen-poor layers (loose lamellae) occurs as a result of the recruitment by groups of osteoblasts, and of the arrangement in a single plane, i.e. that of a loose lamella, of all those belonging to each individual group. If this hypothesis is confirmed by further investigations, the "thickness" of dense lamellae will be found to depend on the interval of time elapsing between the recruitment of the groups of osteoblasts; while the greater or lesser "regularity" of the lamellation depends on the type of frequency with which the recruitments occur. It is worth noting in this connection that the few transversally-structured osteons we occasionally observed with the SEM show the whole wall as a very thick dense lamella and do not seem to contain osteocyte lacunae.

In parallel-fibred bone, the recruitment of osteoblasts probably does not occur in groups like in lamellar bone, and certainly not haphazardly as in woven bone. The osteocyte lacunae are fairly regularly spaced one from another, as in lamellar bone, but not aligned by planes. In term of osteogenesis, parallel-fibred bone seems always to have been the easiest to account for, since in order to lay it down the osteoblasts need neither change orientation nor modify fibrillogenetic activity.

REFERENCES

1. E. Lozupone, Differenze topografiche nella velocità di deposizione del tessuto osseo nella spugnosa di ossa lunghe di cani di età diversa, Arch. ital. Anat. Embriol., suppl.78:54 (1973).
2. G. Marotti, E. Lozupone, A. Favia, and V. Lattanzi, Variazioni topografiche e relative all'età della velocità di apposizione del tessuto osseo sulle trabecole della spugnosa, Boll. Soc. ital. Biol. sper., 45:1017 (1969).
3. J. D. Manson, and N. E. Waters, Maturation rate of osteon cat, Nature (Lond), 200:489 (1963).
4. J. D. Manson, and N.E. Waters, Observations on the rate of maturation of the cat osteon. J. Anat.(Lond), 99.3:539 (1965).
5. G. Marotti, and M. E. Camosso, Quantitative analysis of osteonic bone dynamics in the various periods of life, in: "Les tissus calcifiés", G. Milhaud, M. Owen, and H. J. Blackwood, eds., SEDES, Paris (1968).
6. G. Marotti, Decrement in volume of osteoblasts during osteon formation and its effect on the size of the corresponding osteocytes, in: "Bone histomorphometry", P. J. Meunier, ed., Armour Montagu, Paris (1977).
7. A. Zambonin Zallone, Relationship between shape and size of the osteoblasts and the accretion rate of trabecular bone surfaces, Anat. Embryol., 152:65 (1977).

8. G. Volpi, S. Palazzini, V. Canè, F. Remaggi, and M. A. Muglia, Morphometric analysis of osteoblast dynamics in the chick embryo tibia, Anat. Embryol., 162:393 (1981).

9. C. Palumbo, A three-dimensional ultrastructural study of osteoid -osteocytes in the tibia of chick embryos, Cell Tissue Res., 246:125 (1986).

10. C. Palumbo, S. Palazzini, D. Zaffe, and G. Marotti, Osteocyte differentiation in the tibia of newborn rabbit: An ultrastructural study of the formation of cytoplasmic processes, Acta Anat. (in press).

11. R. V. Talmage, Morphological and physiological considerations in a new concept of calcium transport in bone, Amer. J. Anat., 129:467 (1970).

12. G. Marotti, and M. A. Muglia, A scanning electron microscope study of human bony lamellae. Proposal for a new model of collagen lamellar organization, Arch. ital. Anat. Embriol., 93:163 (1988).

13. G. Marotti, The original contributions of the SEM to the knowledge of bone structure, in: "Ultrastructure of skeletal tissues. Bone and cartilage in normalcy and pathology", E. Bonucci, and P. Motta, eds., Kluwer Academic Publishers, Norwell USA (1989) (in press).

14. W. Gebhardt, Über funktionell wichtige Anordnungsweisen der feineren und gröberen Bauelemente des Wiberltierknochens. II. Spezieller Teil. Der Bau der Haversschen Lamellensysteme und seine funktionelle Bedeutung, Arch. Entw. Mech. Org., 20:187 (1906).

15. A. Boyde, Scanning electron microscope studies of bone, in: "The biochemistry and physiology of bone", G. H. Bourne, ed., Academic Press, New York London (1972).

16. A. Ascenzi, E. Bonucci, and D. S. Bocciarelli, An electron microscope study of osteon calcification, J. Ultrastruct. Res., 12:287 (1965).

17. A. Ascenzi, and A. Benvenuti, Orientation of collagen fibers at the boundary between two successive osteonic lamellae and its mechanical interpretation, J. Biomechanics, 19:455 (1986).

18. M. M. Giraud-Guille M.M., Twisted plywood architecture of collagen fibrils in human compact bone osteons, Calcif. Tissue Int., 42:167 (1988).

19. G. W. Bernard, and D. C. Pease, An electron microscopic study of initial intramembranous osteogenesis, Am. J. Anat., 125:271 (1969).

20. E. Bonucci,(1984) The structural basis of calcification, in: "Ultrastructure of connective tissue matrix", S. Ruggeri, and P. M. Motta eds., Martinus Nijhoff Publisher, Boston (1984).

21. S. J. Jones, A. Boyde, and J. B. Pawley, J.B., Osteoblasts and collagen orientation, Cell Tiss. Res., 159:73 (1975).

ANALYSIS OF EMBRYONIC CARTILAGE AND BONE INDUCTION

IN A DEFINED CULTURE SYSTEM

Harold C. Slavkin, Malcolm L. Snead, Wen Luo, Pablo Bringas, Jr.,
Shigeshi Kikunaga, Yasuyuki Sasano, Conny Bessem, Mark Mayo,
Mary MacDougall, Leslie B. Rall,* Daniel Rappolee* and Zena Werb*

Laboratory for Developmental Biology
Department of Basic Sciences
School of Dentistry
University of Southern California
Los Angeles, California 90089-0191, USA

and

*Laboratory of Radiobiology & Environmental Health
School of Medicine
University of California-San Francisco
San Francisco, California 94143-0750, USA

INTRODUCTION

The primary means by which vertebrate mineralized tissues become determined during development is by interaction between different regions of the embryo, a process known as embryonic induction. Numerous examples of embryonic induction were intensively studied problems in developmental biology during the first 70 years of the 20th century (see reviews by Spemann, 1938, Grobstein, 1967; Hall, 1988). Progress in the last few years has in part been the result of applications of recombinant DNA technology to classical questions in the field of embryonic induction (e.g. see recent reviews by Gurdon, 1987; 1988; Edelman, 1988). The key issues appear to be when, where and which sequence of regulatory factor expression activate signal transduction processes resulting in the allocation, determination and differentiation of specific phenotypes. There are probably multiple signals and multiple receptors required for inductive processes.

Perhaps the most significant finding in this field in recent years was the discovery that particular polypeptide growth factors can substitute for the inducing tissue, resulting, for example, in mesodermal induction in animal cap ectoderm during early amphibian embryogenesis (using an assay of muscle-specific transcription) (see Dale and Slack, 1987). One inductive regulatory factor, which has properties similar to TGF-*beta* (transforming growth factor) was found to be secreted by a *Xenopus* cell line (Smith, 1987; Smith et al., 1988). In another study many different polypeptide growth factors were tested and FGF (fibroblast growth factor) was found to be a potent inducer of mesoderm induction (Slack et al., 1987). An mRNA encoding Vg-1, a TGF-*beta*-like peptide, has been localized in the vegetal region of *Xenopus* embryos, the region likely to be important in induction of mesoderm from surrounding cells (Weeks and Melton, 1987). Signalling by growth factors, competence of responding cells, and response mechanisms have been demonstrated (see critical papers by Sharpe et al., 1987 and Otte et al., 1988). It is becoming apparent that sequential growth factor/receptor signal transduction systems play a central role in embryonic induction.

Whereas the history of bone and cartilage induction is extensive, there has been far less success in the analysis of this problem than with amphibian embryonic mesoderm or neurulation inductions. As with mesoderm induction, bone and cartilage induction is likely to involve more than one inductive signal (see reviews by Hall, 1988; Thorgood, 1988). It is proposed that the induction of mineralized tissues is associated with an architecture which includes the vasculature (see Caplan and Pechak, 1987; Shapiro et al., 1988) and a dependency upon exogenous hormones (see Raisz, 1988). During craniofacial morphogenesis, for example, ectodermally-derived epithelium appears to possess regional specifications for the induction of cartilage, bone and tooth organs (Hall, 1981; Lumsden, 1988). A model proposed by Hall (1988a,b) argues that regulatory factors emanating mainly from a discrete region of the ectoderm induces cranial neural crest-derived ectomesenchymal cells to become chondrogenic and osteogenic structures. This model further proposes that epithelium is the source for several regulatory signals which induce discrete populations of competent ectomesenchyme. At least two regulatory signals are implicated in determining the cranial-caudal or rostral-posterior patterns of chondrogenesis and osteogenesis observed during first branchial arch morphogenesis.

In this review paper we present recent discoveries and strategies related to the inductive processes related to cartilage and bone formation. We offer experimental strategies to investigate the important biological parameters of cartilage and bone induction using a simple explant system of the embryonic mouse first branchial arch in serumless medium, and to identify or suggest early responses to epithelial-mediated induction, competence of ectomesenchyme and potential inducing signals. Because, at present we know so little about the signal transduction mechanisms involved in cartilage and bone induction, many of our hypotheses remain tentative. However, we believe that these approaches should enhance investigations of embryonic cartilage and bone induction.

DEVELOPMENTAL SPECIFICATION OF THE CRANIOFACIAL COMPLEX

The initial form of the embryonic craniofacial complex is determined in three ways: (i) the cranium forms by the relative growth of the developing brain, (ii) the craniofacial region forms by the chondrocranium, and (iii) the mandible forms by the Meckel's cartilage. In each of these regions template structures are initially formed which are subsequently replaced and/or modified by replacement structures—bone forms independent of and adjacent to these transitional chondrogenic templates. It is generally found that both chondrogenesis and osteogenesis are induced as the direct consequence of region specified epithelial-mesenchymal interactions (Hall, 1981; 1982; 1984; 1987; 1988a,b; Smith and Thorogood, 1983; Thorogood, 1988). The key questions are when, where, what and how do these heterotypic tissue interactions mediate cartilage and bone induction. In general, these patterns of embryonic craniofacial cartilage and bone inductions are assumed to be highly conserved throughout vertebrate evolution (Gans, 1988).

SPECIFICATION OF MANDIBULAR CARTILAGE AND BONE INDUCTION

The avian and mammalian mandibular processes are derived from the first branchial arch. Mesencephalic and rhombencephalic cranial neural crest-derived ectomesenchyme cells migrate into the forming branchial arch and become allocated and subsequently determined for a number of different phenotypes including chondrogenesis and osteogenesis (see review by Slavkin, 1978). In general, the vasculature is usually associated with the mineralization of cartilage and bone during *in vivo* development (see Caplan and Pechak, 1987; Shapiro et al., 1988; Thorogood, 1988). Bone formation is also assumed to be dependent upon hormones presumably derived from the vasculature (Raisz, 1988). In long bone formation (i.e. endochondral ossification), a discrete population of mesenchymal cells located within a continuous collar surrounding the cartilage anlage differentiate into osteoblasts which synthesize and secrete the extracellular matrix (ECM) termed osteoid (see extensive review by Caplan and Pechak, 1987). Whereas numerous studies have described the morphogenetic, histochemical and biochemical features of bone formation and remodeling (see recent reviews by Caplan and Pechak, 1987; Hauschka et al., 1988; Raisz, 1988; Rodan, 1988; Termine, 1988; Veis, 1988), knowledge of the allocation and determination of the chondrogenic and osteogenic cell lineages remains unknown. One critical limitation to pursue these studies has been the sparse number of specific molecular markers for progenitor cells of either the chondrogenic or osteogenic lineages. A major challenge to developmental biology, therefore, is to determine when, where and how temporally- and spatially-restricted instructions are signalled and received during embryonic cartilage and bone induction.

Exogenous factors permit mandibular cartilage and bone formation in serum-supplemented organ culture

Jacobson and Fell (1941) cultured 3-7 day embryonic chick mandibular processes using a watch-glass method and a culture medium supplemented with plasma, serum and embryonic chick extract. These culture conditions were permissive for the determination and differentiation of both cartilage and bone *in vitro*. These authors demonstrated that the initiation of osteogenesis was independent of cartilage formation during chick mandibular development. These investigators demonstrated that chondrogenic cells first appear in the avian embryonic mandible as two discrete bilateral aggregates adjacent to the rostral epithelium of the first branchial arch; osteogenic cells presumed determined to form the os angulare, spleniale and supra-angulare appeared to develop from an ectomesenchymal proliferative center immediately adjacent to the presumptive mandibular epidermis at the proximo-lateral extension of the mandible (Jacobson and Fell, 1941). Hall (1980; 1981) reported that the vascularized chick chorioallantoic membrane provided a permissive microenvironment for the initiation of chondrogenesis and osteogenesis using embryonic avian and murine mandibular explants.

Epithelial-derived signals induce cartilage and bone formation

Oral ectodermally-derived epithelium induce mesencephalic and rhombencephalic premigratory neural crest cells to express cartilage and/or bone phenotypes (Tyler and Hall, 1977). In the absence of epithelium no cartilage or bone formed. However, mandibular as well as heterologous sources of epithelia elicit bone formation from appropriately staged first branchial arch ectomesenchyme (see extensive review by Hall, 1988b). In other studies using epithelial-mesenchymal recombination strategies, epithelia was found critical to elicit cartilage and/or bone formation, whereas mesenchyme specificity determined the shape or form of the cartilage or bone (Hall, 1980; 1981; Hall et al., 1983; Smith and Thorogood, 1983). The interaction between mandibular epithelium and ectomesenchyme resulting in the formation of intramembranous bone formation requires a viable epithelium (Hall, 1980). In addition, the proliferative activity (the per cent labeling index after administration of ^{3}H-thymidine) of mandibular or non-mandibular epithelia appears to effect the putative epithelial-derived signals required for ectomesenchyme to express the osteogenic phenotype (Hall, 1980). Another important issue is the time and contact between epithelium and responding ectomesenchyme to form bone. Ectomesenchyme cells require a brief interaction with epithelium, several days in advance of the first osteoid detection, before they condense to elicit bone formation (Tyler and Hall, 1977). In addition, evidence is available to suggest that epithelial-derived signals are retained in the basal lamina for limited periods of time and that these signals are sufficient to induce bone formation (Hall et al., 1983; Smith and Thorogood, 1983; Thorogood, 1988). Transfilter studies have provided evidence that an ECM-mediated interaction promotes epithelial induction of bone formation (see discussion in Hall, 1988b; Smith and Thorogood, 1983). A recent indication of the putative epithelial-derived molecular signal(s) was reported by Hall (1988) who provided preliminary immunohistochemical data suggesting that bone morphogenetic protein (BMP) was

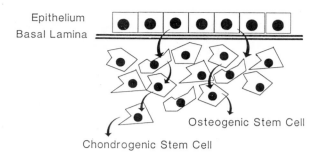

Epithelium
Basal Lamina

Osteogenic Stem Cell

Chondrogenic Stem Cell

Figure 1. Scheme for epithelial-derived signals to induce cartilage and/or bone in competent cranial neural crest-derived ectomesenchyme cells. Two different inductive pathways, signal/receptor transduction mediated, are suggested: (i) allocation and determination of the osteoprogenitor cell lineage, and (ii) allocation and determination of the chondroprogenitor cell lineage.

localized in embryonic chick mandibular epithelium and basement membrane. Hormone-like factors have been identified in epithelial-mesenchymal interactions during embryogenesis (see the excellent review by Rutter and Pictet, 1976) (Figure 1).

Despite these significant advances, however, very little is known regarding (i) the nature, position and timing of the signal(s), (ii) the signal-receptor transduction mechanisms, or (iii) the molecular nature of competency by ectomesenchyme cells which respond to epithelial-derived, cartilage and/or bone-specific signals.

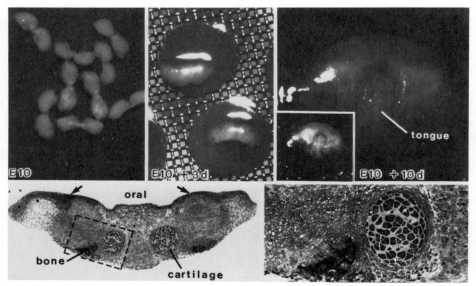

Figure 2. E10 mandibular explants cultured for 10 days *in vitro* produced cartilage, bone, tooth and tongue in a simple culture system using serumless BGJb medium. The histological features shown in the lower panel illustrate molar tooth formation (arrows), cartilage, and bone formation.

Putative intrinsic factors induce cartilage and bone formation in serumless, chemically-defined medium

Of course, the presence of exogenous supplements (e.g. fetal calf sera, chick extracts) for organ culture studies of cartilage and bone induction *in vitro* present a number of confounding and complex variables. Several years ago our laboratory attempted to design a simple culture system for studies of embryonic mouse and avian mandibular development *in vitro* (Slavkin et al., 1982a,b). More recently, we have reported several studies demonstrating that E10-E12 mouse mandibular processes expressed cartilage, bone and tooth inductions using serumless, chemically-defined medium (Slavkin et al., in press) (Figure 2).

The timing, sequence and position for phenotypic expression *in vitro*, albeit smaller in size than *in vivo*, were comparable to those defined for *in vivo* mandibular morphogenesis. Comparison between E10 explants cultured for 10 days *in vitro* and E14 mouse mandibular specimens representing *in vivo* development indicated that the general patterns for bone formation were similar. Embryonic bone induction, osteoblast determination and differentiation, osteoid production and subsequent bone biomineralization were observed in E10 explants developing in the simple culture system (Figure 3A); however, the relative distance between forming Meckel's cartilage and adjacent alveolar bone was diminished in cultured mandibles (Figure 3A). During E14 embryogenesis *in situ* this potential space contained the mandibular division of the fifth cranial nerve observed in transverse sections (i.e. horizontal plane sections) (Figure 3B).

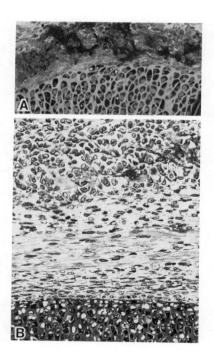

Figure 3. Bone induction in a simple culture system. (A) Meckel's cartilage-bone interface formed *in vitro*. (B) Comparable region during *in vivo* E14 mandibular development indicating the mandibular division of the fifth cranial nerve interposed between Meckel's cartilage and adjacent forming bone (magnification x 200).

Figure 4 illustrates a comparison of growth (based upon cell number and total protein) during embryonic *in vivo* versus *in vitro* mandibular morphogenesis (Figure 4).

We suggest that under these plasma- and serum-deprived conditions early embryonic mouse mandibular processes (E10) produce sequential autocrine and/or paracrine regulatory factors which mediate cartilage and bone induction (Figure 5).

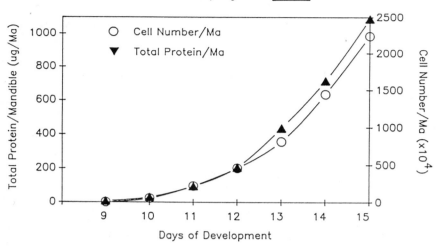

Comparison of Growth During Embryonic Mouse
Mandibular Morphogenesis <u>In Vivo</u>

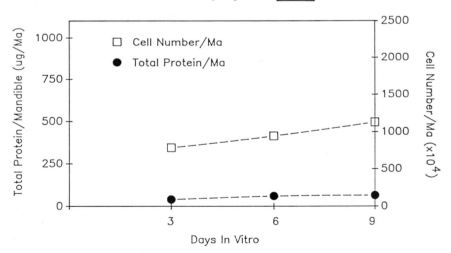

Comparison of Growth During Embryonic Mouse
Mandibular Morphogenesis <u>In Vitro</u>

Figure 4. Comparison of growth during embryonic mandibular morphogenesis *in vivo* and *in vitro*. *In vitro* datasets represent E10 explants cultured for 3, 6 and 9 days *in vitro*. Plotted data represents the mean values of studies performed in triplicate (confidence level > 95%). Ma, mandible.

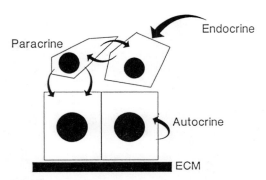

Paracrine

Endocrine

Autocrine

ECM

Figure 5. Putative autocrine and/or paracrine regulatory factors are suggested to control embryonic cartilage and bone inductions when E10 mandibular explants develop in a simple culture system devoid of exogenous growth factors (e.g. serum, plasma, etc.).

Intrinsic Molecular Determinants of Chondrogenesis and Osteogenesis

Table 1 summarizes a number of polypeptides characterized from bone tissues (asterisk indicates those molecules produced locally and assumed to represent the bone phenotype). Fetal cartilage contains a number of growth factors including somatomedin-like peptides (cartilage-derived factor) (Kato et al., 1981) and TGF-*beta* (Seyedin et al., 1987). A number of bone derived growth factors (BDGFs) have been isolated which are nearly identical to PDGF, FGF-*alpha*, FGF-*beta*, TGF-*alpha* and IGF-I (Canalis, 1985; Centrella and Canalis, 1985; Hauschka et al., 1986;1988; Mohan et al., 1987; Pfeilschifter et al., 1986; Robey et al., 1987; Sandy et al., 1989). Bone matrix also contains BMP (see review by Urist et al., 1983). More recent studies indicate that "BMP" consists of three gene products: BMP-1, BMP-2A and BMP-3; BMP-2A and BMP-3 show significant homology to the supergene TGF-*beta* family whereas BMP-1 appears to be a novel regulatory molecule (Wozney et al., 1988). "BMP" irreversibly induces differentiation of perivascular mesenchyme-type cells into osteoprogenitor cells (Urist et al., 1983). The biological functions of these regulatory molecules appears to include chemotaxis, DNA synthesis, cell-cell adhesion resulting in mesenchyme condensations, and the determination of chondrogenic and osteogenic phenotypes.

Recent studies indicate that several substrate adhesion molecules (SAMs) contain motifs which are homologous to several well-defined regulatory molecules. For example, tenascin (also called cytotactin and hexabrachian) is a recently discovered substrate adhesion molecule (SAM) expressed by condensing embryonic mesenchyme cells prior to either cartilage or bone formation (see Mackie et al., 1987; Edelman, 1988). The expression appears to be transitory and was no longer evident when condensing mesenchymal cells established either cartilage or bone phenotypes (Mackie et al., 1987). SAMs presumably guide cranial neural crest-derived ectomesenchyme cell movements towards aggregates or cell condensations which then evolve into discrete pattern formations (histogenesis) such as Meckel's cartilage (see extensive review on cell adhesion and substrate adhesion molecular functions during development by Edelman, 1988). Tenascin synthesis is regulated by TGF-*beta*. Curiously, a single cyotactin gene produces a number of different mRNAs by alternative splicing, resulting in a mechanism for determining tissue-specific cytotactin expression (Jones et al., 1988; 1989). The cDNA sequence contains 13 epidermal-like (EGFL) repeats, 8 consecutive segments that each resemble the type III repeats found in fibronectin, a sequence similar to fibrinogen, a calcium-binding domain, and a single RGD (Arg-Gly-Asp sequence) cell binding sequence (Jones et al., 1988; 1989; Pearson et al., 1988). Therefore, multiple biologically significant regulatory domains are to be found in a single protein SAM molecule. This example is shared with numerous ECM molecules

Table 1. Polypeptides Characterized From Bone Matrix

alpha₁-acid glycoprotein	Hemoglobin
acid phosphatase	IGF-I*
albumin	IgA
alkaline phosphatase*	IgE
anti-thrombin III	IgG
alpha₁-antitrypsin	IgM
apo-I-lipoprotein	Il-1*
bone morphogenetic protein (BMP)*	*beta₂*-microglobulin*
bone phosphoprotein*	osteocalcin*
cholinesterase	osteonectin*
types I and III collagens*	osteopontin*
collagenase*	PDGF*
EGF	prostaglandins (PGE₂)*
FGF-*alpha*★	proteoglycans*
FGF-*beta*★	SGF*
GC-globulin	transferrin
alpha₂-HS-glycoprotein	TGF-*beta*★

*Produced by bone-related tissues
(Data from Centrella and Canalis, 1985; Robey et al., 1987; Hauschka et al., 1986; 1988; Snead et al., in press; Termine, 1988; Veis, 1988)

and could provide a number of growth factor-like motifs which function during chondrogenesis and osteogenesis.

Insulin-like growth factors I and II (i.e. IGF-I and IGF-II), TGF-*beta₁* and c-*fos* are constitutively expressed by cells and implicated in autocrine and paracrine functions during bone formation. Proliferative chondrogenic cells in the growth plate of long bones demonstrate IGF-I intense immunoreactivity whereas hypertrophic cartilage stain only weakly (Nilsson et al., 1986). These studies further indicate that the number of IGF-I staining cells is directly related to the endocrine effects of growth hormone (Nilsson et al., 1986). IGF-II gene transcripts were localized to both mesodermally-derived mesenchyme as well as cranial neural crest-derived ectomesenchyme during embryonic E10-E16 rat craniofacial and body formation using *in situ* hybridization; ectodermally-derived tissues were negative for hybridization (Stylianopoulou et al., 1988). Initial progenitor chondroblasts and chondrocytes expressed IGF-II, whereas this hybridization signal decreased with cartilage and bone mineralization (Stylianopoulou et al., 1988). This pattern of expression was comparable for that described for TGF-*beta*. The highest levels of TGF-*beta* mRNA were associated with osteoblasts in developing bone, whereas TGF-*beta* transcripts decreased in chondroblasts/chondrocytes with increased type II collagen expression (Sanberg et al., 1988). Curiously, proto-oncogene c-*fos* mRNA was localized in chondrocytes adjacent to the joint space of developing human long bones and osteoclasts (Sandberg et al., 1988).

EGF Precursor: A Paradigm for Endogenous Growth Factors

One putative growth factor implicated in cartilage and bone induction is epidermal growth factor (EGF). Whereas EGF precursor has been reported to be produced in both the adult mouse salivary gland and kidney (Rall et al., 1985), Snead and his colleagues (in press) have recently used *in situ* hybridization to localize EGF precursor mRNA expression in fetal mouse Meckel's cartilage and adjacent osteogenic tissues. The regulatory function(s) of precursor EGF or EGF during chondrogenesis or osteogenesis are not known.

The mouse salivary gland EGF precursor is a 1217 amino acid protein which contains mature EGF (aa residues 977-1029) as well as eight EGF-like (EGFL) repeats (Scott et al., 1983). The EGFL repeat motifs also occur in a number of other proteins

Table 2. Relative Expression of Growth Factor mRNA in Developing Embryonic Mouse Mandibles

Growth Factor mRNA	Days In Vivo						Days In Vitro			
	E 8	9	10	11	12	13	E 10	+3	+6	+9
EGF	-	+/-	+	+	+ +	+ + +	+	+ +	+ + +	+ + + +
IGF-I	-	-	+/-	+ +	+ +	+ +	+/-	+	+ +	+ + +
IGF-II	+ +	+ +	+ +	+	+	+	+ +	+	+	+
TGF-α	+	+	+	+	+	+	+	+	+	+
TGF-β1	+	+	+ +	+ +	+ + +	+ + +	+ +	+ +	+ + +	+ + +
β-ACTIN	+	+	+	+	+	+	+	+	+	+

The approximate level of growth factor and *beta*-actin mRNA was measured by the RT-PCR method. The comparisons were made following resolution on agarose gels and ethidium bromide staining.

including (i) the homeotic genes Notch and lin-12 (Greenwald, 1985; Wharton et al., 1985), and (ii) the substrate adhesion molecule cytotactin (tenascin) (Jones et al., 1988; 1989; Pearson et al., 1988), and (iii) domains within laminin also contain EGFL motifs (Panayotou et al., 1989). Both the EGF and the transmembrane domains of the preproEGF sequence are similar to TGF-*alpha* (Derynck, 1988); both EGF and TGF-*alpha* induce a mitogenic response in a variety of cells and both growth factors bind to the same receptor. The 50 amino acid processed form of TGF-*alpha* is synthesized as an internal motif within a 160 amino acid precursor (see review by Derynck, 1988). TGF-*alpha* precursor mRNA is expressed in preimplantation mouse embryos (Rappolee et al., 1988b). EGF, IGF-I, IGF-II, TGF-*alpha* and TGF-*beta* precursor mRNAs are expressed by embryonic mouse mandibular cells both *in vivo* and when E10 mandibular explants are cultured for 3, 6 and 9 days in a simple culture system (unpublished observations) (Table 2). Both EGF and TGF-*beta* transcripts progressively increased *in vivo* as well as *in vitro*, whereas IGF-I and IGF-II were inversely related to one another.

A survey of TGF-*alpha* mRNA expression in E9-E16 mouse embryos reported that TGF-*alpha* is transiently expressed. *In situ* hybridization demonstrated TGF-*alpha* mRNA in E9 and E10 placenta, otic vesicle, oral cavity, pharyngeal pouch, first and second branchial arches and developing kidney (Wilcox and Derynck, 1988); no TGF-*alpha* hybridizing cells were detected after day E10. Insulin-like growth factors I and II (IGF-I and IGF-II) mRNAs were localized uniquely to embryonic rodent mesoderm, ectomesenchyme and endoderm derivatives but were not identified in ectoderm of ectoderm-derived epithelium (Beck et al., 1987). IGF-II mRNA was distributed in the first and second branchial arch ectomesenchyme, and the progenitor chondrogenic cell condensations but was not detected in mature cartilage chondrocytes or mature bone osteocytes (Beck et al., 1987). Comparable observations have been reported for IGF-I and IGF-II mRNA localizations using *in situ* hybridization in human fetal tissues (Han et al., 1987).

Recently, transmembrane TGF-*alpha* precursors were demonstrated to activate EGF/TGF-*alpha* receptors (Brachmann et al., 1989). These studies have established that cell-cell contacts between TGF-*alpha* precursor producing cells and adjacent cells expressing increased levels of EGF/TGF-*alpha* receptors was sufficient to induce the tyrosine autophosphorylation of the receptor (Brachmann et al., 1989; Wong et al., 1989). Therefore, close cell-cell contacts as observed during initial phases of cartilage or bone induction may represent discrete and sequential events mediated by growth factor-receptor signal transduction mechanisms.

PROSPECTUS FOR UNDERSTANDING BONE REGULATORY FACTORS

Embryonic induction is an interaction between one inducing tissue and another responding tissue resulting in the responding tissue pursuing a unique direction of differentiation (Gurdon, 1987). In all examples of embryonic induction, including bone induction, the process is very complex and assumed to represent a series of discrete and sequential reciprocal interactions between the inducing and responding cells and/or tissues. Further, it is reasonable to assume at this point that the molecular signals (e.g. growth factors serving as regulatory molecules) for embryonic bone induction will not be osteogenic specific, but rather the pattern of signal/receptor transduction events will actually serve as the "metabolic code" for osteogenic, for example, rather than myogenic phenotypes (see original hypothesis as developed by Tomkins, 1975).

Embryonic bone induction would appear to begin as both competence and inducing abilities are acquired by spatially and temporally-restricted populations of cells. In the case of mandibular bone induction, reciprocal epithelial-mesenchymal interactions within the forming first branchial arch mediate bone induction. Regionally specified heterotypic (e.g. epithelial-mesenchymal) and/or homotypic (e.g. ectomesenchyme-ectomesenchyme) cell-cell contacts restrict the number of cells that can respond to the putative signals for determining the osteogenic cell lineage—boundaries are determined and pattern formations (histogenesis) are delineated.

The challenge, of course, is to define the progressive expression of regulatory factors and their receptors, to discriminate between permissive and instructive signalling, and to define the specific molecular sequence of events required to irreversibly determine the phenotype for the osteoprogenitor cell lineage.

ACKNOWLEDGEMENTS

The authors thank Valentino Santos for technical assistance, and Michael Brennan for preparing this manuscript. This work was supported by the Office of Health and Environmental Research, U.S. Department of Energy (Contract DE-AC03-76-SF01012), and by grants from the National Institutes of Health (DE-06425, DE-06988, HD-23539 and HD-23651), and by National Institutes of Health Research Career Development Award (M.L.S., DE-00133) and National Research Service Award (5 T32 ES07106).

REFERENCES

Anderson, H.C., 1976, Osteogenic epithelial-mesenchymal cell interactions, *Clin. Orthop. Rel. Res.*, 119:211.

Beck, F., Samani, N.J., Penschow, J.D., Thorley, B., Tregear, G.W., and Coghlan, J.P., 1987, Histochemical localization of IGF-I and -II mRNA in the developing rat embryo, *Development*, 101:175.

Brachmann, R., Lindquist, P.B., Nagashima, M., Kohr, W., Lipari, T., Napier, M., and Derynck, R., 1989, Transmembrane TGF-*alpha* precursors activate EGF/TGF-*alpha* receptors, *Cell*, 56:691.

Canalis, E., 1985, Effect of growth factors on bone cell replication and differentiation, *Clin. Orthop. Relat. Res.*, 193:246.

Caplan, A.I. and Pechak, D.G., 1987, The cellular and molecular embryology of bone formation, *in*: "Bone And Mineral Research/5," W.A. Peck, ed., Elsevier, Amsterdam.

Centrella, M. and Canalis, E., 1985, Transforming and nontransforming growth factors are present in medium conditioned by fetal rat calvariae, *Proc. Natl. Acad. Sci., USA*, 82:7335.

Dale, L. and Slack, J.M.V., 1987, Regional specification within the mesoderm of early embryos of *Xenopus laevis*, *Development*, 100:279.

Derynck, R., 1988, Transforming growth factor *alpha*, *Cell*, 54:593.

Edelman, G.M., 1988, "Topobiology", Basic Books, Inc., New York.

Gans, C., 1988, Craniofacial growth, evolutionary questions, *Development*, 103:3.

Greenwald, I., 1985, Lin-2, a nematode homeotic gene is homologous to a set of mammalian proteins that includes epidermal growth factor, *Cell*, 43:583.

Grobstein, C., 1967, Mechanisms of organogenetic tissue interaction, *Natl. Cancer Inst. Monogr.*, 26:279.

Gurdon, J.B., 1987, Embryonic induction-molecular prospects, *Development*, 99:285.

Gurdon, J.B., 1988, A community effect in animal development, *Nature*, 336:772.

Hall, B.K., 1980, Tissue interactions and the initiation of osteogenesis and chondrogenesis in the neural crest-derived mandibular skeleton of the embryonic mouse as seen in isolated murine tissues and in recombination of murine and avian tissues, *J. Embryol. Exp. Morph.*, 58:251.

Hall, B.K., 1981, The induction of neural crest-derived cartilage and bone by embryonic epithelia: an analysis of the mode of action of an epithelial-mesenchymal interaction, *J. Embryol. Exp. Morph.*, 64:305.

Hall, B.K., 1982, The role of tissue interactions in the growth of bone. *in*: "Factors and Mechanisms Influencing Bone Growth," A.S. Dixon and B.G. Sarnat, eds., Alan R. Liss, Inc., New York.

Hall, B.K., 1984, Genetic and epigenetic control of connective tissues in the cranial structures. *Birth Defects: Original Article Series*, 20(3):1.

Hall, B.K., 1987, Initiation of chondrogenesis from somitic, limb and craniofacial mesenchyme: search for a common mechanism, *in*: "Somites in Developing Embryos," R. Bellairs, D.A. Ede and J.W. Lash, eds., *Plenum*, New York.

Hall, B.K., 1988a, Patterning of connective tissues in the head: discussion report, *Development*, 103:171.

Hall, B.K., 1988b, The embryonic development of bone, *American. Sci.*, 76:174.

Hall, B.K., Van Exan, R., and Brunt, S., 1983, Retention of epithelial basal lamina allows isolated mandibular mesenchyme to form bone, *J. Craniofac. Genet. & Develop. Biol.*, 3:253.

Han, V.K.M., D'Ercole, J., and Lund, P.K., 1987, Cellular localization of somatomedin (insulin-like growth factor)messenger RNA in the human fetus, *Science*, 236:193.

Hauschka, P.V., Mavrakos, A.E., Iafrati, M.D., Doleman, S.E., and Klagsbrun, M., 1986, Growth factors in bone matrix. Isolation of multiple types by affinity chromatography on heparin-Sepharose, *J. Biol. Chem.*, 261:12665.

Hauschka, P.V., Chen, T.L., and Mavrakos, A.E., 1988, Polypeptide growth factors in bone matrix, *in*: "Cell and Molecular Biology of Vertebrate Hard Tissues," G.A. Rodan, ed., Wiley, Chichester.

Jacobsen, W. and Fell, H.B., 1941, The developmental mechanics and potencies of the undifferentiated mesenchyme of the mandible, *Quart. J. Micro. Sci.*, 82:563.

Jones, F.S., Burgoon, M.P., Hoffman, S., Crossin, K.L., Cunningham, B.A., and Edelman, G.M., 1988, A cDNA clone for cytotactin contains sequences similar to epidermal growth factor-like repeats and segments of fibronectin and fibrinogen, *Proc. Natl. Acad. Sci., USA*, 85:2186.

Jones, F.S., Hoffman, S., Cunningham, B.A., and Edelman, G.M., 1989, A detailed structural model of cytotactin: protein homologies, alternative RNA splicing and binding regions, *Proc. Natl. Acad. Sci. USA*, 86:1905.

Kawamura, M. and Urist, M.R., 1988, Growth factors, mitogens, cytokines and bone morphogenetic protein in induced chondrogenesis in tissue culture, *Develop. Biol.*, 130:435.

Kimelman, D. and Kirschner, M., 1987, Synergistic induction of mesoderm by FGF and TGF-*beta* and the identification of an mRNA coding for FGF in the early Xenopus embryo, *Cell*, 51:869.

Lian, J., Stewart, C., Puchacz, E., Mackowiak, S., Shalhoub, V., Collart, D., Zambetti, G., and Stein, G., 1989, Structure of the rat osteocalcin gene and regulation of vitamin D-dependent expression, *Proc. Natl. Acad. Sci, USA*, 86:1143.

Lumsden, A.G.S., 1988, Spatial organization of the epithelium and the role of neural crest cells in the initiation of the mammalian tooth germ, *Development*, 103:155.

Mackie, E.J., Thesleff, I., and Chiquet-Ehrismann, R., 1987, Tenascin is associated with chondrogenic and osteogenic differentiation *in vivo* and promotes chondrogenesis *in vitro*, *J. Cell Biol.*, 105:2569.

Mohan, S., Linkhart, T.A., Jennings, J.C., and Baylink, D.J., 1987, Identification and quantitation of four distinct growth factors stored in human bone matrix, *J. Bone Miner. Res.*, 2(Suppl. 1):44.

Nakano, T., Kimoto, S., Tanikawa, K., Kim, K.T., Higaki, M., Kawase, T., and Saito, S., 1989, Identification of osteoblast-specific monoclonal antibodies, *Calcif. Tiss Int.*, 44:220.

Nilsson, A., Isgaard, J., Lindahl, A., Dahlstrom, A., Skottner, A., Isaksson, O.G.P., 1986, Regulation by growth hormone of number of chondrocytes containing IGF-I in rat growth plate, *Science*, 233:571-574.

Otte, A.P., Koster, C.H., Snoek, G.T., and Durston, A.J., 1988, Protein kinase C mediates neural induction in *Xenopus laevis*, *Nature*, 334:618.

Panayotou, G., End, P., Aumailley, M., Timpl, R., and Engel, J., 1989, Domains of laminin with growth-factor activity, *Cell*, 56:93.

Pearson, C.A., Pearson, D., Shibahara, S., Hofsteenge, J., and Chiquet-Ehrismann, R., 1988, Tenascin: cDNA cloning and induction by TGF-beta, *EMBO J.*, 7:2977.

Pechak, D.G., Kujawa, M.J., and Caplan, A.I., 1986, Morphology of bone development and bone remodeling in embryonic chick limbs, *Bone*, 7:459.

Pedersen, R.A., 1988, Early mammalian embryogenesis, *in*: "The Physiology of Reproduction," E. Knobil and J. Neill et al., eds., Raven Press, Ltd., New York.

Pfeilschifter, J., D'Souza, S., and Mundy, G.R., 1986, Transforming growth factor *beta* is released from resorbing bone and stimulates osteoblast activity, *J. Bone Miner. Res.*, 1(Suppl.):294.

Rappolee, D.A., Mark, D., Banda, M.J., and Werb, Z., 1988a, Wound macrophages express TGF-*alpha* and other growth factors *in vivo*: analysis by mRNA phenotyping, *Science*, 241:708.

Rappolee, D.A., Brenner, C.A., Schultz, R., Mark, D., and Werb, Z., 1988b, Developmental expression of PDGF, TGF-*alpha* and TGF-*beta* genes in preimplantation mouse embryos, *Science*, 241:1823.

Rappolee, D.A., Wang, A., Mark, D., and Werb, Z., 1989, Novel method for studying mRNA phenotypes in single or small numbers of cells, *J. Cell. Biochem.*, 39:1.

Raisz, L.G., 1988, Hormonal regulation of bone growth and remodelling, *in*: "Cell and Molecular Biology of Vertebrate Hard Tissues," G.A. Rodan, ed., Wiley, Chichester.

Rall, L.B., Scott, J., Bell, G.I., Crawford, R.J., Penschow, J.D., Niall, H.D., and Coghlan, J.P., 1985, Mouse prepro-epidermal growth factor synthesis by the kidney and other tissues, *Nature*, 313:228

Robey, P.G., Young, M.F., Flanders, K.C., Roche, N.S., Kondaiah, P., Reddi, A.H., Termine, J.D., Sporn, M.B., and Roberts, A.B., 1987, Osteoblasts synthesize and respond to transforming growth factor-type *beta* (TGF-*beta*) *in vitro*, *J. Cell Biol.*, 105:457.

Rodan, G.A., Heath, J.K., Yoon, K., Noda, M., and Rodan, S.B., 1988, Diversity of the osteoblastic phenotype, *in*: "Cell and Molecular Biology of Vertebrate Hard Tissues," G.A. Rodan, ed., Wiley, Chichester.

Rutter, W.J., and Pictet, R.L., 1976, Hormone-like factor(s) in mesenchymal-epithelial interactions during embryonic development, *in*: "Embryogenesis in Mammals," K.Elliot and M. O'Connor, eds., Wiley, New York.

Sandberg, M., Vuorio, T., Hirvonen, H., Alitalo, K., and Vuorio, E., 1988, Enhanced expression of TGF-*beta* and c-*fos* mRNAs in the growth plates of developing human long bones, *Development*, 102:461-470.

Sandy, J.R., Meghji, S., Scutt, A.M., Harvey, W., Harris, M., and Meikle, M.C., 1989, Murine osteoblasts release bone-resorbing factors of high and low molecular weights: stimulation by mechanical deformation, *Bone and Mineral*, 5:155.

Scott, J., Urdea, M., Quiroga, M., Sanchez-Pescador, R., Fong, N., Selby, M., Rutter, W.J., and Bell, G.I.,1983, Structure of a mouse submaxillary messenger RNA encoding epidermal growth factor and seven related proteins, *Science*, 221:236.

Seyedin, S.M., Segarini, P.R., Rosen, D.M., Thompson, A.Y., Bentz, H., and Graycar, J., 1987, Cartilage-inducing factor-B is a unique protein structurally and functionally related to transforming growth factor-*beta*, *J. Biol. Chem.*, 262:1946.

Shapiro, I.M., Golub, E.E., Chance, B., Piddington, C., Oshima, O., Tuncay, O.C., and Haselgrove, J.C., 1988, Linkage between energy status of perivascular cells and mineralization of the chick growth cartilage, *Develop. Biol.*, 129:372.

Sharpe, C.R., Fritz, A., De Robertis, E.M., and Gurdon, J.B., 1987, A homeobox-containing marker of posterior neural differentiation shows the importance of predetermination in neural induction, *Cell*, 50:749.

Slack, J.M.W., Darlington, B.G., Heath, J.K., and Godsave, S.F., 1987, Mesoderm induction in early *Xenopus* embryos by heparin-binding growth factors, *Nature*, 326:197.

Slavkin, H.C., 1978, Mandibular morphogenesis, *in*: "Reconstruction of Jaw Deformities," L.A. Whitaker, ed., C.V. Mosby Co., St. Louis.

Slavkin, H.C., Bringas, P., Cummings, E.C., and Grodin, M.S., 1982a, Murine mandibular chondrogenesis and osteogenesis in a serumless, chemically-defined medium, *in*: "Chemistry and Biology of Mineralized Connective Tissues," A. Veis, ed., Elsevier/North holland, New York.

Slavkin, H.C., Honig, L.S., and Bringas, P., 1982b, Experimental dissection of avian and murine tissue interactions using organ culture in a serumless medium free from exogenous (nondefined) factors, *in*: "Factors and Mechanisms Influencing Bone Growth," A.D. Dixon and B.G. Sarnat, eds., Alan R. Liss, Inc., New York.

Slavkin, H.C., Bringas, P., Sasano, Y., and Mayo, M., (in press) Early embryonic mouse mandibular morphogenesis and cytodifferentiation in serumless, chemically-defined medium: A model for studies of autocrine and/or paracrine regulatory factors, *J. Craniofac. Genet. & Develop. Biol.*

Slavkin, H.C., Sasano, Y., Kikunaga, S., Bessem, C., Bringas, P., Mayo, M., Luo, W., Mak, G., Rall, L., and Snead, M.L. (in press) Cartilage, bone and tooth induction during early embryonic mouse mandibular morphogenesis using serumless, chemically-defined medium, *Conn. Tiss. Res.*

Smith, J.C., 1987, A mesoderm-inducing factor is produced by a *Xenopus* cell line, *Development*, 99:3.

Smith, L. and Thorogood, P., 1983, Transfilter studies on the mechanism of epithelio-mesenchymal interaction leading to chondrogenic differentiation of neural crest cells, *J. Embryol. Exp. Morph.*, 75:165.

Smith, J.C., Yaqoob, M., and Symes, K., 1988, Purification, partial characterization and biological effects of the XTC mesoderm-inducing factor, *Development*, 103:591.

Snead, M.L., Luo, W., Oliver, P., Nakamura, M., Don-Wheeler, G., Bessem, C., Bell, G.I., Rall, L.B., and Slavkin, H.C., (in press) Localization of epidermal growth factor precursor in tooth and lung during embryonic mouse development, *Develop. Biol.*

Spemann, H, 1938, "Embryonic Induction and Development, " Yale University Press, New Haven.

Stylianopoulou, F., Efstratiadis, A., Herbert, J., and Pintar, J., 1988, Pattern of the insulin-like growth factor II gene expression during rat embryogenesis, *Development*, 103:497-506.

Termine, J.D., 1988, Non-collagen proteins in bone, *in*: "Cell and Molecular Biology of Vertebrate Hard Tissues," G.A. Rodan, ed., Wiley, Chichester.

Thorogood, P., 1988, The developmental specification of the vertebrate skull, *Development*, 103:141.

Tomkins, G.M., 1975, The metabolic code, *Science*, 189:760.

Tyler, M.S. and Hall, B.K., 1977, Epithelial influences on skeletogenesis in the mandible of the embryonic chick, *Anat. Rec.*, 188:229.

Urist, M.L., DeLange, R.J., and Finerman, G.A.M., 1983, Bone cell differentiation and growth factors, *Science*, 220:680.

Wahl, M.I., Nishibe, S., Suh, P.G., Rhee, S.G., and Carpenter, G., 1989, Epidermal growth factor stimulates tyrosine phosphorylation of phopholipase C-II independently of receptor internalization and extracellular calcium, *Proc. Natl. Acad. Sci. USA*, 86:1568.

Weeks, D.L. and Melton, D.A., 1987, A maternal mRNA localized to the vegetal hemisphere in *Xenopus* eggs codes for a growth factor related to TGF-*beta*, *Cell*, 51:861.

Wharton, K.A., Johansen, K.M., Xu, T., and Artavanis, T., 1985, Nucleotide sequence from the neurogenic locus Notch implies a gene product that shares homology with proteins containing EGF-like repeats, *Cell*, 43:567.

Wilcox, J.N. and Derynck, R., 1988, Developmental expression of transforming growth factors alpha and beta in mouse fetus, *Molecular & Cellular Biology*, 8:3415.

Wong, S.T., Winchell, L.F., McCune, B.K., Earp, H.S., Teixido, J., Massague, J., Herman, B., and Lee, D.C., 1989, The TGF-*alpha* precursor expressed on the cell surface binds to the EGF receptor on adjacent cells, leading to signal transduction, *Cell*, 56:495.

Wozney, J.M., Rosen, V., Celeste, A.J., Mitsock, L.M., Whitters, M.J., Kriz, R.W., Hewick, R.M., and Wang, E.A., 1988, Novel regulators of bone formation: molecular clones and activities, *Science*, 243:1528

THE ROLE OF CELLS IN THE CALCIFICATION PROCESS

J.N.M. Heersche*, H.C. Tenenbaum**, C.S. Tam***,
C.G. Bellows*, and J.E. Aubin*

  *MRC Group in Periodontal Physiology, Faculty of Dentistry
 **Mt. Sinai Hospital Research Institute and Faculty of Dentistry
***Queen Elizabeth Hospital Research Institute and
  Dept. of Pathology
  University of Toronto, Toronto, Ontario, Canada

Although the vertebrate body contains an abundance of potential sites for mineralization, not every tissue calcifies, which indicates that regulatory processes are operative. The mechanisms responsible for stimulating and inhibiting the initiation and progression of mineralization are likely to be cell-mediated, and various experimental systems have been used to study the involvement of cells, the function of which may be regulated systemically or locally. In this chapter, we will discuss experiments in which we studied the role of vitamin D metabolites as regulators of bone matrix calcification in rats in vivo and experiments designed to analyse the factors involved in regulation of de novo mineralization of bone formed in vitro. First, however, we present a brief overview of the matrix constituents associated with calcification.

Mechanisms of Tissue Calcification

The discussion will be limited to mineralization of bone, dentine and cartilage. In the other mineralizing connective tissues, ie. tendon and cementum, the mechanisms may be similar, but fewer data are available for these.

In both bone and dentine, the tissue surface is covered by a continuous layer of cells; cells of the osteoblast lineage in the case of bone, and odontoblasts in the case of dentine. Synthesis of the organic matrix in both tissues is followed by a lag period (of a duration characteristic for each species), after which the matrix becomes mineralized. It is likely that the cells possess specific means to transfer the large amounts of calcium and phosphate required for calcification from the extracellular fluid into the bone or dentine matrix. The same cells presumably also produce and release molecules responsible for the orderly progression of mineralization at sites in the organic matrix that are usually several um removed from the nearest cell surface. The presence of such molecules may be responsible for the fact that in demineralized sections of bone and dentine the mineralization front can be visualized using specific staining procedures.

Although the organic matrix of bone and dentine consists principally of collagen (~90%), the remaining 10% of organic molecules (glycoproteins and proteoglycans) have been suggested to be the major regulators of the calcification process (see review by Boskey, 1989). The concept of other proteins being involved in the mineralization of collagen fibres seems attractive in view of the poor nucleating properties of pure collagen and the observation that most of the mineral in bone and dentine is clearly associated with the collagen fibres. There is no shortage of proteins that may play such a role in the mineralization process. Dentine phosphoryn, the major soluble phosphoprotein of dentin (50% of noncollagenous protein), was the first molecule shown to bind strongly and specifically to native collagen (Dickson et al., 1975) and to calcium ions. Later, Termine et al. (1981) isolated a protein (osteonectin) from bone tissue, comprising 23% of the non-collagenous proteins of bone, that also bound to both collagen and hydroxyapatite. Although osteonectin now appears not to be unique for bone tissue, and rather abundant in platelets (Stenner et al., 1986) as well as in non-mineralizing tissues (Wasi et al., 1984; Engel et al., 1987), it's abundance in bone would suggest a specific function in this tissue to be likely. Also abundant in the non-collagenous bone protein fraction are osteopontin or BSP I (8-12%), bone gla protein or osteocalcin (15-20%), bone proteoglycan I (4-10%) and bone phosphoprotein (~8%) (for review, see Boskey, 1989). All may be involved in mineralization, but firm evidence to support a definite role for any of these proteins in the mineralization process is not available.

The role of noncollagenous bone proteins in the mineralization process may be two-fold: they may function as nucleators or as inhibitors of crystal growth, depending on whether they are attached to a solid support, i.e. a collagen molecule or are in solution (Linde et al., 1989). If nucleating molecules were to bind specifically to certain areas of the molecule as suggested by Dickson et al. (1975) and by Termine et al. (1981) and Arsenault (1989), one might expect initiation of mineral deposition on the collagen fibre to occur in such areas. Of interest in this regard are observations by Arsenault (1989) that mineral is deposited in both the gap zone and the overlap zone of collagen fibres. He suggested that localization of non-collagenous proteins using immunoelectron microscopical techniques would probably reveal specific correlations between nucleation and localization of such molecules.

The cells at the bone surface involved in the active deposition of organic matrix possess a high content of the membrane bound enzyme alkaline phosphatase (AP). A layer of AP positive cells (stratum intermedium) is also situated adjacent to the ameloblasts in the enamel organ. Primarily because of this spatial association, AP has long been associated with mineralization (Robison, 1923), although the mechanism of this association is still not known. More direct evidence supporting a role for AP in the mineralization process will be discussed later.

Although in mature bone and in circumpulpal dentine the majority of the mineral is associated with collagen fibres, collagen does not seem to be associated with the initiation of mineralization in woven bone, mantle dentine and hypertrophic cartilage. In these latter sites, mineral appears first in matrix vesicles, small membrane bounded structures discovered by Bonucci (1967) and Anderson (1967) in which calcium and phosphate accumulate and probably precipitate initially as octacalcium phosphate (for review, see Wuthier, 1988). In the second phase of matrix vesicle associated mineralization, the mineral is transformed into hydroxyapatite. The crystal ruptures the membrane, thus becomes exposed to the extra-vesicular fluid, and from this initial crystal a wave of mineralization then proceeds, possibly propagated by collagen fibres.

Matrix vesicles are rich in AP, and several lines of evidence (Wuthier, 1988) suggest that this enzyme is closely associated with matrix vesicle mineralization. Thus, AP appears to be associated both with initiation of mineralization in matrix vesicles and with calcification occurring at sites where mineralization progresses presumably independently of the presence of matrix vesicles.

Regulation of Mineralization In Vivo by Vitamin D Metabolites

The most striking effect of vitamin D deficiency in adult mammals is the development of widened osteoid seams. Despite the rapid expansion of knowledge concerning vitamin D actions on target organs, numerous questions remain regarding the direct effects of the various vitamin D metabolites on osteoblasts and matrix mineralization. For example, $1,25(OH)_2D_3$ has been shown to have opposite effects on the synthesis of several constituents of the bone matrix: synthesis of collagen type I by osteoblasts is clearly inhibited (Raisz et al., 1978; Harrison et al., 1989) whereas synthesis of osteocalcin (Price and Baukol, 1980) and of osteopontin (Prince and Butler, 1987) is markedly increased. The plasma concentration of osteocalcin correlates with histomorphometric parameters of bone formation (Delmas et al., 1985), and is generally considered a good parameter of osteoblastic activity. Considering, however, that collagen comprises about 90% of the organic matrix of bone, one might expect that collagen synthesis would similarly correlate with overall matrix synthesis in the osteoblast. The opposite effects of $1,25(OH)_2D_3$ on collagen synthesis (decreased) and osteocalcin synthesis (increased) thus seem difficult to interpret. The possibility that collagen synthesis may reflect osteoid production only, whereas osteocalcin production might be associated mainly with mineralization, seems of interest and requires further investigation.

We have attempted to clarify the effects of vitamin D metabolites on mineralization by investigating their effects on the rate of bone mineral apposition (BMAR) in adult vitamin D-deficient rats. By giving three doses of tetracycline at 48-h intervals, and by measuring sites in which all doses can be identified, the mean linear BMAR can be estimated without the interference of activation of new osteoblasts (Tam et al., 1981; 1986). The linear BMAR measurements were made on the trabecular bone of the lower metaphysis of the right femur. We studied the secondary spongiosa only. Fifteen to 20 sites were measured in each experimental animal, and the arithmetic mean of these was taken as the mean rate for the respective rats.

The effects of vitamin D-depletion on the bone mineral apposition rate (BMAR) and on circulating vitamin D metabolites are shown in Table 1. Vitamin D-depletion reduced the mineral apposition rate. Whereas serum calcium, phosphate and $1,25(OH)_2D_3$ levels were normal, levels of $25OHD_3$ and $24,25(OH)_2D_3$ were clearly decreased. These results agree with clinical observations showing that serum concentrations of $1,25(OH)_2D_3$ are generally not decreased even in severely D-deplete patients (Eastwood et al., 1979), and strongly suggest that circulating levels of either $25(OH)D_3$ or $24,25(OH)_2D_3$ are important in maintaining a normal mineralization rate in newly formed bone. Of course, the decrease in BMAR in D-depleted rats might be a consequence of, or secondary to, decreased apposition of organic bone matrix, or could be a consequence of decreased serum Ca or P levels. We therefore measured the rate of organic matrix apposition in rats maintained for 5 weeks on

71

a D-deficient diet or on the same diet with added vitamin D3 (5IU/gram bw) (Shimizu et al., 1989) by labelling the animals with 2 doses of ^{3}H proline at a 72-hour interval. The results clearly eliminate changes in serum Ca or P or a decreased organic matrix apposition rate as the cause of the decreased BMAR (Table 2). The results also show a discrepancy between effects of vitamin D-deficiency on the BMAR and the OMAR. It is not clear at the present time whether these two phenomena are causally related, but experiments to analyse this further are in progress.

Table 1. Serum concentrations of D metabolites and BMAR in adult vitamin D-sufficient and D-restricted rats

| | Duration (days) | Serum D Metabolites | | | BMAR (um/h) |
		25OHD3 (ng/ml)	1,25(OH)2D3 (pg/ml)	24,25(OH)2D3 (ng/ml)	
Control	0	66.4±15.1	50.6±2.9	33.3±3.4	0.074±0.001
	7	18.6±11.1	60.4±13.0	68.5±10.8	0.075±0.003
	14	67.6±11.9	53.5±18.3	54.4±5.9	0.061±0.002
	28	93.7±38.2	42.9±7.2	64.2±9.3	0.061±0.002
D-	7	8.4±2.6	81.6±8.5	8.6±0.6	0.058±0.003*
	14	4.2±0.9	61.7±7.7	5.5±0.5	0.047±0.004*
	28	3.4±0.6	61.2±7.2	1.8±0.5	0.044±0.003*

The vitamin D-restricted groups were fed a D-deficient diet (Teklad, catalog no. 74800) which contained 1% Ca and 1% P. The control groups were given the same diet supplemented with 1000 IU D3/day. BMAR correlated well with the serum concentrations of either 25OHD3 or 24,25(OH)2D3, but not of 1,25(OH)2D3. n = 6 in the D-restricted groups, and n= 3 in the control groups. Results represent the mean±standard error. *: significantly different from control, $p < 0.05$.

Table 2. BMAR, organic matrix apposition rate (OMAR) and serum concentrations of calcium, phosphorus and of vitamin D metabolites in vitamin D sufficient and vitamin D restricted rats

	Ca (mg/dl)	P (mg/dl)	25OHD3 (ng/ml)	1,25(OH)2D3 (pg/ml)	BMAR (um/d)	OMAR (um/d)
D+	9.6±0.5	9.5±0.7	11.6±2.5	51.3±14.7	2.3±0.2	2.9±0.1
D-	9.4±0.2	9.3±1.4	<0.2*	44.3±14.0	1.9±0.1*	3.9±0.2*

Results are mean±SD based on 5 animals per group.
*Significantly different from vitamin D sufficient group, P<0.05.

In the next series of experiments, D-depleted rats were repleted with 50 ng/day of either 1,25(OH)2D3, 25OHD3 or 24,25(OH)2D3. Several aspects of the results (Table 3) merit further discussion. Firstly, both 25(OH)2D3 and 24,25(OH)2D3 restored the BMAR while 1,25(OH)2D3 did not, suggesting that either the former metabolites or further metabolites of them are required for the normal apposition of bone mineral. Secondly, however, it appeared that both the osteoid-seam width and the mineralization lag time were restored by all metabolites. Thus, administration of all three metabolites results in mineralization of existing osteoid. The observation that $1,25(OH)_2D_3$ has no effect on the BMAR, whereas administration of the other metabolites does restore the BMAR, may imply that $1,25(OH)_2D_3$ administration reduces the organic matrix apposition rate, whereas administration of $24,25(OH)_2D_3$ or $25(OH)_2D_3$ may not.

Table 3. Mean osteoid seam, mineralization lag time (MLT), and bone mineral apposition rate (BMAR), in D-restricted rats supplemented with various metabolites of vitamin D

Supplementation	Mean Osteoid Seam (um)	M.L.T. (days)	B.M.A.R. (um/h)
Nil	7.6*	8.5 (1.3)*	0.041 (0.001)
25OHD$_3$ (50 ng/day)	2.5	2.0 (0.3)	0.052 (0.002)**
$1,25(OH)_2D_3$ (50 ng/day)	3.0	3.1 (0.2)	0.042 (0.001)
$24,25(OH)_2D_3$ (50 ng/day)	2.8	2.1 (0.1)	0.058 (0.002)**

Male Sprague-Dawley rats were made D deficient by feeding with a vitamin D-deficient diet (Teklad catalog no. 74800) for 8 weeks from a time when they weighed 50 g. Six weeks after the start of this dietary treatment they were divided into groups of 5 and were given either no further additional treatment or one of the D metabolites indicated, orally, from day 43 to 56. Tetracycline labelling was started on day 52. Standard errors of the mean are shown in parentheses.
*Significantly different from treated groups, P<0.01.
**Significantly different from non-treated groups, P<0.01.

The data support the concept that $24,25(OH)_2D_3$ deficiency is the major factor responsible for the observed mineralization defect in vitamin D-deficiency. Interestingly, additional results (Tam et al., 1986) have shown that restoration of the mineralization rate to normal by $24,25(OH)_2D_3$ administration requires the presence of Parathyroid hormone. Thus, the question whether the effect of $24,25(OH)_2D_3$ on mineralization represents a direct effect on osteoblasts or is indirect is as yet unanswered. Experiments in in vitro systems are more likely to resolve this question, and will be briefly discussed in the next section.

Mineralization of newly formed bone in vitro

Formation of bone in vitro from populations of osteoprogenitor cells has been analysed in a variety of systems: cultures of limb mesenchymal cells (Osdoby and Kaplan, 1979), membrane bone periosteal cells (Thorogood, 1979), embryonic chick femora (Endo, 1960; Ito et al., 1963) and folded periostea from 17-day-old chick calvariae (Nijweide, et al., 1975). Although the authors of all the cited reports observed various degrees of osteodifferentiation in their cultures, the precise factors controlling osteogenesis and differentiation of osteogenic precursor-cells were difficult to analyze. In addition, reproducible mineralization of the osteoid formed was not observed. Of the systems used, that of Nijweide and colleagues appeared to be the most reproducible for obtaining osteodifferentiation (Nijweide et al., 1975). Using their culture system as our basic model, we have pursued a number of questions related to osteoblast differentiation and mineralization of bone.

When periosteum from the calvariae of 17-day-old fetal chick embryos was cultured on a medium containing embryonic extract and fowl plasma, mineralization of newly formed bone occurred consistently when β-glycerophosphate was added to the culture medium (Tenenbaum and Heersche, 1982). The requirement for additional organic phosphate to achieve mineralization of the osteoid formed in vitro was interpreted by us as indicating that organic phosphate availability, but not necessarily inorganic phosphate availability, was the major limiting factor preventing mineralization. We hypothesized that degradation or metabolism of organic phosphate by AP associated with either cell or matrix vesicle membranes was the major mechanism whereby this phosphate would be made available in the vicinity of cells and not elsewhere.

Further experimentation by Tenenbaum et al. has provided additional evidence that AP activity is likely to be involved in the mineralization process in this system. Firstly, organic phosphates which could be physiological substrata for the enzyme, such as for example phosphoethanolamine, were equally effective in inducing mineralization in this system (Tenenbaum and Palangio, 1987). Secondly, inhibition of AP activity by the addition of levamisole inhibited mineralization (Tenenbaum, 1987). Since in the folded periosteum bone forming system mineralization of the osteoid deposited in vitro occurs mainly on day 5 and 6 in culture, but appears to be initiated during day 4 of culture, levamisole was added at different times of culture to study its effects on initiation and progression of mineralization. When levamisole was present during day 4 of culture, mineralization was inhibited. However, adding it at day 5 of culture had no effect on mineralization, suggesting that AP activity was required for the initiation of mineralization but not for its progression.

If this interpretation is correct, the abundance of AP activity in osteoblasts, particularly in osteoblast processes in the vicinity of the mineralization front (see chapter by Bonucci), may not be related to the progression of mineralization. The observation that pre-osteoblasts and stratum intermedium cells also have a high AP content and are both not adjacent to mineralized tissue similarly suggests another role for the enzyme in these cells. It could be that other aspects of AP, for example its role as a calcium binder (de Bernard et al., 1986) or as a hydrolase for inhibitors of apatite crystal growth (Neuman et al., 1951, Wuthier et al., 1972) are important at these sites. Results showing that inorganic pyrophosphate (PPi) was capable of inhibiting mineralization regardless of when it was added during culture (Tenenbaum, 1987) would support this latter possibility. Other aspects of the role of AP in mineralizing tissues have been reviewed recently (Wuthier and Register, 1985; Whyte, 1989).

The folded periosteum bone forming system has allowed us to probe some of the mechanisms involved in mineralization of newly formed osteoid. To obtain additional information on the relationship between mineralization and synthesis of the non-collagenous proteins thought to be involved in the mineralization process, and on the direct effects of vitamin D metabolites on the mineralization process, we have started to study mineralization of bone nodules formed in vitro from enzymatically released rat calvaria cell populations (Bellows et al., 1986; Nefussi et al., 1985). In this system, discrete three dimensional nodular struc-tures are formed reproducibly when fetal rat calvaria cells are cultured in the presence of 15% serum, 50 ug/ml of ascorbic acid and 10 mM Na glycerophosphate. The nodules formed resemble woven bone histologically, and immunolabelling has documented the presence of type I and III collagen and osteonectin as well as the absence of type II collagen (Bellows et al., 1986). To use this system as a model for studies of regulation of osteogenesis and mineralization, we felt it important to verify that the nodular structures exhibited features closely resembling bone formed in vivo. Thus, we have analyzed nodules by transmission electron microscopy, X-ray diffraction analysis and electron microprobe analysis (Bhargava et al., 1988). All the ultrastructural features observed indicated that nodules resemble true bone: a mineralization front was detectable in which small, discrete structures resembling matrix vesicles and feathery mineral crystals were evident, and electron microprobe and electron or X-ray diffraction analysis confirmed the mineral to be hydroxyapatite.

We have studied the effects of $1,25(OH)_2D_3$ and $24,25(OH)_2D_3$ on the formation of bone nodules in this system (Ishida et al., 1988). Both metabolites inhibited nodule formation when present continuously during a 21-day culture period, the effects were dose-dependent for each metabolite and they correlated with the biological effectiveness of these metabolites in other systems, i.e. $1,25(OH)_2D_3$ was more effective than $24,25(OH)_2D_3$. Addition of a maximally effective concentration of $1,25(OH)_2D_3$ (10^{-9}M) at days 0,2,4,6, etc. of culture until the end of the culture period revealed that $1,25(OH)_2D_3$ inhibited nodule formation when added at the earlier times, but had no effect on either number or size or the degree of calcification of the bone nodules when added at day 10 or later. The results suggest that $1,25(OH)_2D_3$ inhibits proliferation and/or differentiation of osteogenic progenitor cells, but appears to have no direct effect on bone formation and mineralization by differentiated osteoblasts.

Further investigation of the role of $1,25(OH)_2D_3$ and $24,25(OH)_2D_3$ in this system was clearly desirable, but required a quantitative evaluation of the mineralization process. Quantitation of mineralization has been achieved by varying the time at which β glycerophosphate is added to the system, using ^{45}Ca uptake as an indication of mineralization. When β glycerophosphate is omitted from the culture system, nodules still develop but fail to mineralize. Upon the addition of sodium β glycerophosphate (βGP), mineralization occurs after approximately a 24-h delay (Table 4). We hypothesize that, within this 24-h lag period, organic phosphate induces synthesis of factors necessary to initiate mineralization, be they factors involved in removing inhibitors of mineralization or matrix molecules required for initiation or progression of mineralization.

Table 4.   The ^{45}Ca content of bone nodules (cpm)

Time (h)	Continuous	2 h pulses
4	1,189	760
8	1,123	478
24	23,335	1,814
48	37,114	12,906

Rat calvaria cells (populations II-V) were grown for 17 d in αMEM containing 10% FBS, 50 ug/ml ascorbic acid and 10 nM Dexamethasone. After unmineralized nodules had formed, 10 mM βGP was added to all cultures. 0.1 uCi ^{45}Ca was added either at the same time as βGP (continuous exposure) or at the time points indicated for a 2 h period. ^{45}Ca uptake was measured either at the end of the 48 h culture period (continuous) or at the end of the 2 h pulse period (2 h pulse). Numbers represent the net CPM of 4 mineralizing cultures. Background counts (non-mineralizing cultures) were subtracted.

Analysis of the factors involved in initiation and progression of mineralization using this assay system is now in progress, with particular emphasis on the appearance of messenger RNA for noncollagenous matrix proteins thought to be associated with the mineralization process. Preliminary results (Lee et al., 1989) show that increased amounts of mRNA for some non-collagenous bone matrix proteins are detectable within 24 hrs of the addition of βGP, thus suggesting that the mineralization induced by βGP may be related to the synthesis of these proteins. It is anticipated that study of the effects of vitamin D metabolites in this system may clarify whether these metabolites directly affect mineralization of bone.

References

Anderson, H.C. Electron microscopic studies of induced cartilage development and calcification. J. Cell Biol. 35:81-101, 1967.

Arsenault, L.E. personal communication.

Bellows, C.G., Aubin, J.E., Heersche, J.N.M. and Antosz, M.E. Mineralized bone nodules formed in vitro from enzymatically released rat calvaria cell populations. Calcif. Tiss. Int. 38:143, 1986.

Bhargava, U., Bar-Lev, M., Bellows, C.G. and Aubin, J.E. Ultrastructural analysis of bone nodules formed in vitro by isolated fetal rat calvaria cells. Bone 9:155-163, 1988.

Bonucci, E. Fine structure of early cartilage calcification. J. Ultrastruc. Res. 20:33-50, 1967.

Boskey, A.L. Noncollagenous marix proteins and their role in mineralization. Bone and Mineral 6:111-123, 1989.

de Bernard, B., Bianco, P., Bonucci, E., Constantine, M., Lunazzi, G.C., Martinuzzi, P., Modricky, C., Moro, L., Panfili, E., Pollesello, P., Stagni, N. and Vittur, F. Biochemical and immunohistochemical evidence that in cartilage an alkaline phosphatase is a Ca^{2+}-binding glycoprotein. J. Cell Biology 103:1615-1623, 1986.

Delmas, P.D., Malaval, L., Arlot, M.E. and Meunier, P.J. Serum bone gla protein compared to bone histomorphometry in endocrine disease. Bone 6: 339, 1985.

Dickson, I.R., Dimuzio, M.T., Volpin, D. Ananthanarayanan, S. and Veis, A. The extraction of phosphoproteins from bovine dentin. Calcified Tissue Research 9:51-61, 1975.

Eastwood, J.B., de Wardemen, H.E., Gray, R.W. and Lemann, Jr. L. Normal plasma $1,25(OH)_2$ vitamin D concentration in nutritional osteomalacia. Lancet 1:1377, 1979.

Endo, H. Ossification in tissue culture. I. Histological development of the femur of chick embryo in various liquid media. Exp. Cell Res. 21:151-163, 1960.

Engel, J., Taylor, W., Paulsson, M., Sage, H., and Hogan, B. Calcium binding domains and calcium-induced conformational transition of SPARC/BM-40/osteonectin an extracellular glycoprotein expressed in mineralized and non-mineralized tissues. Biochemistry 26:6958-6965, 1987.

Harrison, J.R., Petersen, D.N., Lichtler, A.C., Mador, A.T., Rowe, D. and Kream, B. 1,25-dihydroxyvitamin D_3 inhibits transcription of type I collagen genes in the rat osteosarcoma cell line ROS 17/2.8. Endocrinology 125: 327-333, 1989.

Ishida, H., Bellows, C.G., Aubin, J.E. and Heersche, J.N.M. Effects of vitamin D_3 metabolites on formation of bone nodules from isolated rat calvaria cells in vitro. J. Dent. Res. 67. Special Issue 350 (Abstract), 1988.

Ito, Y., Endo H., Enomoto, H., Wakabayashi, K. and Takamura, K. Ossification in tissue culture II. Chemical development of the femur of chick embryo in various liquid media. Exp. Cell Res. 31:119-127, 1963.

Lee, K.L., Bellows, C., Aubin, J.E. and Heersche, J.N.M. Work in progress. 1989.

Linde, A., Lussi, A. and Crenshaw, M.A. Mineral induction by immobilized polyanionic proteins. Calcif. Tiss. Int. 44:286-295, 1989.

Manolagas, S.C., Burton, D.W. and Deftos, L.J. 1,25-dihydroxyvitamin D_3 stimulates the alkaline phosphatase activity of osteoblast-like cells. J. Biol. Chem. 256:7115-7117, 1981.

Nefussi, J.-R., Boy-Lefebre, M.L., Boulebacke, H. and Forest, N. Mineralization in vitro of matrix formed by osteoblasts isolated by collagenase digestion. Differention 29:160, 1985.

Neuman, W.F., DiStefano, V. and Mulryan, B.J. The surface chemistry of bone. III. Observations on the role of phosphatase. J. Biol. Chem. 193:227-235, 1951.

Nyweide, P.J. Embryonic chicken periosteum in tissue culture, osteoid formation and calcium uptake. Proc. K. Ned. Akad. Wet. C78:410, 1975.

Ornoy, A.D., Goodwin, D., Noff, D. and Edelstein, S. 24,25-Dihydroxyvitamin D is a metabolite of vitamin D essential for bone formation. Nature 276:5, 1978.

Osdoby, P. and Kaplan, A.J. Osteogenesis in cultures of limb mesenchymal cells. Dev. Biol. 73:84-102, 1979.

Price, P.A. and Baukol, S.A. 1,25-dihydroxyvitamin D_3 increases synthesis of the vitamin K-dependent bone protein by osteosarcoma cells. JBC 255:11660-11663, 1980.

Prince, C.W. and Butler, W.T. 1,25-dihydroxyvitamin D_3 regulates the biosynthesis of osteopontin, a bone-derived cell attachment protein. Collagen Related Research 7:305-313, 1987.

Raisz, L.G., Maina, G.M., Gworek, S.C., Dietrich, J.W. and Canalis, E.M. Hormonal control of bone collagen synthesis in vitro. Inhibitory effect of 1-hydroxylated vitamin D metabolites. Endocrinology 102:731-735, 1978.

Robison, R. The possible significance of hexose phosphoric esters in ossification. Biochem. J. 17:286-293, 1923.

Shimizu, N., Vieth, R., Reimers, S. and Heersche, J.N.M. The effects of vitamin D restriction on bone and dentin apposition in the rat. J. Dent. Res. 67: p. 148 (abstract), 1988.

Stenner, D.D., Tracy, R.P., Riggs, B.L., and Mann, K.G. Human platelets contain and secrete osteonectin, a major protein of mineralized bone. Proc. Natl. Acad. Sci. USA 83:6892-6896, 1986.

Tam, C.S., Heersche, J.N.M., Jones, G., Murray, T.M. and Rasmussen, H. The effect of vitamin D on bone in vivo. Endocrinology 118:2217-2224, 1986.

Tam, C.S., Jones, G., and Heersche, J.N.M. The effect of vitamin D restriction on bone apposition in the rat and its dependence on parathyroid hormone. Endocrinology 101:1448, 1981.

Tenenbaum, H. and Heersche, J.N.M. Differentiation of osteoblasts and formation of mineralized bone in vitro. Calcif. Tiss. Int. 34:76-79, 1982.

Tenenbaum, H. Levamisole and inorganic pyrophosphate inhibit B-glycerophosphate induced mineralization of bone formed in vitro. Bone and Mineral 3:13-26, 1987.

Tenenbaum, H.C. and Palangio, K. Phosphoethanolomine and fructose 1,6-diphosphate induced calcium uptake in bone formed in vitro. Bone and Mineral 2:201-210, 1987.

Termine, J.D., Kleinman, H.D., Whitson, S.W., Conn, K.M., McGarvey, M.L. and Martin, G.R. Osteonectin, a bone-specific protein binding mineral to collagen. Cell 26:99-105, 1981.

Thorogood, P. In vitro studies on skeletogenic potential of membrane bone periosteal cells. J. Embryol. Exp. Morphol. 54:185-207, 1979.

Wasi, S., Otsuka, K., Yao, K.L., Tung, P.S., Aubin, J.E., Sodek, J. and
   Termine, J.D. An osteonectin-like protein in porcine periodontal
   ligament. Can. J. Biochem. and Cell Biol. 62:470-478, 1984.

Whyte, M.P. Alkaline phosphatase: physiological role explored in
   hypophosphatasia. In: Bone and Mineral Research/6. W.A. Peck,
   editor. Elsevier, Amsterdam-New York-Oxford, 1989. p. 175-218.

Wuthier, R.E. and Register, T.C. Role of AP, a polyfunctional enzyme,
   in mineralizing tissues. In: Butler, W.T., ed. The chemistry and
   biology of mineralized tissues. Birmingham, Alabama. Ebsco Media.
   113-24, 1985.

Wuthier, R.E., Bisaz, S., Russell, R.G.G. et al. Relationship between
   pyrophosphate, amorphous calcium phosphate, and other factors in the
   sequence of calcification in vitro. Calcif. Tiss. Res. 10:198-206,
   1972.

BIOCHEMISTRY OF THE INTERCELLULAR MATRIX IN CARTILAGE CALCIFICATION

Benedetto de Bernard and Franco Vittur

Dipartimento di Biochimica, Biofisica e Chimica delle Macro-
molecole-Universita' degli Studi di Trieste-Italy

INTRODUCTION

Calcification is a process which takes place in the extracellular matrix, although strictly dependent on the biochemical activity of cells.

The aim of this paper is to briefly consider the components of cartilage matrix which are in some way involved in the process (the actors).

Cartilage is a good model in this respect since it is possible to study the mineralization steps in the tissue (the action), through the analysis of the extracellular matrix of the resting, transforming, hypertrophic and calcifying zones.

By comparing the results of this analytical study, information is expected on the alterations which the actors undergo during the phenomenon. In the final scene, when calcification is complete, new actors may be seen, while others may have disappeared.

From the general survey of the phenomena, the mechanism of the process may receive some elucidation.

THE ACTORS

a) Collagen

Among the connective tissues, cartilage is unique as it is endowed with a specific set of collagens: types II, IX and XI. Collagen X is predominantly found in hypertrophyc cartilage (Mendler et al. 1989).

A single population of fibrils is admitted in chick embryo cartilage, containing 10% of collagen IX and XI, the rest being represented by collagen II (Mendler et al. 1989).

Collagen II is formed by three identical alpha 1 (II) chains and is similar to collagen I and III of other connective tissues.

The C- propetide of type II procollagen has been found identical with chondrocalcin (Van der Rest, 1986), a protein regarded with great inte= rest for its calcium affinity (Choi et al. 1983). More recently, Hinek and Poole (1988) report that the molecule accelerates the rate of mineral growth and increases the activity of alkaline phosphatase.

Collagen XI is a heterotrimer, the alpha 3 (XI) chain being similar if

not identical to an over glycosylated form of the alpha 1 (II) chain
(Mendler et al. 1989).

Type IX collagen is also assembled from three polypetides, alpha 1
(IX), alpha 2 (IX) and alpha 3 (IX) chains, stabilised by disulfide
bridges. Alpha 2 (IX) chain may be considered a proteoglycan since it has a
covalently bound glycosaminoglycan chain. Biochemical studies demonstrate
that type IX and II collagens are covalently attached through trivalent
hydroxypyridinium cross-links (Wu and Eyre,1984). In general, collagen
fibrils present specific surface properties which allow them to interact
with themselves and with other matrix components such as proteoglycans and
glycoproteins.

b) Proteoglycans

Large chondrointinsulfate rich proteoglycans are also components of
cartilage extracellular matrix. These molecules include a core protein,
which covalently anchors chondroitinsulfate, keratan sulfate glycosamino-
glycans, forming a highly negatively charged monomer. These structures
frequently interact with hyaluronic acid (HA) to produce supramolecular
aggregates.

Several functional domains have been recognized in the core protein.
These include the region near the NH_2- end which interacts with hyaluronic
acid and link protein, followed by a region of keratan sulfate attachment
and a region of chondroitin sulfate attachment which extends almost to
the COOH terminus of the polypeptide.

An additional cysteine-containing segment of about 200 aminoacids is
identified at the COOH terminus of the core protein (Doege et al. 1986).
Proteoglycan core protein contains also a domain which has the ability to
interact with glucides (Halberg et al. 1988). The target for this lectin-
like activity in cartilage is still to be identified. Collagen II or some
other minor cartilage glycoprotein may be good candidates. It is quite
possible that a multiplicity of such interactions exist in cartilage contri-
buting to the general properties of the tissue (Scott, 1988).
Proteoglycans produce a large effect on the chemical potential of water due
to their high concentration of negatively charged sulfate and carboxylate
groups. They are able therefore to control not only the extent of hydration
of the tissue, but also the packing density of collagen molecules
(Katz et al. 1986). Ca^{2+} affinity by cartilage proteoglycans has been measured
by Vittur et al.(1977b). The affinity is not high (10^{-4} M) but their capacity
is remarkable. These polyelectrolytes are surrounded by large amounts of
structural water which exclude other ions, positively charged, but of lower
valence. This may explain the fact that 81 μ Eq of Ca^{2+} are segregated within
the molecular domain of 20 mg of proteoglycan aggregates in the presence of
1200 μEq of sodium (Dziewiatkowski and Mayznerski, 1985). Also recent reports
underline the properties of Ca^{2+} affinity to proteoglycans (Dziewiatkowski,
1987; Hunter et al. 1988).

c) Glycoproteins

A special review was dedicated to the glycoproteins of cartilage by one
of the A. of this article (de Bernard, 1982). Glycoproteins with structural
function, Ca $^{2+}$ affinity and enzymatic activity have been identified in

cartilage. Among the latter, alkaline phosphatase (AP) is generally accepted as the most relevant to the calcification process. (For a review see Wuthier and Register, 1985).

d) Circulating fluid

The properties and composition of the fluid circulating in the extracellular space of cartilage have been studied intensively by the Howell's group (Howell et al. 1978). These investigators have found a pH slightly higher than the usual physiological value in fluid aspirated from the hypertrophic zone of epiphyseal cartilage. An organic acid-resistant nucleating agent for Ca-Pi mineral, as well as proteoglycan aggregates, inhibitors of calcification, were also identified in this fluid.

The presence of matrix vesicles (M.V.) or at least of cell membrane lipids was suggested by Boskey (1978) and by Wuthier and Gore (1977). The fluid contains also collagen. Alkaline phosphate activity, marker of M.V., was measured in some fractions of the fluid: this finding is perhaps the best experimental evidence that this multipurpose enzyme is present not only in cells or M.V., but also circulates in the fluid which baths cells and subcellular structures. Among the possible substrates of this phospho-hydrolase, nucleotides such as ATP have been identified in the fluid, on the basis of the 260/280 nm absorbance ratio measurements (Howell, 1978). More recently this finding has been confirmed (Shapiro et al. 1982; Kakuta et al. 1986): the different extent of phosphorylation of the adenine nucleotides has been also measured as well as the ratio of reduced over oxidized pyridine nucleotides (Matsumoto et al. 1988).

THE ACTION: THE PROCESS OF MINERALIZATION

In preosseous cartilage, the early site of mineral deposition is ascribed to the matrix vesicles (Bonucci, 1967).

These structures which derive from the fragmentation of chondrocytes processes, detachment of the swollen tips of them and fragmentation of whole cells, are identified in high number in the longitudinal septa of calcifying cartilage.

From the biochemical point of view, M.V. may be described as small parts of cytosol of chondrocytes surrounded by a membrane, containing glycoproteins and different amounts of calcium and phosphate.

The alkaline phosphatase, an integral membrane protein, is considered the marker enzyme; it is not however the only enzyme identified in M.V. Their membrane is replete with a certain number of phosphatase activities (Anderson,1985) and a neutral protease activity has been also reported by Hirschman et al. (1983). A Ca^{2+}, Mg^{2+} ATPase has been histochemically identified by Akisaka and Gay (1985).

Crystallites formed inside these M.V. will eventually extend outside these globules, in the matrix , forming a calcification nodule. As mineralization continues, the nodules grow by the addition of other crystallites and fuse with other nodules till the whole area becomes masked by a mineral phase (Bonucci, 1987).

This picture suggests that although M.V. are the initial loci of calcium phosphate precipitation, the whole process is not ruled only by them.

Of special interest are the studies by Bonucci on the nature of the material which is trapped within the inorganic phase of the early crystallites. Upon post-embedding decalcification and staining of the area, structures appear which reproduce at the e.m. the images of the original crystals (ghosts). Histochemical analysis reveals the nature of the organic phase as composed by acid polysaccharides and glycoproteins. Interestingly, collagen structures are not revealed. Only the final scene, when calcification is complete, shows that the mineral substance forms electron-dense bands which reinforce the collagen periodicity (Bonucci and Reurink, 1978).

From this rapid survey of the phenomenon, the following important questions deserve an accurate examination:

a) the fact that M.V. appear at the level of a specific zone, immediately before the calcifying area, does suggest a modification of cells metabolic activity, of the matrix or of both ?;

b) which are the matrix components more involved in the events, which eventually lead to the calcium salts formation ?

MODIFICATION OF THE ACTORS DURING THE ACTION

A) Modification of chondrocytes

Cell proliferation, hypertrophy and matrix vesicles production represent the main stages of chondrocytes modification, which occur before tissue calcification. These alterations are the consequence of or are accompanied by biochemical modifications of the cells structures.

The number and amounts of proteins and glycoproteins of the plasma membrane of cells is modified in the transition from the resting to the ossifying region. Alkaline phosphatase, a 70 Kda glycoprotein, identified by the western blot analysis and by immuno-precipitation (Fig. 1) with a specific polyclonal antibody, is synthesised in higher amount in the Oc cells than in the cells of the resting region (Rc cells), (Vittur et al. submitted).

Upon PTH stimulation, Oc cells produce more cAMP than the Rc cells, which indicates that the two types of cell membrane may differ also for the number of receptors to the hormone (Vittur et al, in press).

Finally steady state fluorescence anisotropy measurements indicate that Oc plasma membrane has a higher fluidity than Rc, possibly on the account of a different lipid composition (Vittur et al. submitted).

By approaching the calcification zone, additional modifications are detectable. M.V. which derive from plasma membrane of cells, show a simplified pattern of proteins and glycoproteins. This finding is the proof that an intense proteolysis occurs during the process which originates the vesicles. Alkaline phosphatase is not only a 70Kda glycoprotein but a 52 Kda molecule, although the catalytic properties are maintained (de Bernard et al. 1986).

B) Modification of the cartilage constituents

A summary of the modifications of the tissue passing from the resting region to that of the calcifying area is given by Table 1.

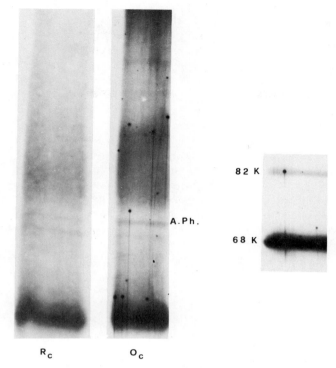

Fig. 1. Alkaline Phosphatase (AP) in resting (Rc) and ossifying (Oc) chondrocytes. 4.10^6 Rc and 2.10^6 Oc were homogenized and the enzyme was immuno-precipitated with the specific antibody. The complex was solubilized in sodium dodecyl sulphate (SDS), fractionated on 10-20% polyacrylamide gel electrophoresis (PAGE) and silver stained.

Table 1. Nucleotides and matrix components of normal epiphyseal cartilage

	Zones		
	Resting-Proliferating	Hypertrophic	Calcifying
ATP (a)	10.54	2.89	1.29
GTP (a)	4.81	2.13	1.16
Collagen (b)	35.30	25.70	26.49
n.coll. prot. (c)	49.50	27.12	38.06
Glycosaminoglycans (d)	20.56	17.63	13.73
Mineral (e)	2.91	7.18	14.58

a) from Matsumoto et al.1988: nmoles of nucleotide/mg dry weight.
b) from hydroxyproline x 7.14; c) non collagenous nitrogen x 6.25;
d) (uronic ac. + hexosamines)/2 x 2.69; e) phosphorus x 5.40.
from de Bernard et al, 1977: % of dry weight.

It appears that the amount of ATP and GTP is higher in the resting region than in the area of calcification (Matsumoto et al. 1988). This important information has to be correlated with another finding, i.e. with the increment of NADH over NAD^+ ratio in the latter region, as reported by Shapiro et al., 1982. The fact that a certain degree of oxygen deficiency exists in this area, explains not only the diminished capacity of the tissue to synthesize ATP in that zone, but also other phenomena which will be described later.

Concomitantly with the mineral deposition, we observe a removal of the organic phase of the matrix: the process involves in particular glycosamino-glycans, 34% of them being removed (de Bernard et al. 1977).

Since the decrement of glycosamino-glycans is accompanied by a comparable diminution of non collagenous proteins, it is legitimate to infer that proteoglycan is the component which is removed during the preparation of cartilage matrix to the process of calcification. This finding is now widely accepted and has been confirmed also by recent reports (Ehrlich et al.1982; Campo and Romano, 1986; Buckwalter et al. 1987).

The involvement of proteoglycans in this process is shown also by the variations of their rheological properties. Both proteoglycan crude extracts and proteoglycan subunits (PGs) show different elution profiles, when applied in associative conditions to a column of Sepharose 2 B., if they derive from resting region or from the calcifying area.

Eluted molecules may be followed by measuring uronic acid. Aggregated proteoglycans (PGC) of high molecular weight are eluted with the void volume, when extracted either from nasal septum or from resting cartilage (Fig. 2,A). On the contrary, from the ossifying cartilage, a population of proteoglycans is obtained which is largerly eluted in the inner volume, indicating a low degree of association (Fig. 2,A). It is interesting the fact that upon addition of hyaluronic acid to the proteoglycans subunits, (Fig. 2 (C versus B) experiments of gel permeation show that molecules of proteoglycans do associate when they are derived from nasal septum or resting cartilage, whereas those extracted from the ossifying cartilage do not recognize the hyaluronic acid (Vittur et al 1977b; Vittur et al. 1979).

This finding is also suggestive for a modification of the hyaluronic acid binding domain of the core protein of proteoglycans to the point that HA does not bind to them. *

A significant amount of collagen has been identified by chemical analysis in the guanidinium extracts of the two types of cartilage (Vittur et al., 1977a). Upon digestion of this collagen with a highly purified collagenase, a significant alteration of the elution profile of proteoglycans derived from the ossifying region of scapula cartilage is obtained (Vittur et al. 1977a). As shown in Fig. 3, proteoglycans shift from a high degree of association to an evident dissociation in monomers. In the case of PGs from nasal and resting cartilages, the profiles of elution from the Sepharose 2B columns do not appear to be affected by the digestion with the collagenase.

The importance of this finding is enhanced if correlated with the experimental evidence that collagen binds to alkaline phosphatase and that this interaction is inhibited by proteoglycans (Vittur et al. 1984).

Development and maturation of epiphyseal cartilage is dependent upon adequate amounts of dietary vitamin D. In its absence, young animals show

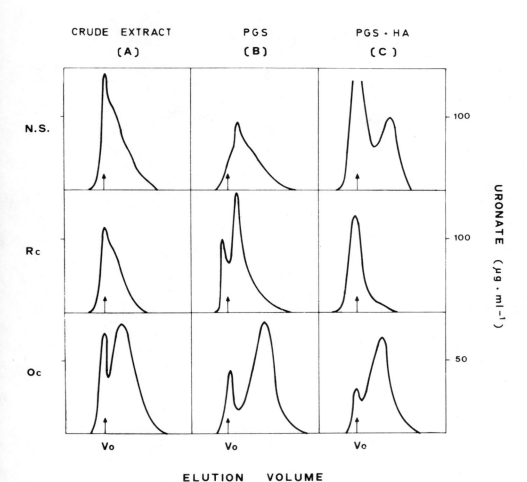

CRUDE EXTRACT
(A)

PGS
(B)

PGS · HA
(C)

N.S.

Rc

Oc

URONATE (μg · ml⁻¹)

100

100

50

Vo   Vo   Vo

ELUTION   VOLUME

Fig. 2. Comparison of Sepharose 2B elution profiles of guanidinium
extracts (A), proteoglycan subunits (B) and proteoglycan
subunits additioned with hyaluronic acid (C), derived from
nasal septum (N.S.), resting (Rc) and ossifying (Oc) zones
of pre-osseous scapula cartilage.
Crude extracts: proteoglycans extracted in 4 M guanidinium
chloride-0.05 M Tris-HCL pH 7.4, dialyzed before chromatography; PGS: proteoglycan subunits, obtained from the 4 M
guanidinium chloride extracts, by CsCL density gradient
centrifugation; HA: 1% (w/w) hyaluronic acid.

---

* When this manuscript was sent for publication, an article appeared
(Q. Nguyen et al. Biochem J. 259, 61-67, 1989) showing that inability
of proteoglycans fragments to interact with hexogenous hyaluronic acid
is due to the activation of a metallo-proteinase, identical with stro-
melysin, previously characterized from fibroblasts.

enlargement of the growth plate and bone fails to form.

If the macromolecular components of the matrix are involved in the mineralization process, an analysis of the epiphyseal plate of rachitic animals may reveal which of the components are the most altered.

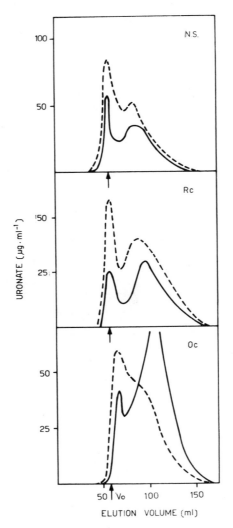

Fig. 3. Gel chromatography on Sepharose 2B of proteoglycans after
collagenase digestion of the crude extracts from nasal
septum (N.S.), resting cartilage (Rc) and Ossifying
cartilage (Oc).

----------------- untreated extracts

_____ after digestion with collagenase

Table 2 illustrates the composition of the rachitic cartilage of rats kept on a diet deficient in vitamin D and low in phosphate. The rachitic cartilage is characterized by a high amount of collagen and a low amount of glycosamino-glycans and of non collagenous proteins (Stagni et al. 1979). The recovery from the rachitic state as shown from the deposition of minerals coincides with the removal of the excess of collagen, the increment of proteoglycans of appropriate structure, since the ratio hexosamine/uronate shifts from 1.33 to 1.0.

A detailed study on the type of collagen sinthesized by rachitic cartilage has shown that concentrations and relative proportions of type X and XI collagens are markedly increased (Reginato et al. 1988).

From the data presented in the Table 2, it appears that in proteoglycans of rachitic cartilage, the uronate moieties are decreased with respect to the hexosamine residues, thereby suggesting that the chains of keratan sulphate are prevailing over those of chondroitin sulphate. Proteoglycans in which chondrointin sulphate-rich regions are short and keratosulphate-rich regions are of normal length are described by other investigators.

The lack of vitamin D causes therefore reduced and abnormal proteoglycans and for compensation high amount of collagen. This conclusion seems to be sustained by the fact that the physico-chemical properties of the proteoglycans of rachitic cartilage are different from those of the normal counterpart. (See Fig. 4).

C) Alkaline phosphatase (AP)

There is little doubt that among the different factors which play a role in the mechanism of calcification, AP appears of paramount importance. Various roles have been postulated for the enzyme but its true function is still elusive.

Some facts however appear to lay on a solid ground.

It is known that AP is attached to plasma membrane by a strong interaction with phosphatidyl inositol via a glycan moiety (Low and Saltiel, 1988). The fact that the enzyme is bound to phospholipids may explain some aspects of mineralization: a) the presence of lipids in the calcified areas; b) the calcium affinity of AP (Vittur et al. 1972); c) the different Mr attributed to the enzyme.

Indeed the native molecule may be split at different levels and released from the plasma membrane of cells or of M.V. A specific phospholipase C (a true phosphoinositidase) is responsible for the release of the enzyme as a big molecule, characterized by the association with the glycan moiety (Low and Saltiel,1988). But the enzyme may be released also through the intervention of proteolytic enzymes. In the latter case, a lower Mr AP should be found.

It is expected that the Ca^{2+} binding property of AP is more evident when the large molecule is studied, including the glycosyl phosphatidyl inositol portion; since M.V. are doomed to dissolution, in calcifying areas AP should operate predominantly in this form. Its presence in the mineralized zones has been recently assessed with immuno-histochemical techniques by de Bernard et al. (1986), who were also the first to demonstrate that in that area the phosphatase activity of the enzyme is not detectable. This important finding has been recently confirmed by

Table 2. Matrix components of preosseous cartilage from rachitic and healing rats

	Rachitic	Healing vit.D	Healing phosphate
Collagen (a)	34.8	22.8	24.1
non coll. protein (b)	30.1	45.0	33.7
Glycosaminoglycans (c)	15.7	19.6	22.9
Mineral (d)	3.3	16.9	15.4
Hexosam/Uronate	1.3	1.2	1.0

a) from hydroxyproline x 7.14; b) from non collagenous nitrogen x 6.25;
c) from uronate x 2,69; d) from phosphorus x 5.40.

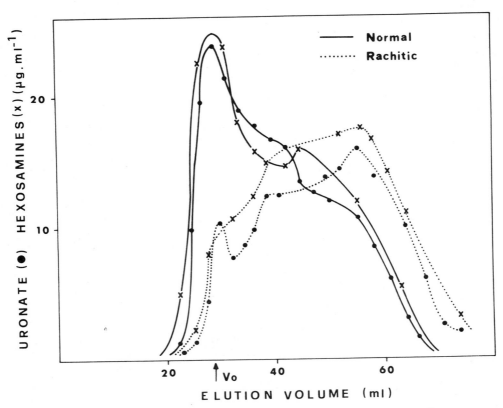

Fig. 4. Gel chromatography on Sepharose 2B of proteoglycans from normal and rachitic cartilage: proteoglycans were extracted from chicken cartilage by 4 M guanidinium chloride pH 7.5 and, after removal of the dissociative reagent, the extracts were subjected to the gel filtration (pH 6.8).

Genge et al. (1988a), who report the correlation between loss of APase activity and accumulation of calcium during mineralization.

The enzyme should be considered also from another point of view: it has a strong capacity to interact with other macromolecules.

The ability of AP to interact with collagen was first demonstrated by Vittur et al. (1984). It was part of that work also the evidence that proteoglycan subunits inhibit the binding of AP to type II collagen.

Recently some interesting structural relationship between AP and proteins of the extracellular space have been identified (Tsonis et al. 1988): with complement factor B, with cartilage matrix protein, with von Willebrand factor. Actually the region of the latter factor which shows homology to AP is known to be included in the collagen binding domain of the molecule.

The observations made by Vittur et al. (1984) receive therefore new support.

THE FINAL PICTURE

It appears then, that, at least in preosseous cartilage, the process of mineralization may be explained in the near future at the molecular level. It will however include different components and different events. It seems likely that a cascade of reactions will be identified, each of them dominated by one of the matrix components we have been analyzing in this article.

It is not impossible to imagine that the initial event is represented by an impairment of the metabolic activity of chondrocytes in the hypertrophic-ossifying region of the tissue. O_2 deficiency has been found in this district, accompanied by increased ADP/ATP and $NADH/NAD^+$ ratios.

It has been demonstrated in vitro by Lemasters et al. (1987) that in these conditions, a disturbance of membrane-cytoskeleton connection ensues with focal weakening of the cell surface (small blebs). This is exactly what happens in that region of cartilage, where the formation of M.V. is observed as the consequence of fragmentation of cell processes.

From the biochemical point of view the event means also the discharge in the extracellular matrix of various enzymes, partly associated with M.V., such as AP and proteases, and partly free in the extracellular fluids.

The fact that the early steps of mineralisation take place within M.V. may be explained by the presence in a microenvironment of more than one factor acting as heterogenous nucleator of calcium phosphate precipitation: in primis AP which binds Ca^{2+} and provides phosphate from its substrates. Significant amounts of Ca^{2+} become available during the partial degradation of proteoglycans, which are an important extracellular reservoir of the cation (Hunter et al. 1988). Due to the collapse of ionic gradients caused by the lack of ATP, an important Ca^{2+} inflow in M.V. is to be expected (Zanetti et al. 1982).

Obviously, mineralisation cannot be limited to the M.V.: AP and the Ca^{2+} binding proteins described by Genge et al. (1988b), both associated with phospholipids, can permit the circulation of a preformed mineral phase, from the sites of the initial deposition of minerals, to other matrix constituents.

It is to consider the possibility the Ca^{2+} - and phosphatidyl serine-binding proteins identified by Genge et al (1988b) are components of the membranes of cells or of M.V. or fragments of AP itself. It is in the calcified areas, in fact, that the enzyme loses its catalytic activity and acquires that of a mineral template (see de Bernard et al. 1986, and Genge et al., 1988a).

It is in the lane of these ideas that we are moving for the future investigations.

ACKNOWLEDGEMENTS

Research supported by the Italian Ministery of Public Education and by the Italian National Research Council. The collaboration of Dr. P. D'Andrea in the experiments illustrated by Fig. 1. is gratefully acknowledged.

REFERENCES

Akisaka T. and Gay C.V. 1985. Ultrastructural localisation of calcium activated adenosin triphosphatase (Ca^{2+}-ATPase) in growth plate cartilage. J. Histochem. Cytochem. 33, 925.

Anderson H.C. 1985. Matrix vesicles calcification: Review and update. Bone and Mineral Res. 3, 109.

de Bernard B. 1982. Glycoproteins in the local mechanism of calcification. Clin. Orthop. Rel. Res. 162, 233.

de Bernard B., Stagni N., Coluatti I., Vittur F. and Bonucci E. 1977. Glycosaminoglycans and endochondral calcification. Clin. Orthop. Rel. Res. 126, 285.

de Bernard B., Bianco P., Bonucci P., Costantini M., Lunazzi G.C., Martinuzzi P, Modricky C., Moro L., Panfili E., Pollesello P., Stagni N. and Vittur F. 1986. Biochemical and immunohistochemical evidence that in cartilage an alkaline phosphatase is a Ca^{2+} binding glycoprotein. J. Cell Biol. 103, 1615.

Bonucci E. 1967. Fine structure of early cartilage calcification. J. Ultrastruct. Res. 20, 33.

Bonucci E. 1987. Is there a calcification factor common to all calcifying matrices? Scanning Microscopy 1, 1089.

Bonucci E. and Reurink J. 1978. The fine structure of decalcified cartilage and bone: a comparison between decalcification procedures performed before and after embedding. Calcif. Tissue Res. 25, 179.

Boskey A.L. 1978. The role of calcium-phospholipid-phosphate complexes in tissue mineralisation. Met. Bone Dis. 1, 137.

Buckwalter J.A., Rosenberg L.C. and Ungar R. 1987. Changes in proteoglycan aggregates during cartilage mineralization. Calcif. Tissue Int. 41, 228.

Campo T.D. and Romano J.E. 1986. Changes in cartilage proteoglycans associated with calcification. Calcif. Tissue Int. 39, 175.

Choi H.V., Tang L.H., Johnson T.L., Pal S., Rosenberg L.C., Reiner A. and Poole A.R. 1983, Isolation and characterisation of a 35,000 molecular weight subunit fetal cartilage matrix protein. J. Biol. Chem. 258, 655.

Doege K., Fernardez P., Hassel J.R., Sasaki M. and Yamada Y., 1986,

Partial cDNA sequence encoding a globular domain at the C terminus of the rat cartilage proteoglycan. J. Biol. Chem. 261, 8108.

Dziewiatkowski D.D. and Majznerski L.L. 1985. Role of proteoglycans in endochondral ossification: inhibition of calcification. Calcif. Tissue Int. 37, 560.

Dziewiatkowski D.D. 1987. Binding of calcium by proteoglycans in vitro. Calcif. Tissue Int. 40, 265.

Ehrlich M.G., Armstrong A.L., Neuman R.G., Davis M.W. and Mankin H.J. 1982. Patterns of proteoglycan degradation by a neutral protease from human growth-plate epiphyseal cartilage. J. Bone Joint Surgery, 64-A, 1350.

Genge B.R., Sauer G.R., Wu L.N.Y., McLean F.M. and Wuthier R.E. 1988a. Correlation between loss of alkaline phosphatase activity and accumulation of calcium during matrix vesicle-mediated mineralization. J. Biol. Chem. 263, 18513.

Genge B.R., Wu L.N.Y. and Wuthier R.E. 1988b. Identification of three major matrix vesicles proteins as Ca^{2+}- and phosphatidyl serine binding proteins (CAPSBP). III Int. Conference on the chemistry and biology of mineralized tissues. Chatham, Mass. pag. 194.

Halberg D.F., Proulx G., Doege K., Yamada Y. and Drickamer K. 1988, A segment of the cartilage proteoglycan core protein has lectin-like activity. J. Biol. Chem., 263, 9486.

Hinek A. and Poole A.R. 1988. The influence of vitamin D metabolites on the calcification of cartilage matrix and the C-propeptide of Type II collagen (chondrocalcin). J. Bone Min. Res. 3, 421.

Hirschman A., Deutsch D., Hirschman M., Bab A., Sela J. and Muhlrad A. 1983. Neutral peptidase activities in matrix vesicles from bovine fetal alveolar bone and dog osteosarcoma. Calcif. Tissue Int. 35, 791.

Howell D.S., Blanco L., Pita J.C. and Muniz O. 1978. Further characterization of a nucleational agent in hypertrophic cell extracellular cartilage fluid. Met. Bone Dis. 1, 155.

Hunter G.K., Wong K.S. and Kim J.J. 1988. Binding of calcium to glycosaminoglycans: an equilibrium dialysis study. Archiv. Biochem. Biophys. 260, 161.

Kakuta S., Golub E.E., Haselgrove J.C., Chance B., Frasca P. and Shapiro I.M. 1986. Redox studies of the epiphyseal growth cartilage: pyridine nucleotide metabolism and the development of mineralization. J. Bone Min. Res. 1, 433.

Katz E.P., Wachtel E.J. and A. Maroudas. 1986, Extrafibrillar proteoglycans osmotically regulate the molecular packing of collagen in cartilage. Biochim. Biophys. Acta. 882, 136.

Lemasters J.L., Digiuseppi J., Nieminen A.L. and Herman B. 1987. Blebbing, free Ca^{2+} and mitochondrial membrane potential preceding cell death in hepatocytes. Nature,325,78.

Low M.G. and Saltiel A.R. 1988. Structural and functional roles of glycosyl-phosphatidyl inositol in membranes. Science, 239, 268.

Matsumoto H., DeBolt K. and Shapiro I.M. 1988. Adenine, gauanine and inosine nucleotides of chick growth cartilage: relationship between energy status and the mineralization process. J. Bone Min. Res. 3, 347.

Mendler M., Eich-Bender S.G., Vaughan L., Wintherhalter K.H. and Bruckner P. 1989. Cartilage contains mixed fibrils of collagen Types II, IX, and XI. J. Cell Biol. 108, 191.

Reginato A.M., Shapiro I.M., Lash J.W. and Jimenez S.A. 1988. Type X collagen alterations in rachitic chick epiphyseal growth cartilage. J. Biol. Chem. 263, 9938.

Scott. J.E. 1988. Proteoglycan-fibrillar collagen interactions. Biochem.J. 252, 313.

Shapiro I.M., Golub E.E., Kakuta S., Hazelgrove J., Havery J., Chance B. and Frasca P. 1982. Initiation of endochondral calcification is related to changes in the redox state of hypertrophic chondrocytes. Science 217,950.

Stagni N., Camerotto R., de Bernard B., Vittur F., Zanetti M. and Rovis L. 1979. Proteoglycans in rachitic cartilage. Bull. Mol. Biol. Med. 4,294.

Tsonis P.A., Argraves W.S. and Millan J.L. 1988. A putative functional domain of human placenta alkaline phosphatase predicted from sequence comparisons. Biochem. J. Lett. 254, 623.

Van der Rest M., Rosenberg L., Olsen B.R. amd Poole A.R. 1986. Chondrocalcin is identical with the C-propeptide of type II procollagen. Biochem.J., 237, 923.

Vittur F., Pugliarello M.C. and de Bernard B. 1972. The calcium binding properties of a glycoprotein isolated from pre-osseous cartilage. Biochem. Biophys. Res. Comm. 48, 143.

Vittur F., Zanetti M., Stagni N. and de Bernard B. 1977a. Are newly synthetized proteoglycans responsible for calcification in cartilage? Bull. Mol. Biol. Med. 2, 189.

Vittur F. Stagni N., Zanetti M., de Bernard B. and Rovis L. 1977b. Some properties of proteoglycans derived from non calcifying and calcifying cartilage. Bull. Mol. Biol. Med. 2, 40.

Vittur F., Zanetti M., Stagni N. and de Bernard B. 1979. Further evidence for the participation of glycoproteins to the process of calcification. in: Perspectives in inherited metabolic diseases. vol. 2. Berra B., Balduini C., Di Donato S. and Tettamanti G. Eds. Edi.ermes Milano, p. 13.

Vittur F., Stagni N., Moro L. and de Bernard B. 1984. Alkaline phosphatase binds to collagen; a hypothesis on the mechanism of extravesicular mineralization in epiphyseal cartilage. Experientia 40, 836.

Vittur F., Pollesello P., Figueras T. and de Bernard B. 1989. Different sensitivity of cultured chondrocytes and ROS 17/2 cells to polyamines. Bull. Mol. Biol. Med. in press.

Wu J.J. and Eyre D.R. 1984. Cartilage type IX collagen is cross-linked by hydroxypyridinium residues. Biochem. Biophys. Res. Comm. 123, 1033-1039.

Wuthier R.E. and Gore S.T. 1977. Partition of inorganic ions and phospholipids in isolated cell, membrane and matrix vesicle fractions: Evidence for Ca:Pi acidic phospholipid complexes. Calcif. Tissue Res. 24, 163.

Wuthier R.E. and Register T.C. 1985. Role of alkaline phosphatase, a polyfunctional emzyme, in mineralizing tissues. in: "The chemistry and biology of mineralized tissues " (Butler W.T. ed.) EBSCO Media Inc., Birmingham AL, p. 113.

Zanetti M., Camerotto R., Romeo D. and de Bernard B. 1982. Active extrusion of Ca^{2+} from epiphyseal chondrocytes of normal and rachitic chickens. Biochem. J. 202, 303.

THE VITAMIN D ENDOCRINE SYSTEM AND BONE

Anthony W. Norman

Division of Biomedical Sciences and Department of
Biochemistry, University of California
Riverside, CA 92521

Vitamin D is generally accepted as being essential for
life in higher animals. It is one of the most important
biological regulators of calcium and phosphorus metabolism.
Along with the two peptide hormones PTH and calcitonin,
vitamin D is responsible for the minute-to-minute as well as
the day-to-day establishment and maintenance of calcium
homeostasis.

The past 20 years of vitamin D_3 research have established the fact that $1\alpha,25$-dihydroxyvitamin D_3 $[1,25(OH)_2D_3]$
is the most potent metabolite of vitamin D_3 in stimulating
the intestinal absorption of calcium and phosphorus and in
mobilization of these minerals from bone. The classical
target organs for this secosteroid hormone are intestine,
bone, and kidney, but in recent years the radioactive
hormone or its receptor has been localized in many tissues
in vertebrate organisms (see Table 1), including numerous
cancer cell lines. Examples of the nonclassical target
tissues include pituitary, skin, reproductive organs,
pancreas, and brain, to mention a few. These newly
identified target tissues for $1,25(OH)_2D_3$ have raised the
possibility of unforeseen functions for the vitamin D_3
endocrine system. One of the novel functions to have
recently emerged is the participation of $1,25(OH)_2D_3$ in the
regulation of the immune system. The purpose of this
article is to review recent developments in our understanding of the vitamin D endocrine system and to identify
as well as suggest possible mechanisms and actions on bone.

Figure 1 presents a summary of the structure of
vitamin D, its precursor 7-dehydrocholesterol, and its major
daughter metabolites, $1,25(OH)_2D_3$ and $24R,25(OH)_2D_3$.

Vitamin D_3 and all of its metabolites are structurally
related to cholesterol as well as to other conventional
steroid hormones (see inset box for the structure of the
steroid hormone corticosterone). The numbering system for
identifying all the carbon atoms is identical amount
cholesterol, steroid hormones, and vitamin D compounds.

Table 1

TISSUE DISTRIBUTION OF 1,25 (OH)$_2$D$_3$ RECEPTORS

Tissues	Specific cell type
Adipose	Adipocytes
Bone	Osteoblast
Bone marrow	Monocyte/T-lymphocyte (activated)
Brain	Hippocampus/selected neurons
Breast	Epithelial
Cartilage	Chondrocyte
Colon	Epithelial
Eggshell gland	?
Epididymus	?
Intestine	Epithelial
Kidney	Epithelial (proximal and distal)
Liver (fetal)	?
Lung	?
Muscle, cardiac	Cardiac muscle cell
Muscle, (embryonic)	Myoblast
Muscle, smooth	Smooth muscle cell
Ovary	?
Pancreas	B cell
Parathyroid	Chief
Parotid	Acinar
Pituitary	Somatomammotroph
Placenta	?
Retina	?
Skin	Epidermal and fibroblasts
Testis	Sertoli/seminiferous tubule
Thymus	T lymphocytes
Thyroid	C cell
Uterus	?
Yolk sac (bird)	?
Cancer cells	Melanoma, breast carcinoma, leukemia, osteosarcoma, fibrosarcoma, colon carcinoma, medullary thyroid carcinoma, pancreatic adenocarcinoma, bladder carcinoma, cervical carcinoma, pituitary adenoma

7-Dehydrocholesterol (structure 1, the provitamin D with its characteristic Δ 5,7 conjugated double bond system in the B-ring), which is present in skin, is transformed by a photo-chemical reaction initiated by u.v. light (sunlight) into previtamin D$_3$ (structure not shown), which then promptly thermally equilibrates (in the absence of u.v. light) into vitamin D$_3$ (compounds 2, 3, 4, and 5, which are all different representations of the same compound). In this photochemical reaction the 9,10 carbon-carbon bond is broken, which produces a secosteroid. A secosteroid is a steroid that has one broken ring; for vitamin D, it is the B-ring. Structures 2, 3, 4, and 5 summarize the evolution of the conformational representations of vitamin D$_3$. Structure 2 resulted from the original chemical structure determination. Here, the seco nature of the steroid was

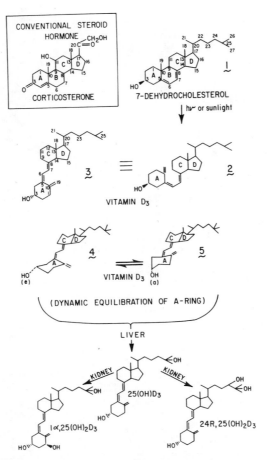

Figure 1. Structure of vitamin D₃ and its key metabolites.

apparent, and the remainder of the ring structure and the
relative orientation of ring A to rings C and D were implied
to be identical to that of the provitamin or cholesterol
(top row). However, after X-ray crystallographic analysis
was completed, it was thought that a more accurate depiction
of the vitamin D secomolecule was the one that is shown in
structure 3. This structure more clearly emphasizes the
consequences of breaking the 9,10 carbon bond. In particular, the A-ring is inverted from rings C and D with rotation
occurring around the bond between C-7 and C-8. As a result,
the α or β designations for substituent groups on the A-ring
must be drawn with reverse notation due to the inversion of
the A-ring. The bottom line of the figure indicates the
structure of the three principal metabolites of the parent
vitamin D_3, namely $25(OH)D_3$, $1,25(OH)_2D_3$ and $24,25(OH)_2D_3$.
hu, u.v. light irradiation.

Figure 2 summarizes the structures of the some 37
metabolites of vitamin D_3 which have been isolated and
chemically characterized. This figure organizes these

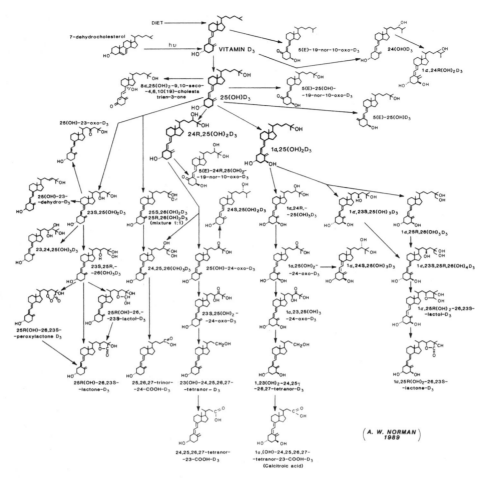

Figure 2. Summary of vitamin D₃ metabolism. This figure
    lists the structure of all metabolites of vitamin D₃
    which have been isolated and chemically characterized.
    For access to reference citations for this work see
    Henry & Norman (4).

metabolites into metabolic pathways. It is important to
appreciate that only four of these metabolites to date have
been extensively studied to evaluate their capability for
producing unique biological responses; these are 25(OH)D₃,
1,25(OH)₂D₃, 24R,25(OH)₂D₃ and 1,25R(OH)₂-26,23S-lactone D₃.
It is quite conceivable that any of the other metabolites
may possess the capability to produce unique biological
responses; however, this will be deduced after appropriate
experimentation.

    As a consequence of intensive efforts in many laborato-
ries over the past 20 years, a new model has emerged for the
mechanism of action of fat-soluble vitamin D (see Fig. 3).
This model is based on the concept that, in terms of its
structure and mode of action, the daughter metabolite

$1,25(OH)_2D_3$ is similar to the classic steroid hormones, e.g., aldosterone, testosterone, estradiol, cortisol, and ecdysone. Current understanding of the mechanism of action of steroid hormones is that it occurs through interaction of a hormone-receptor complex with the genetic substance in the nucleus of target cells (Fig. 3).

The discovery of the $1,25(OH)_2D_3$ receptor dates back to 1969, when Haussler and Norman (23) provided evidence for the existence of a chromosomal protein capable of binding the biologically active metabolite of vitamin D with high affinity. The molecular mass of the avian receptor is now known to be 60,000 daltons, with a Stokes radius of 36Å, whereas the mammalian receptors range in mass from 52,000 to 56,000 daltons (17).

One of the astonishing developments in the field of vitamin D endocrinology has been the plethora of reports describing the detection of receptors for $1,25(OH)_2D_3$ in so-called "nonclassical target organs." These results are summarized in Table 1. At the present time there is clear biochemical evidence to support the existence of $1,25(OH)_2D_3$ receptors in no less than 25 tissues as well as many cancer cell lines. In the context of bone, it is noteworthy that only osteoblasts, but not osteoclasts, have been shown to possess $1,25(OH)_2D_3$ receptors.

The principal mode of study of the $1,25(OH)_2D_3$ receptors, which is reported in the entries provided in Table 1, has been by one of three techniques: (a) 5-20% sucrose density gradient analysis, where by definition a $1,25(OH)_2D_3$ receptor should have a mobility of approximately 3.2-3.7S; (b) by formal Scatchard analysis, where a $1,25(OH)_2D_3$ receptor would be presumed to have a high affinity, i.e. $K_d = 1-10 \times 10^{-11}$ M; and (c) by chromatography on columns of DNA-cellulose, which is reflective of the intrinsic interaction of steroid hormone receptors with chromatin-derived material.

One inescapable conclusion of the information presented in Table 1 related to the wide distribution of receptors for $1,25(OH)_2D_3$ is that the vitamin D endocrine system extends far beyond the three classical target organs of the intestine, bone, and kidney. Inherent in this statement is the presumption that the presence of specific binding proteins/receptor for $1,25(OH)_2D_3$ would be correlated with some biological response that is dependent upon the hormone.

One intriguing aspect related to the biochemical properties of the $1,25(OH)_2D_3$ receptor is the presence of "cooperativity" in the binding of its ligand $1,25(OH)_2D_3$. Similar mechanisms have been previously reported for the estrogen and progesterone receptors. In all these systems the modulation of the cooperativity may regulate the affinity of the ligand for the receptor and in turn the affinity of the ligand-receptor complex for selected DNA sequences.

Certainly one of the unique aspects of the $1,25(OH)_2D_3$ receptor in relation to other steroid receptors is the

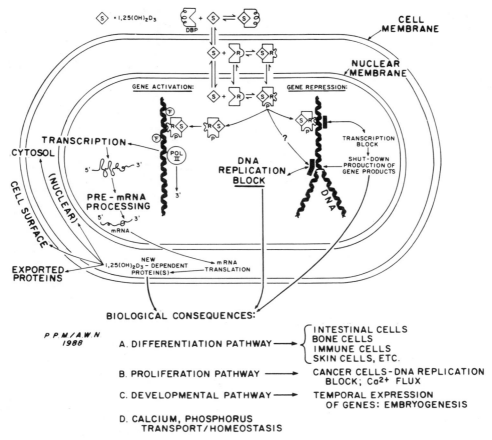

BIOLOGICAL CONSEQUENCES:

A. DIFFERENTIATION PATHWAY ⟶ INTESTINAL CELLS
BONE CELLS
IMMUNE CELLS
SKIN CELLS, ETC.

B. PROLIFERATION PATHWAY ⟶ CANCER CELLS-DNA REPLICATION
BLOCK; Ca^{2+} FLUX

C. DEVELOPMENTAL PATHWAY ⟶ TEMPORAL EXPRESSION
OF GENES: EMBRYOGENESIS

D. CALCIUM, PHOSPHORUS
TRANSPORT/HOMEOSTASIS

Figure 3. Model for the interaction of $1,25(OH)_2D_3$ with
its nuclear receptor and generation of biological
responses via gene activation and gene repression.
Also shown is the DNA replication block by direct or
indirect action of the $1,25(OH)_2D_3$ receptor complex.
The biological consequences of these actions are
indicated at the bottom. DBP, serum vitamin D binding
protein; R, $1,25(OH)_2D_3$ receptor; S the $1,25(OH)_2D_3$
steroid; P, phosphorus; POL II, RNA polymerase II; F,
transcription factor, DNA deoxyribonucleic acid; mRNA,
messenger ribonucleic acid.

ability of the $1,25(OH)_2D_3$ receptor to efficiently and
effectively bind the conformationally mobile A-ring of this
seco-steroid. It is not yet known with certainty whether
the conformer with the equatorial or axial orientation of
the key 1-alpha hydroxyl group is bound to the $1,25(OH)_2D_3$
receptor (See Fig. 4, top line).

A major recent advance in our understanding of the
$1,25(OH)_2D_3$ receptor in relation to the other steroid receptors has occurred as a consequence of the molecular cloning
of the avian receptor. It is now apparent that the $1,25-$
$(OH)_2D_3$ receptor is a member of the nuclear transacting
receptor family and shares amino acid sequence homology with
the chicken estrogen and progesterone receptors and also
with the v-erb A oncogene product. Comparison of the

structure of the 1,25(OH)$_2$D$_3$ receptor with other nuclear receptors such as the estradiol, thyroxine (T$_3$), progesterone, cortisol, aldosterone and retinoic acid receptors is shown in Fig. 4. Note that the DNA-binding domain is the most conserved portion of these receptor molecules whereas the ligand-binding domain is considerably less conserved. The high degree of sequence homology between these receptors especially in the DNA-binding domain suggests that they evolved from a common ancestral molecule. The sequence homology also implies that their interaction with specific DNA sequence motifs occurs through a similar hormone-receptor mediated mechanism.

The 1,25(OH)$_2$D$_3$ receptor is a DNA-binding protein capable of up-regulating or down-regulating the transcription of RNA polymerase II genes. Furthermore, putative DNA-binding loops or "fingers" have been proposed for the avian receptor and the other steroid receptors similar to the "zinc-fingers" proposed for the 5S transcription factor TFIIIA.

1,25(OH)$_2$D$_3$ receptors preferentially bind to double-stranded DNA rather than single-stranded DNA or RNA. This binding property is sensitive to sulfhydryl blocking agents, indicating the involvement of cysteine residues associated

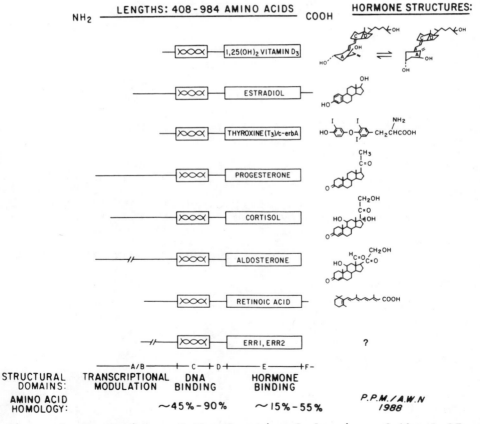

Figure 4. Comparison of the functional domains of the 1,25-(OH)$_2$D$_3$ receptor with other known nuclear receptors. See Minghetti and Norman (2) for a detailed discussion.

with the proposed DNA-binding "fingers" of the receptor. In addition, when the 1,25(OH)$_2$D$_3$ hormone associates with its unoccupied receptor an increase in affinity of the receptor for DNA occurs.

Available evidence suggests that the expression of the eukaryotic genome is being altered by 1,25(OH)$_2$D$_3$ (Table 2). The growing list of genes in which their expression is either up- or down-regulated by this hormone is very extensive (Table 2). Undoubtedly this list will continue to grow as new cDNA probes become available and as molecular measurements of 1,25(OH)$_2$D$_3$ induced genomic changes become more sensitive.

The diversity in biological activities governed by 1,25(OH)$_2$D$_3$ clearly suggest that the seco-steroid is involved in a wide array of gene regulatory events. As an example in the transformation of chicken fibroblast cells by v-src (differentiation--->proliferation) it has been estimated that the expression of 1000 genes are up-regulated by this transforming gene product. Similarly it can be postulated that approximately the same number of genes could be affected in the 1,25(OH)$_2$D$_3$ mediated differentiation of a myeloid stem cell to a mature macrophage (proliferation --->differentiation), one of its known immunoregulatory roles. We postulate that there must be a significant reprogramming of genetic information by 1,25(OH)$_2$D$_3$ and its receptor to mediate the proliferative--->differentiation transition that is inevitably associated with these cells as they undergo a dramatic change in their biological destiny. In our minds this represents a dramatic change in the genome and could account for many of the alterations in gene expression reported in Table 2.

An overview of the vitamin D endocrine system is presented in Figure 5. This figure summarizes the events which (i) support the production of vitamin D (upper left), (ii) are involved with its metabolism to its hormonally active form, namely 1,25(OH)$_2$D$_3$, in the kidney (upper center) including the regulatory involvement of a number of other classical hormones (upper right), (iii) describe the interaction of 1,25(OH)$_2$D$_3$ in its classical target organs of intestine, bone and kidney (lower center), (iv) describe the interaction of 1,25(OH)$_2$D$_3$ in a lengthy list of "new" target organs/cells, some of which produce calbindin-D (lower right), and (v) describe the existence of a paracrine system for the production and interaction of 1,25(OH)$_2$D$_3$ in cells of hematopoiesis.

24,25(OH)$_2$D$_3$ is a second dihydroxylated metabolite of vitamin D$_3$ which is produced by the kidney (Fig. 1). There is emerging evidence that 24,25(OH)$_2$D$_3$ has the capability to generate selected physiological responses different from 1,25(OH)$_2$D$_3$. A discussion of this topic is beyond the scope of this review.

While the majority of biological responses generated by 1,25(OH)$_2$D$_3$ are believed to occur as a consequence of occupied receptor interaction with selected genes (see Fig. 2) it is unlikely that absolutely all 1,25(OH)$_2$D$_3$-mediated biological responses are achieved through this mechanism.

Table 2

GENES REGULATED BY $1,25(OH)_2D_3$[#]

$1,25(OH)_2D_3$ Receptor	Interleukin-I
Calbindin-D_{28K}	GM-colony stim. factor
Calbindin-D_{9K}	Interferon-γ
Carbonic anhydrase	EGF Receptor
IMCAL$_{20.5K}$	TGF-β
Alkaline Phosphatase	TNF-α
Metallothionein	Protein Kinase C
Osteocalcin	Parathyroid Hormone
Collagen, type I	Prolactin
Fibronectin	TSH
c-myc	Calcitonin
c-myb	Ornithine Decarboxylase
c-fos	Cell Surface Antigens
c-fms	Spermidine-N-acetyl transferase
c-KI-ras	Tyrosinase
Histone-H_4	25(OH)D-1-Hydroxylase
	25(OH)D-24-Hydroxylase

[#] Abstracted from Minghetti & Norman, FASEB J. 2:3043 (1988) which supplies appropriate reference citations.

There are a number of reports describing biological responses to $1,25(OH)_2D_3$ which occur too rapidly to be consistent with gene activation; for example, very rapid (within seconds) effects of $1,25(OH)_2D_3$ on modulating the intracellular concentration of calcium have been reported. It is also believed in the case of the other classical steroid hormones, that they too are pleiotropic in their actions and produce biological effects both by genome-dependent and genome-independent actions.

In 1981, Suda and colleagues (27) showed that $1\alpha,25(OH)_2D_3$ induced mouse myeloid leukemia cells (M1) to differentiate to mature monocyte/macrophages. Likewise, $1\alpha,25(OH)_2D_3$ promoted monocytic differentiation of HL-60 promyelocytic leukemia cells (28). Upon incubation with

$1\alpha,25(OH)_2D_3$ (10^{-10} - 10^{-7} M, ED_{50} about 5×10^{-9} M), the cells changed morphologically and became adherent to charged surfaces, acquired the ability to phagocytize yeast, reduced nitroblue tetrazolium, increased the expression of macrophage-related antigens, produced lysozyme and stained positively for nonspecific acid esterase. Furthermore, a proportion of HL-60 cells (30-50%) became multinucleated and gained the ability to bind and degrade bone matrix. Simultaneously, the proliferation of myeloid cell lines was inhibited by $1\alpha,25(OH)_2D_3$. HL-60 cells possess $1\alpha,25$-$(OH)_2D_3$-receptors (ca. 4000 copies/cell) (5). Indirect evidence for mediation of differentiation through $1\alpha,25$-$(OH)_2D_3$ cellular receptors was provided by the demonstration that the potency of various vitamin D_3 metabolites to induce HL-60 differentiation paralleled their known ability to bind to the $1\alpha,25(OH)_2D_3$-receptor.

Normal human myeloid stem cells also have been shown to have the capability to differentiate to macrophages after exposure to $1\alpha,25(OH)_2D_3$. After treatment with 5×10^{-9} $1\alpha,25(OH)_2D_3$ for five days, monocytes and macrophages in liquid cultures of human bone marrow cells increased approximately five-fold (to ca. 68% of total cells) as compared to flasks which did not contain $1\alpha,25(OH)_2D_3$. Colony-forming assays with normal human bone marrow in the presence of granulocyte-macrophage colony-stimulating factor (GM-CSF) showed that $1\alpha,25(OH)_2D_3$ caused granulocyte-macrophage colony-forming cells (GM-CFC) to preferentially form colonies containing macrophages (8). This effect was associated with an increase in the absolute number of

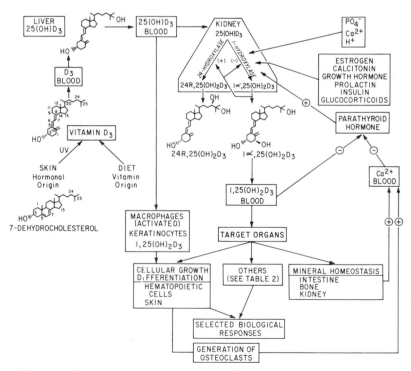

Figure 5. Summary of the vitamin D endocrine system.

macrophage colonies and was not due to selective inhibition of GM-CSF-mediated granulocytic differentiation by $1\alpha,25(OH)_2D_3$.

Cellular $1\alpha,25(OH)_2D_3$-receptors have been discovered in activated, but not in resting, circulating human lymphocytes and in circulating monocytes (29). Recently, regulation of both lymphocyte and monocyte/macrophage functions by $1\alpha,25-(OH)_2D_3$ has been demonstrated. Low $1\alpha,25(OH)_2D_3$ concentrations (10^{-11} - 10^{-10} M) inhibited in vitro proliferation and interleukin-2 (IL-2) synthesis of lectin-activated normal human lymphocytes. Expression of IL-2 receptors was not altered by the hormone. Probably, the anti-proliferative effects on lymphocytes are exerted through both IL-2 dependent and IL-2 independent mechanisms. Moreover, $1\alpha,25(OH)_2D_3$ reduced specifically both the mRNA and protein accumulation of interferon-γ and GM-CSF in both normal human mitogen-activated T-lymphocytes and T-lymphocytes from a cell line (S-LB1) transformed with human T-lymphotropic leukemia virus-1 (HTLV-1) (30). The modulation of IFNγ and GM-CSF gene expression apparently occurred independently of IL-2 regulation as addition of high concentrations of recombinant IL-2 could not reverse the $1\alpha,25(OH)_2D_3$ effects.

During the last three years, several workers have demonstrated that human macrophages have the ability to synthesize $1\alpha,25(OH)_2D_3$ from the precursor $25(OH)D_3$. Extra renal $25(OH)D_3$-1α-hydroxylase activity was first detected in alveolar macrophages from hypercalcemic sarcoidosis patients (24). Normal human alveolar and bone marrow-derived macrophages also have been shown to synthesize $1\alpha,25(OH)_2D_3$ in vitro after activation by IFNγ or bacterial lipopolysaccharide (25). These results suggest the existence of a vitamin D autocrine/paracrine system involving $1\alpha,25(OH)_2D_3$ derived from activated macrophages and hematopoietic target cells in the bone marrow or at the site of an inflammation, e.g. the alveolitis in the sarcoid lung (see Fig. 6).

One provocative recent development concerning the application of new vitamin D metabolites to bone cells concerns the effects of the $1,25(OH)_2D_3$-26,23-lactone.

$1\alpha,25$-Dihydroxyvitamin D_3-26,23-lactone [$1\alpha,25(OH)_2D_3$-26,23-lactone] has been isolated and identified as the main metabolite of $1\alpha,25$-dihydroxyvitamin D_3 [$1\alpha,25(OH)_2D_3$] in the serum of rats and dogs. Recently we succeeded in chemically synthesizing the four diastereoisomers of $1\alpha,25-(OH)_2D_3$-26,23-lactone. The stereochemical configurations of the naturally occurring $1\alpha,25(OH)_2 D_3$-26,23-lactone at the C-23 and C-25 positions have unequivocally been determined to be 23(S) and 25(R), respectively (see Fig. 2). This naturally occurring $1\alpha,25(OH)_2D_3$-26,23-lactone was found to slightly stimulate intestinal calcium absorption and decrease serum calcium levels in vitamin D-deficient rats fed a low calcium diet. Furthermore, the $1\alpha,25(R)(OH)_2D_3$-26,23(S)-lactone also inhibits bone resorption induced by $1\alpha,25(OH)_2D_3$ in vivo and in vitro. More recently we have found that the 23(S),25(S)- and 23(R),25(R)-$1\alpha,25(OH)_2D_3$-26,23-lactones stimulate bone resorption, but that the 23(S),25(R)- and 23(R),25(S)-$1\alpha,25(OH)_2D_3$-26,23-lactones inhibit bone resorption.

Studies using a variety of *in vivo* and *in vitro* systems have indicated that osteoclast precursors are present among bone marrow cells and have suggested that osteoclasts are formed by their fusion. More recent reports arising from experiments employing long-term culture of bone marrow cells state that immature monocytes may undergo fusion induced by $1\alpha,25(OH)_2D_3$, resulting in multinucleated cells with several characteristics of osteoclasts.

Therefore we have tested the effect of the four diastereoisomers of $1\alpha,25(OH)_2D_3$-26,23-lactone on mouse bone marrow cultures and report here that the 23(S),25(R)- and 23(R),25(S)-$1\alpha,25(OH)_2D_3$-26,23-lactones inhibit rather than stimulate multinucleated cell formation induced by $1\alpha,25(OH)_2D_3$, while the 23(S),25(S)- and 23(R),25(R)-$1\alpha,25(OH)_2D_3$-26,23-lactones alone can stimulate multinucleated cell formation (see reference 21).

Unfractionated mouse bone marrow cultures were stimulated by treatment by $1\alpha,25(OH)_2D_3$ to form multinucleated cells with several characteristics usually associated with bone-resorbing osteoclasts as reported previously. The cells were multinucleated, responded to calcitonin, and contained tartrate-resistant acid phosphatase, a marker enzyme for osteoclasts. These data support the hypothesis that the precursors of osteoclasts are non-adherent mononuclear bone marrow cells. However, the time required for the effect of $1\alpha,25(OH)_2D_3$ on the multinucleated cell formation varied with the preparation of the unfractionated cells. These differences may reflect the fact that the hormone stimulates the fusion of already differentiated osteoclast progenitors present in the unfractionated population.

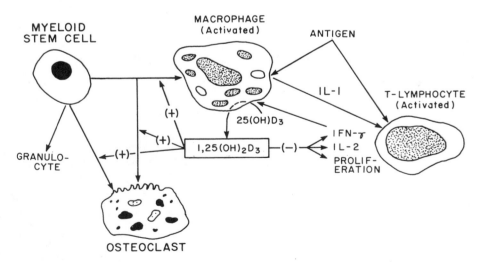

Figure 6. Proposed vitamin D paracrine/autocrine system involving $1\alpha,25(OH)_2D_3$ from activated macrophages. IL-1, interleukin-1; IL-2, interleukin-2; IFNγ, interferon-γ. See Reichel and Norman (1) for a more detailed discussion.

Fig. 7 shows the effects of the four diastereoisomers of $1\alpha,25(OH)_2D_3$-26,23-lactone on multinucleated cell formation induced by 10^{-8}M $1\alpha,25(OH)_2D_3$ in mouse bone marrow cell cultures. Addition of 10^{-8}M $1\alpha,25(OH)_2D_3$ increased the number of multinucleated cells (Fig. 7A). The number of multinucleated cells was slightly increased by the addition of 10^{-7}M of the 23(S),25(S)- or 23(R),25(R)-$1\alpha,25(OH)_2D_3$-26,23-lactones. However, these 23(S),25(S)- or 23(R),25(R)-$1\alpha,25(OH)_2D_3$-26,23-lactones had little effect on the multinucleated cell formation induced by 10^{-7}M $1\alpha,25(OH)_2D_3$ (Fig. 7B). On the other hand, the multinucleated cell number remarkably decreased when 10^{-8}M to 10^{-7}M of the 23(S),25(R)- or 23(R),25(S)-$1\alpha,25(OH)_2D_3$-26,23-lactone was added simultaneously with 10^{-8}M or 10^{-7}M $1\alpha,25(OH)_2D_3$ (Fig. 7, A and B). Also, the number of nuclei per multinucleated cell was decreased (data not shown). The activity of the 23(R),25(S)-$1\alpha,25(OH)_2D_3$-26,23-lactone was almost the same as that of the natural 23(S),25(R)-$1\alpha,25(OH)_2D_3$-26,23-lactone. Moreover, 24,25-dihydroxyvitamin D_3 failed to cause multinucleated cell formation and also did not inhibit the cells induced by $1\alpha,25(OH)_2D_3$ (data not shown), thus indicating the presence of a specificity in the action of the 23(S),25(R)- and 23(R),25(S)-$1\alpha,25(OH)_2D_3$-26,23-lactones. These results imply the existence of a receptor for $1\alpha,25R(OH)_2D_3$-26,23S-lactone in the multinucleated cells.

The 23(S),25(R)- and 23(R),25(S)-$1\alpha,25(OH)_2D_3$-26,23-lactones are the first vitamin D_3 analogues found to directly inhibit $1\alpha,25(OH)_2D_3$-induced multinucleated cell formation. In addition, our results strongly indicated that the 23(S),25(R)- and 23(R),25(S)-$1\alpha,25(OH)_2D_3$-26,23-lactones suppress bone resorption _via_ inhibition of osteoclast formation, while the 23(S),25(S)- and 23(R),25(R)-$1\alpha,25(OH)_2D_3$-26,23-lactones may actively stimulate bone resorption _via_ stimulation of osteoclast formation, as does $1\alpha,25(OH)_2D_3$ (25,26). These data taken together with our previous reports (22,23), these results indicate the possible roles of the 23(S),25(R)- and 23(R),25(S)-$1\alpha,25(OH)_2D_3$-26,23-lactones as stimulators of osteoblastic cell function and as inhibitors of osteoclastic cell function have important implications in the hormonal control of bone metabolism. The effective concentrations which stimulate increases in alkaline phosphatase activity and collagen synthesis in clone MC3T3-El cells are the same levels observed in beagle dog plasma, around 100 pg/ml (unpublished data). Thus, the 23(S),25(R)-$1\alpha,25(OH)_2D_3$-26,23-lactone is suggested to be involved in bone formation _in vivo_. Greater concentrations of the 23(S),25(R)-$1\alpha,25(OH)_2D_3$-26,23-lactone were needed to inhibit multinucleated cell formation induced by $1\alpha,25$-$(OH)_2D_3$ than that observed in beagle dog plasma. However, this isomer is a major metabolite of $1\alpha,25(OH)_2D_3$ and is relatively stable as compared to other vitamin D_3 metabolites under _in vivo_ or _in vitro_ condition. Thus, the 23(S),25(R)-$1\alpha,25(OH)_2D_3$-26,23-lactone could act as an inhibitor of bone resorption _in vivo_ as well.

In steroid hormone-like fashion, the action of $1\alpha,25(OH)_2D_3$ is thought to be mediated by its binding to specific cellular receptors. The activities of other vitamin D_3 metabolites involved in calcium metabolism

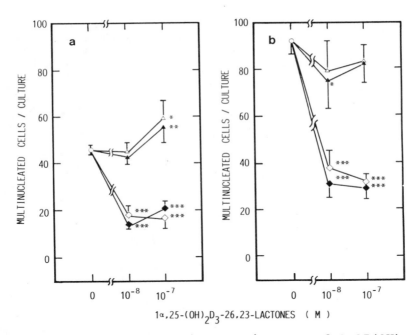

Figure 7. Effects of four diastereoisomers of $1,25(OH)_2$-26,23-lactone on multinucleated cell formation induced by $1\alpha,25(OH)_2D_3$ in mouse bone marrow cell cultures. Mouse bone marrow mononuclear cells were cultured with 10^{-8} M (A) or 10^{-7} M (B) $1\alpha,25(OH)_2D_3$ in the absence (O) or presence ($\triangle$, $\blacktriangle$, $\diamondsuit$, and $\blacklozenge$) 10^{-8} or 10^{-7} M of each of the four diastereoisomers of $1\alpha,25(OH)_2D_3$-26,23-lactone for 8 days as described in Fig. 1.
$\triangle$, 23(S),25(S)-$1\alpha,25(OH)_2D_3$-26,23-lactone;
$\blacktriangle$, 23(R),25(R)-$1\alpha,25(OH)_2D_3$-26,23-lactone;
$\diamondsuit$, 23(S),25(R)-$1\alpha,25(OH)_2D_3$-26,23-lactone;
$\blacklozenge$, 23(R),25(S)-$1\alpha,25(OH)_2D_3$-26,23-lactone. Results are presented as the mean $\pm$ SEM for quadruplicate determinations in two independent determinations. *, $P < 0.05$; **, $P < 0.01$; ***, $P < 0.001$ [vs. $1\alpha,25(OH)_2D_3$ alone].

usually are correlated with their binding affinities for the receptor, suggesting that they also act through binding to the $1\alpha,25(OH)_2D_3$ receptor, although receptors for $24,25(OH)_2D_3$ have been described in parathyroid glands, chondrocytes and limb bud mesenchymal cells. However, the inhibitory action of the 23(S),25(R)-$1\alpha,25(OH)_2D_3$-26,23-lactone on bone resorption induced by $1\alpha,25(OH)_2D_3$ can not be simply explained by ligand-receptor interactions, because the binding affinity of this diastereoisomer makes it the poorest competitor relative to $1\alpha,25(OH)_2D_3$. Moreover, the 23(S),25(R)- and 23(R),25(S)-$1\alpha,25(OH)_2D_3$-26,23-lactone have a biphasic stimulative effect on alkaline phosphatase activity in osteoblastic clone MC3T3-El cells; the isomers may also act on the osteoblastic cells through another pathway independent from that of the $1\alpha,25(OH)_2D_3$ receptor.

Finally, osteoclasts are known to possess receptors for calcitonin but not for $1\alpha,25(OH)_2D_3$.

It is not yet known whether $1\alpha,25(OH)_2D_3$ and the four diastereoisomers of $1\alpha,25(OH)_2D_3-26,23$-lactone act on bone marrow cells through the $1\alpha,25(OH)_2D_3$ receptor. The $23(S),25(R)-$ and $23(R),25(S)-1\alpha,25(OH)_2D_3-26,23$-lactones inhibited the $1\alpha,25(OH)_2D_3$-induced multinucleated cell formation, while the $23(S),25(S)-$ and $23(R),25(R)-$ $1\alpha,25(OH)_2D_3-26,23$-lactones did not, indicating that the former isomers may also act on the cell through a pathway different from that used by the latter isomers and $1\alpha,25(OH)_2D_3$.

SUMMARY

Current evidence supports the concept that the classical biological actions of vitamin D in mediating calcium homeostasis are supported by the combined presence of two dihydroxylated metabolites, namely $1,25(OH)_2D_3$ and $24,25-(OH)_2D_3$. In addition there is recent evidence to support the specific actions of $1\alpha,25R(OH)_2D_3-26,23S$-lactone in osteoclasts. A complex endocrine system coordinates the metabolism of vitamin D into these hormonally active forms. It is now clear that the vitamin D endocrine system embraces many more target tissues than simply the intestine bone and kidney. Notable additions to this list include the pancreas, the pituitary, breast tissue, placenta, eggshell gland and cells of the immune system. Key advances in understanding the diversity of the vitamin D endocrine system, particularly with respect to the interaction of $1,25(OH)_2D_3$, have been made through study of the tissue distribution of specific receptors for this ligand. Both the $1,25(OH)_2D_3$ receptors as well as the vitamin D-dependent proteins are widely disbursed in many target tissues.

The second dihydroxylated metabolite, $24,25(OH)_2D_3$, has been reported to be capable of inducing a variety of specific biological effects: some when the steroid is administered alone and some in the presence of its companion dihydroxylated metabolite. There is emerging evidence of the presence of specific receptors for $24,25(OH)_2D_3$, particularly in chondrocytes and parathyroid glands. These observations collectively demonstrate the widespread involvement of vitamin D in both cellular, particularly bone, as well as whole animal calcium metabolism.

REFERENCES

Listed below are a selection of reference citations which should allow the interested reader to gain access to the appropriate scientific literature.

Review Articles

1. Reichel, H., H. P. Koeffler and A. W. Norman. The role of the vitamin D endocrine system in health and disease. New Engl. J. Med. 320:980-991 (1989).
2. Minghetti, P. P. and A. W. Norman. $1,25(OH)_2$-vitamin D_3 receptors: Gene regulation and genetic circuitry. FASEB J. 2, 3043-3053 (1988).

3. Norman, A. W. and H. Reichel. Effects of $1\alpha,25$-dihydroxyvitamin D_3 on leukemia cells. ISI Atlas Science 1, 249-253 (1988).
4. Henry, H. L. and A. W. Norman. Vitamin D: Metabolism and biological actions. Ann. Rev. Nutr. 4, 493-520 (1984).
5. Haussler, M. R. Vitamin D receptors: Nature and function. Ann. Rev. Nutr. 6, 527-562 (1986).
6. Brommage, R. and H. F. DeLuca. Evidence that 1,25-dihydroxyvitamin D_3 is the physiologically active metabolite of vitamin D_3. Endocr. Rev. 6, 491-511 (1985).
7. Norman, A. W., J. Roth and L. Orci. The vitamin D endocrine system: Steroid metabolism, hormone receptors and biological response (calcium binding proteins). Endocr. Rev. 3, 331-366 (1982).
8. Rigby, W. F. C. The immunobiology of vitamin D. Immunol. Today 9, 54-58 (1988).
9. Norman, A. W. (1979) Vitamin D: The Calcium Homeostatic Steroid Hormone, Academic Press, New York, 490 pp.
10. Norman, A. W. (1984) The role of receptors in mediating the biological responses to 1,25-dihydroxyvitamin D_3-- the hormonally active form of vitamin D, p. 479-493. In, J. A. Gustafsson and H. Eriksson (eds.), Steroid Hormone Receptors: Structure and Function, Elsevier Biomedical Press, Amsterdam, The Netherlands.
11. Pike, J. W. Intracellular receptors mediate the biological action of 1,25-dihydroxyvitamin D_3. Nutr. Rev. 43, 161-168 (1985).

Research Papers

12. Wilhelm, F., A. W. Norman. Studies on the mode of action of calciferol. LVI. Biochemical characterization of positive cooperativity in the binding of $1\alpha,25$-dihydroxyvitamin D_3 to its chick intestinal crude chromatin receptor. J. Biol. Chem. 260, 10087-10092 (1985).
13. Green, S., P. Chambon. A superfamily of potentially oncogenic hormone receptors. Nature 324, 615-617 (1986).
14. Giguere, V, N. Yang, P. Segui and R. M. Evans. Identification of a new class of steroid hormone receptors. Nature 331, 91-94; 1988.
15. Arriza, J. L., C. Weinberger, G. Cerelli, T. M. Glaser, B. L. Handelin, D. E. Housman, and R. M. Evans. Cloning of human mineralocorticoid receptor complementary DNA: structural and functional kinship with the glucocorticoid receptor. Science 237, 268-275 (1987).
16. Petkovich, M., N. J. Brand, A. Krust and P. A. Chambon. A human retinoic acid receptor which belongs to the family of nuclear receptors. Nature 330, 444-450 (1987).
17. McDonnell, D. P., D. J. Mangelsdorf, J. W. Pike, M. R. Haussler and B. W. O'Malley. Molecular cloning of complementary DNA encoding the avian receptor for vitamin D. Science 235, 1214-1217 (1987).
18. Miller, J., A. D. McLachlan and A. Klug. Repetitive zinc-binding domains in the protein transcription factor IIIA from xenopus oocytes. The EMBO J. 4, 1609-1614 (1985).

19. Pike, J.W. and N. W. Sleator. Hormone-dependent phosphorylation of the 1,25-dihydroxyvitamin D_3 receptor in mouse fibroblasts. _Biochem. Biophys. Res. Commun._ 131, 378-385 (1985).

20. Theofan, G., A. P. Nguyen and A. W. Norman. Regulation of calbindin-D_{28K} gene expression by 1,25-dihydroxyvitamin D_3 is correlated to receptor occupancy. _J. Biol. Chem._ 261, 16943-16947 (1986).

21. Ishizuka, S., N. Kurihara, S. Hakeda, N. Maeda, K. Ikeda, M. Kumegawa and A. W. Norman. $1\alpha,25$-Dihydroxyvitamin D_3 $[1\alpha,25-(OH)_2D_3]$-26,23-lactone inhibits 1,25-$(OH)_2D_3$-mediated fusion of mouse bone marrow mononuclear cells. _Endocrinology_ 123, 781-786 (1988).

22. Okamura, W. H., A. W. Norman and R. M. Wing. Vitamin D: concerning the relationship between molecular topology and biological function. _Proc. Natl. Acad. Sci. USA_ 71, 4194-4197 (1974).

23. Haussler, M. R. and A. W. Norman. Chromosomal receptor for a vitamin D metabolite. _Proc. Natl. Acad. Sci. USA_ 62, 155-162 (1969).

24. Ishizuka, S., J. Oshida, H. Tsuruta and A. W. Norman. The stereochemical configuration of the natural $1\alpha,25$-dihydroxyvitamin D_3-26,23-lactone. _Arch. Biochem. Biophys._ 242, 82-89 (1985).

25. Ishizuka, S. and A. W. Norman. The difference of biological activity among four diastereoisomets of $1\alpha,25$-dihydroxyvitamin D_3-26,23-lactone. _J. Steroid Biochem._ 25, 505 (1986).

26. Merke, J. and A. W. Norman. Studies on the mode of action of calciferol. XXXII. Evidence for a $24(R),25(OH)_2$-vitamin D_3 receptor in the parathyroid gland of the rachitic chick. _Biochem. Biophys. Res. Commun._ 100, 551 (1981).

27. Abe, E., C. Miyaura, H. Sakagami, M. Takeda, K. Konno et al. Differentiation of mouse myeloid leukemia cells induced by $1\alpha,25$-dihydroxyvitamin D_3. _Proc. Natl. Acad. Sci. USA_ 78, 49904994 (1981).

28. Mangelsdorf, D. J., H. P. Koeffler, C. A. Donaldson, J. W. Pike and M. R. Haussler. 1,25-Dihydroxyvitamin D_3-induced differentiation in a human promyelocytic leukemia cell line (HL-60). Receptor-mediated maturation to macrophage-like cells. _J. Cell Biol._ 98, 391 (1984).

29. Provvedini, D. M., K. D. Tsoukas, L. J. Deftos and S. C. Manolagas. 1,25-Dihydroxyvitamin D_3 receptors in human leukocytes. _Science_ 221, 1181-1183 (1983).

30. Reichel, H., H. P. Koeffler, A. Tobler and A. W. Norman. $1\alpha,25$-Dihydroxyvitamin D_3 inhibits interferon-γ synthesis by normal human peripheral blood lymphocytes. _Proc. Natl. Acad. Sci. USA_ 84, 3385-3389 (1987).

ROLE OF PARATHYROID HORMONE IN BONE FORMATION

AND RESORPTION

Roger Smith

Nuffield Orthopaedic Centre and
John Radcliffe Hospital, Headington
Oxford, U.K.

Introduction

One of the most striking effects of parathyroid hormone (PTH) is
that on bone. Osteitis fibrosa cystica was early recognised as a
characteristic feature of bone in patients with hyperparathyroidism
(Hunter and Turnbull, 1932). The main pathological changes which lead to
this include an increase in number (and apparently activity) of osteoclasts,
marrow fibrosis, and sometimes the formation of expanded cyst-like lesions,
or brown tumours. Although excess bone resorption predominates, and is
well documented radiologically at particular sites, such as the phalanges
and ends of the long bones, there is often an increase in bone formation.
This is exemplified by the osteosclerosis of secondary hyperparathyroidism
in renal glomerular osteodystrophy.

Such clinical and pathological observations show that in vitro PTH
has important effects on bone, and these can be demonstrated in vitro and
in bone culture systems. The question which this article addresses is what
are these effects and how are they brought about? The answer includes
consideration of the factors controlling synthesis of PTH (and related
compounds), the effects of PTH on the 1 alpha hydroxylation of 25 hydroxy
vitamin D to produce 1,25 dihydroxy vitamin D, (a potent bone resorber),
the determination of which type of cell (or cells) in bone is the main
receiver of the PTH and 1,25 dihydroxy vitamin D message, the modulating
effect of other growth factors on the cellular response to these hormones,
the question of how cells talk to each other, and consideration of the way
in which osteoclasts eventually resorb bone.

Some years ago PTH-mediated bone resorption was considered to be a
simple osteoclastic event but now the effects of PTH on bone are known to be
very complex, and it is possible only to give an outline of them
(Smith, 1984). In what follows it must constantly be recalled that much
recent work is concerned with isolated or transformed bone cells, sometimes
with mixed populations and often with cells of uncertain origin. The
findings from such artificial systems cannot be transferred uncritically
to interpret the effect of PTH on bone as a tissue in vivo which is highly
heterogeneous (Wong, 1986; Raisz, 1988). The apparent effects of PTH differ
according to the systems studied. In complex systems such as organ cultures
in addition to the mixture of cell populations there are many local
messengers; these are largely absent in culture systems consisting

111

predominantly of one cell type. Such messengers may be produced by bone cells in response to PTH so that the eventual effects of PTH in bone tissue can reflect secondary interchanges between cells. The extracellular matrix cannot be regarded as inert in this respect. The mixed cell populations include large multinucleated osteoclasts, plump osteoblasts lining the newest bone matrix, osteocytes within the mineralised bone, and small fibroblast-like cells lining the bone surfaces. In organ culture PTH appears to resorb bone directly by increasing the number and activity of the osteoclasts, but has little or no effect on isolated osteoclast preparations (Chambers, 1988). Comparison of the effect of PTH in these differing environments has led to the idea that the main bone cell receptor for the action of PTH is the osteoblast (or its precursor).

Synthesis and secretion of PTH

PTH is manufactured as a large precursor molecule (in the manner of proteins destined for export), preproPTH, under the control of a gene on chromosome 11. The gene for PTH related protein (PTHrP), which has many of the features of PTH (see below) is on chromosome 12. Despite this separation it is considered that in evolutionary terms the genes have only recently diverged.

PreproPTH is converted to native PTH by the successive removal of its extensions (MacIntyre, 1986). PTH itself is an 84 amino acid polypeptide of which only the 1-34 amino terminal fragment is biologically active. The receptor binding site resides within the 3-34 fragment. PTH is secreted either as the whole molecule or as amino terminal or carboxy terminal components and is subsequently fragmented and metabolised. In vivo the production of PTH is increased by a reduction in plasma ionised calcium. The parathyroids are unusual endocrine glands since their activity increases when the circulating level of calcium decreases. The exact mechanism for this is unknown and may be multiple; in human parathyroid adenomata an increase in calcium concentration leads to a reduction in mRNA for PTH (Farrow et al, 1988), and there is also evidence for post-transcriptional control.

There are two main pathological situations in which there is a sustained increase in PTH. The first results from persistent hypocalcaemia (as in vitamin D-deficient osteomalacia or in renal glomerular failure), with secondary hyperparathyroidism. This overactivity reflects an increase in the size of the glands as well as in their activity. In the second situation, overactivity of the parathyroid cells occurs without a known stimulus - primary hyperparathyroidism. This is most commonly in the form of an adenoma, which may be monoclonal (Arnold et al, 1988) or less frequently as hyperplasia.

Effects of PTH on tissues

Biologically active PTH produces its effects on calcium metabolism via three tissues, the small intestine, the kidney and the skeleton. Other tissues, such as dermal fibroblasts, have sensitive PTH adenyl cyclase activity but the significance of this is unknown (Pun et al, 1988). PTH increases small intestinal calcium absorption mainly (or entirely) by stimulating the 1-alpha hydroxylation of 25 hydroxyvitamin D, but its effects on the renal tubular cell (increasing reabsorption of calcium) and on bone cells are also direct. The separate effect of PTH on TmP/GFR has only an indirect effect on plasma calcium concentration.

Although it can be shown experimentally that PTH increases the synthesis of 1,25 dihydroxyvitamin D, its concentration in primary hyperparathyroidism is not always elevated, and any increase is often modest (Lalor et al,

1989). Thus in the intact subject with hyperparathyroidism, the bone cells may be influenced by increased PTH alone, or by an increase in both PTH and 1,25 dihydroxyvitamin D (see below). In hypoparathyroid states bone disease is unusual apart from the skeletal abnormalities of pseudohypoparathyroidism, such as short metacarpals, which are not closely related to the underlying defect.

PTH related protein

Recent investigations of hypercalcaemia in patients with non-metastatic solid tumours (humoral hypercalcaemia of malignancy) have identified a PTH related protein (PTHrP) as an important cause (Mundy, 1988; Meikle, 1989). The amino terminal sequence of this protein shows considerable similarities to that of PTH. The gene for this protein has been identified and cloned; and the biological effects of PTHrP are almost identical to those of PTH, including those on bone cells. PTHrP may be a naturally occurring calciotrophic hormone in the foetus (Care and Abbas, 1987). Its production by malignant cells may be analogous to the ectopic production of other hormones by tumours. Recent comparisons between the effects of synthetic amino terminal sequences of PTH and PTHrP on cAMP by cultured osteosarcoma cells show the close similarity between the two hormones (Fukayama et al, 1988).

Effects of PTH on bone

Indirect, via 1,25 dihydroxyvitamin D

a) On bone cells

Dihydroxyvitamin D produces its effects by controlling the expression of the genes of the receptor cell. A large number of cells can be shown to contain the vitamin D receptor, albeit in low concentration, and this includes the osteoblast. The receptor has been isolated and its gene cloned. It has a 1,25 and a DNA binding region and belongs to the steroid-receptor super family (Evans, 1988). The mode of action of the 1,25 receptor has been well elucidated by studies on Type II vitamin D dependent rickets in which the end organ resistance to 1,25 dihydroxyvitamin D may be due to single point mutations in the exon coding for the DNA binding region (Lancet, 1989). It is now acknowledged that the effects of 1,25 dihydroxyvitamin D are not limited to calcium metabolism, and that this hormone has effects on many tissues. The complexity and multiplicity of these actions on the eukaryotic genome have been classified into those associated with classic mineral homeostasis, with regulation of bio-synthesis and catabolism of vitamin D secosteroids, with differentiation events in the immune system and skin, and with regulating DNA replication and cellular proliferation (Minghetti and Norman, 1988). Of particular relevance is the effect on cell proliferation and maturation. Thus 1,25 dihydroxyvitamin D has a number of effects on the skeleton via its influence on bone cells. These are 1) Effects on many of the genes of the osteoblast, increasing for instance the synthesis of alkaline phosphatase and decreasing the production of collagen; 2) Effects on cell maturation. One well recognised effect of 1,25 dihydroxyvitamin D is to reduce the proliferation and increase the differentiation of responsive cells. This has naturally led to the attempted therapeutic use in neoplastic diseases such as leukemia and breast cancer (Colston et al, 1989). 3) Effects on the immune system 1,25 dihydroxyvitamin D causes differ-entiation of committed precursors with the characteristics of mature osteoclasts in vitro and has many other effects on modulating the immune effects on T cells and cytokine production in the marrow environment. Recent work makes it likely that 1,25 dihydroxyvitamin D is an essential hormone for the differentiation of bone resorbing cells. 4) An increase in osteoclast resorption. This may occur by two mechanisms, namely an increase in number of osteoclasts, and a facilitation by osteoblasts of osteoclastic bone resorption. It is widely considered (see below) that osteoblasts prepare the way for osteoclastic bone resorption by producing a collagenase (initially in an inactive form) which locally removes the unmineralised bone matrix normally present as a thin layer over mineralised bone. This exposes mineralised bone to resorption by osteoclasts (and possibly other mononuclear cells). The exact way in which such resorption is carried out is unknown, but it is thought that the osteoclast extensions form a tight seal on the bone surface isolating the osteoclastic milieu from that outside. Within the private and acidic environment bone is resorbed by lysosomal enzymes.

b) On mineralisation

Lack of vitamin D causes defective mineralisation and rickets and osteomalacia is cured by giving 1,25 dihydroxyvitamin D or its precursors. The mechanism of this therapeutic effect is still disputed, since it is not yet known whether it follows passively from the increased intestinal absorption of calcium or whether 1,25 dihydroxyvitamin D has a direct effect on the mineralisation process. Vitamin D deficiency leads to hypocalcaemia and secondary hyperparathyroidism, itself leading to bone resorption.

Direct effects of PTH on bone

a) on bone cells

The main cells of bone, the osteoblasts (and osteocytes) and the osteo-clasts have a separate lineage and separate characteristics (Owen, 1985). Of the calciotrophic hormones the osteoclasts appear to possess receptors for calcitonin only, and it is currently supposed that any change in the activity of the osteoclasts induced by PTH is in response to messages from the osteoblasts. What these messages are is only dimly perceived.

Early studies on bone tissues using tritiated thymidine showed that PTH increased the activity of the osteoblasts as well as the osteoclasts suggesting at least an initial anabolic effect of PTH; whether osteoblasts or preosteoblasts are the main target of PTH has been questioned (Rouleau et al, 1988).

The way in which osteoblasts (or preosteoblasts) are stimulated by PTH is complex, and involves at least some of the newly described mechanisms of intracellular signalling (see below). The apparent effect of PTH on bone depends on the system studied. In organ cultures where bone population is mixed and osteoblasts and osteoclasts coexist, PTH increases the activity and number of osteoclasts by an undefined mechanism. Again in organ culture the effects of PTH on the formation of bone are variable, depending on time, dose and method of administration. High concentrations of PTH inhibit collagen synthesis by osteoblasts and reduce alkaline phosphatase activity. The osteoblasts become stellate, secrete collagenase and plasminogen activator, and perhaps prepare the bone for osteoclast resorption. In contrast intermittent low concentrations of PTH increase the number and activity of osteoblasts. Of the many possible hypotheses to explain this, none is entirely satisfactory, but it is possible that in such organ systems (and in vitro) PTH can stimulate the release of anabolic cytokines from bone. The anabolic effects of PTH itself could have therapeutic relevance in osteoporosis (see below). Exposure of bone tissue directly to PTH shows dramatic changes in osteoclast morphology within 10-60 minutes with the activation of existing osteoclasts as well as increases in their number. The anabolic effects which have been shown to occur with continuous or intermittent low dose infusion of PTH are of slower onset and may thus represent secondary effects of PTH, although they may be direct.

114

In cultures of differing bone populations, specifically osteoblasts and osteoclasts the separate effects of PTH may be more clearly defined. Studies on primary cultures or freshly isolated osteoblasts, or transformed osteoblasts, or osteosarcoma cells, have begun to define a role for such cells in addition to their function in bone formation. Importantly they have shown that the osteoblast contains enzymes capable of degrading the organic matrix of bone. Thus bone resorption stimulating hormones (including PTH, PGE_2, 1,25 dihydroxyvitamin D and epidermal growth factor) stimulate plasminogen activator in cultured osteoblasts. This protease converts plasminogen to plasmin which can activate latent collagenase. These (and other) biochemical changes are associated with morphological changes in the osteoblast which retract when exposed to PTH (in bone and in primary cultures) producing gaps in the cell layer providing access for the osteoclasts to the underlying matrix. Such changes are mediated through effects on the osteoblast cytoskeleton.

Another result of the study of bone cell cultures has been to suggest that the osteoclastic response to PTH is mediated through the osteoblast, although the way this is brought about is unknown. Similarly there is little information on the possible effects of PTH on preosteoclasts and osteoprogenitor cells.

Interestingly osteoblasts and their immature precursors appear to have PTH receptors whereas their derivatives the osteocytes do not (and in this way they resemble osteoclasts).

b) Cellular signals

The best known effect of PTH on its receptor cells is stimulation of the adenyl cyclase pathway (Rasmussen, 1986), but work on cultured osteoblasts suggests that PTH also has a direct independent effect on one of the other major cellular signalling mechanisms, that is the phosphoinositol system (Farndale et al, 1988).

The action of PTH on the production of cAMP is well defined and resembles that of other peptide hormones acting through receptors on the external surface of the target cell. (The response of the osteoclast to calcitonin is also mediated through the cAMP mechanism). The receptors induce changes on the inner surface of the cell membrane leading to alterations in activity within the cell. The cell membrane receptor is a lipoprotein complex linked to a transducer unit and a catalytic unit. The transducer unit, the nucleotide regulatory complex (N complex) has three components (in the case of PTH these are referred to as guanyl (G) proteins; Hosking and Kerr, 1988). Activation involves dissociation of the alpha component of this complex which binds to and activates the catalytic unit. The catalytic unit (which is an enzyme) mediates the action of various hormones, and in the case of PTH the enzyme is adenyl cyclase and the product is cyclic AMP. This itself acts as a second messenger to transmit the hormone signal into stimulation within the cell (Mitchell, 1987). This is done by activating protein kinases which phosphorylate a number of proteins, using ATP as a substrate. The cellular effects of PTH on osteoblast-like cells include stimulation of proliferation, (inhibition of proliferation at high doses), increase of cellular calcium (in some cell lines) and the activation of adenyl cyclase. Although the importance of the adenyl cyclase system in the stimulation of the osteoblast by PTH is not denied, some observations make it difficult to accept that cyclic AMP is the major or only secondary messenger for the PTH response. Thus analogues which block PTH stimulation of adenyl cyclase do not stop bone resorption, and PTH analogues which have little effect on cAMP production can nevertheless stimulate bone resorption.

The relative importance of cAMP compared with other second messenger signals in mediating the different biological responses to PTH is being examined by the use of mutant osteosarcoma cell lines in which the consequences of activation of the adenyl cyclase system may be specifically inhibited by brief exposure to Zn^{2+} (Bringhurst et al, 1989). Additionally work on neonatal mouse osteoblasts suggests that PTH (like PGE_2) can stimulate phosphoinositide turnover; and recent experiments on cultured osteoblasts suggest that PTH (and prostaglandins) may also act by modulating the activity of phospholipase C responsible for the production of diacylglycerol and inositol triphosphate. Phospholipase C may also produce diacylglycerol from phosphatidylcholine providing an alternative pathway of phospholipid turnover (Pelech and Vance, 1989). These mechanisms could account for the observed increase in intracellular calcium.

In vivo the effect of PTH on osteoblasts via these mechanisms is likely to be influenced by other bone resorbing factors; for instance in culture systems the adenylate cyclase response of clonal osteoblast-like cells to PTH is decreased by transforming growth factor alpha epidermal growth factor and other cytokines (Gutierrez et al, 1987). This may be of importance in the intact organism, particularly to explain the different changes in the skeleton due to primary hyperparathyroidism (where bone formation may be increased) and to humoral hypercalcaemia of malignancy (where bone formation is often suppressed).

Mechanism of bone resorption

Osteoblasts are closely concerned with osteoclast activity by a number of complex mechanisms. Since these have been elucidated largely by the study of isolated cell systems the interpretation of the experimental findings varies. It appears that osteoclastic bone resorption can be regulated on at least three different levels. Differentiation of osteo-clasts is exclusively an effect of 1,25 dihydroxyvitamin D which probably bypasses the osteoblast (although it may use an intermediate cell): induction of bone resorption requires collaboration with collagenase producing osteoblasts; and modulation of osteoclastic activity is carried out by signals from the osteoblast (with the exception of calcitonin).

The way in which the osteoblast and osteoclast actually set about resorbing bone is complex (Sakamoto and Sakamoto, 1986; Thompson et al, 1989). It is currently proposed that the osteoclast cannot itself resorb the thin layer of unmineralised osteoid which covers mature bone, and this is removed by collagenase produced from the osteoblast, initially in an inactive form. The production of active collagenase by the osteoblast appears to depend on a complex cascade which involves plasminogen activator, plasmin, and metalloproteinases and which is regulated by a tissue inhibitor of metalloproteinases (TIMP) and a plasminogen activator inhibitor. The osteoclast then applies itself to the exposed mineralised surface forming a tight seal around the circumference of this area of attachment within which digestion of bone occurs mainly by the action of lysosomal enzymes acting at an acid pH. The events which occur within this sealed zone are complex; they involve special adhesive structures, cytoskeletal elements which define the clear zone, and elaborate mechanisms which allow digestion of bone in an acid environment. This resorbing activity depends inter alia on the presence of a ruffled border and also the effectiveness of the proton pump, itself depending on the activity of carbonic anhydrase isoenzyme 11. Deficiency of either produces osteosclerotic bone disease.

Clinical relevance

Pseudohypoparathyroidism (PHP)

This disorder is very rare but provides valuable insight into the way in which PTH acts on cells (Hosking and Kerr, 1988). The clinical and biochemical manifestations are undoubtedly heterogeneous, but two main subtypes are recognised; in Type I an abnormality of the PTH-receptor-adenylate cyclase complex reduces cAMP production by target cells, and in Type II cAMP production is adequate but the intracellular expression of PTH directed events is deficient.

The general structure of the adenylate cyclase system has been described. Many patients with PHP have reduced levels of the stimulatory sub component of the guanyl-nucleotide-binding proteins (Gs) although the inhibitory protein (Gi) appears to be normal in amount. This is probably not enough to account for the resistance to PTH (and other hormones) and is not constantly associated with the typical phenotype - short stature, mental simplicity, short metacarpals and ectopic (subcutaneous and cerebral) calcification.

Vitamin D dependent rickets

Detailed study of patients with the rare condition of vitamin D dependent rickets (hypocalcaemic vitamin D resistant rickets) has defined at least two conditions: Type I with an inherited deficiency of 1 alpha hydroxylase, and Type II with end-organ resistance to 1,25 dihydroxy-vitamin D. In the second disorder early and severe hypocalcaemic rickets coexists with secondary hyperparathyroidism and raised circulating concentrations of 1,25 dihydroxyvitamin D; alopecia is also a feature. Although the study of fibroblasts from various kindreds shows that the intracellular abnormality is heterogeneous, it now appears that this disorder is often due to a mutation (or mutations) in the gene coding for the 1,25 dihydroxyvitamin D receptor protein. This protein belongs to the steroid receptor super family. The hormone binding domain is at the carboxy terminus and the DNA binding domain has two 'finger' structures that complex zinc-zinc fingers (Struhl, 1989). Described point mutations occur in the DNA binding site at the tip of the zinc fingers (Malloy et al, 1989; Lancet, 1989).

Osteopetrosis

The rare experiments of nature which result in osteopetrosis illuminate the mechanisms by which osteoclasts resorb bone. Generally divided into a severe recessively inherited disorder and a dominantly inherited mild disorder, further differences are described. In the dominant disease radiographs show diffuse symmetrical osteosclerosis but in some patients there are characteristic alternating areas of dense bone (giving a striated or endobone appearance). It is this latter group which has a marked increase in acid phosphatase (and significant slight increase of plasma calcium and PTH), presumably reflecting abnormal osteoclastic activity (Bollerslev et al, 1988). Severe infantile osteopetrosis is likewise known to be heterogeneous in man and electron microscopy shows that in some, but not all, subjects with osteopetrosis, the osteoclasts lack their characteristic ruffled border. Likewise only some respond to bone marrow transplantation. Interestingly the circulating concentrations of 1,25 dihydroxyvitamin D may be increased suggesting a cellular resistance to this hormone.

Humoral hypercalcaemia of malignancy (HHM)

Hypercalcaemia is commonly associated with malignant disease and has many causes. That associated with non-metastatic solid tumours has been investigated in detail (Mundy, 1988; Meikle, 1988). Such work has demonstrated the importance of PTHrP and identified the multiple factors both pathological and physiological which regulate osteoclastic bone resorption.

Further understanding of hypercalcaemic malignant disease is one compelling reason to continue investigation of the action of PTH and related hormones on bone. Another is the possibility of using PTH and its analogues in the treatment of bone loss, discussed elsewhere in this symposium.

References

Arnold A, Staunton C E, Kim H G, Randall A B, Gaz D, Kronenberg H M. Monoclonality and abnormal parathyroid genes in parathyroid adenomas. N Eng J Med 1988; 318: 658-662

Bollerslev J, Nielsen H K, Larsen H F, Mosekilde L. Biochemical evidence of disturbed bone metabolism and calcium homeostasis in two types of autosomal dominant osteopetrosis. Acta Med Scand 1988; 244: 747-83.

Bringhurst F R, Zajac J D, Daggett A S, Skurat R N, Kronenberg H M. Inhibition of parathyroid hormone responsiveness in clonal osteoblastic cells expressing a mutant form of 3', 5'-cyclic adenosine monophosphate dependent protein kinase. Mol End 1989; 3: 60-67.

Care A D, Abbas S K. Calcium homeostasis in the adult and foetus. Front Horm Res 1987; 17: 203-210.

Chambers T J. The regulation of osteoclastic development and function. Ciba Found Symp 1988; 136: 92-107.

Colston K W, Berger U, Coombes R C. Possible role for vitamin D in controlling breast cancer proliferation. Lancet 1989; i 188-191.

Evans R M. The steroid and thyroid hormone receptor super family. Science 1988; 240: 889-895.

Farndale R W, Sandy J R, Atkinson S J, Pennington S R, Meghi S, Meikle M C. Parathyroid hormone and prostaglandin E_2 stimulate both inositol phosphates and cyclic AMP accumulation in mouse osteoblast cultures. Biochem J 1988; 252: 263-268.

Farrow S M, Karmali R, Gleed J H, Hendy G N, O'Riordan J L H. Regulation of preparathyroid hormone messenger RNA and hormone synthesis in human parathyroid adenomata.Endocrinol 1988; 117: 133-138.

Fukayama S, Bosma T J, Goad D L, Voelkel E F, Tashjian A H. Human parathyroid hormone (PTH)-related protein and human PTH: Comparative biological activities on human cells and bone resorption. Endocrinol 1988; 123: 2841-2848.

Gutierrez G E, Mundy G R, Derynck R, Hewlett E L, Katz M S. Inhibition of parathyroid hormone-responsive adenylate cyclase in clonal osteoblast-like cells by transforming growth factor alpha and epidermal growth factor. J Biol Chem 1987; 262: 15845-15850

Hosking D J, Kerr D. Mechanism of parathyroid hormone resistance in pseudohypoparathyroidism. Clin Sci 1988; 74: 561-566.

Hunter D, Turnbull H M. Hyperparathyroidism: Generalised osteitis fibrosa. Br J Surg 1932; 19: 203-284

Lalor B C, Mawer E B, Davies M, Lumb G A, Hunt L, Adams P H. Determinants of the serum concentration of 1,25 dihydroxy vitamin D in primary hyperparathyroidism. Clin Sci 1989; 76: 81-86.

Lancet Zinc fingers and vitamin D resistance. 1989; i: 478.

MacIntyre I. The hormonal regulation of extra-cellular calcium. Br Med Bull 1986; 42: 343-352.

Malloy P J, Hochberg Z, Pike J W, Feldman D. Abnormal binding of vitamin D receptors to deoxyribonucleic acid in a kindred with vitamin D dependent rickets, Type II. Clin Endocrinol 1989; 68: 263-269.

Meikle M C. Hypercalcaemia of malignancy. Nature 1988; 336: 311.

Michell R H. How do receptors at the cell surface send signals to the cell interior? Br Med J 1987; 295: 1320-1323.

Minghetti P P, Norman A W. 1,25(OH)$_2$ Vitamin D$_3$ receptors: gene regulation and genetic circuitry. FASEB J 1988; 2: 3043-3053.

Mundy G R. Hypercalcaemia of malignancy revisited. J Clin Invest 1988; 82: 1-6.

Owen M. Lineage of osteogenic cells and their relationship to the stromal system. Bone and Mineral Research 1985; 3: 1-25.

Pelech S L, Vance D E. Signal transduction via phosphatidylcholine cycles. TIBS 1989; 14: 28-30.

Pun K K, Arnaud C D, Nissenson R A. Parathyroid hormone receptors in human dermal fibroblasts. J Bone Min Res 1988; 3: 453-460.

Raisz L G. Hormonal regulation of bone growth and remodelling. Ciba Found Symp 1988; 136: 226-238.

Rasmussen H. The calcium messenger system. N Eng J Med 1986; 314: 1094-1101, 1164-1170.

Rouleau M F, Mitchell J, Goltsman D. In vivo distribution of parathyroid hormone receptors in bone: evidence that a predominant osseous target cell is not the mature osteoblast. Endocrinology 1988; 123: 187-191.

Sakamoto S, Sakamoto M. Bone collagenase, osteoblasts and cell mediated bone resorption. Bone and Mineral Research 1986; 4: 49-102.

Smith R. Recent Advances in the Metabolism and Physiology of Bone in Recent Advances in Physiology. (Ed P F Baker) 1984; 10: 317-348.

Struhl K. Helix-turn-helix, zinc finger, and leucine-zipper-motifs for eukaryotic transcriptional regulatory proteins. TIBS 1989; 14: 137-140.

Thomson B M, Atkinson S J, McGarrity A M, Hembry R M, Reynolds J J, Meikle M C. Type I collagen degradation by mouse osteoblasts stimulated with 1,25(OH)$_2$ Vitamin D$_3$; evidence for a plasminogen activator-plasmin-metalloproteinase cascade. Bone and Tooth Society, April 1989 (Abstract).

Wong G L. Skeletal effects of parathyroid hormone. Bone and Mineral Research 1986; 4: 103-119.

CALCITONIN: MOLECULAR BIOLOGY, PHYSIOLOGY, PATHOPHYSIOLOGY AND ITS THERAPEUTIC USES

Sunil J Wimalawansa

Endocrine Unit, Dept. Chemical Pathology
Royal Postgraduate Medical School
Du Cane Road, London W12 ONN

INTRODUCTION

Discovery and distribution of CT

Calcitonin (CT) is a 32 amino acid peptide hormone, and its existence was postulated in 1962 by Copp and colleagues (Copp et al, 1962) (for review see Queener & Bell, 1975; MacIntyre et al, 1988; Wimalawansa & MacIntyre, 1989b). Initial studies on sheep suggested the parathyroid gland as the source of CT (Copp & Henze, 1964). Later, the source of this calcium lowering factor was identified as the thyroid gland (Foster et al, 1964a). CT is synthesised by the parafollicular cells (C-cells) of the thyroid in mammals (Foster et al, 1964b; Pearse, 1966; Bussolati and Pearse, 1967); and by C-cells associated with the ultimobranchial gland in lower vertebrates (Copp et al, 1967; Tauber, 1967). The C-cells derive from the neural crest (Le Dourain and Le Leivre, 1970) and migrate forward to become the ultimobranchial body in lower vertebrates and the parafollicular cells in man (Pearse & Polak, 1971) and related species (Pearse and Carvalheira, 1967). During migration, C-cells may concentrate in regions other than the thyroid and ultimobranchial body, and the localisation of C-cells also may vary in different species, for example as in Kulchitsky cells of human lung (Becker et al, 1980) and alimentary tract of *Ciona Intestinalis* (Fritsch et al, 1980). Ultimobranchial glands have been shown as the source of CT in dogfish, chicken (Copp et al, 1967) and in other avian species (Culter et al, 1977), whereas the lung is the major source of CT in the lizard (Ravazzola et al, 1981). Two different CTs have been identified in birds (Perez Cano et al, 1982a), reptiles and mammals (Perez Cano et al, 1982b). Immunoreactive-human CT (i-hCT)-like molecule has been demonstrated in the nervous system of protochordates and cyclostome *myxine* (Girgis et al, 1980), in neural ganglia of *Ciona Intestinalis* , an immediate ancestor of the vertebrate, but lacking any skeleton (Girgis et al, 1980; Fritsch et al, 1979, 1982) and in the ultimobranchial body of amphibia *Rana pipiens* (Perez Cano et al, 1981). i-CT has also been shown in the central nervous system of pigeon (Galan Galan et al, 1981). Although CT has been shown in the pituitary by both immuno-fluorescent studies (Deftos et al, 1978a) and radio-immunoassay (RIA) of pituitary extracts (Deftos et al, 1978b; Flynn et al, 1981), demonstration of CT synthesis in the pituitary by cDNA probes has not been successful (Jacobs et al, 1982).

Structure and Chemistry of CT

CT has been relatively conserved during evolution. At present CT from eight different species have been identified generating 11 known sequences (Fig. 1). Six of the invariant amino acid residues are clustered at the amino terminal and two are at the carboxy terminal end of the molecule. Furthermore, all CT has a 1-7 disulphide bridge and prolinamide at the C-terminus. CT so far identified can be divided into three groups: the primate-rodent (human & rat), the artiodactyl (ox, pig and sheep) and the teleost (salmon and eel). Human CT (Figure 2) was isolated from a medullary thyroid carcinoma, a tumour of C-cells, (Neher et al, 1968) and synthesised in the same year (Sieber et al, 1968). Porcine (Baghdiantz et al, 1964; Potts et al, 1968; Findlay et al, 1984), bovine (Brewer & Ronan, 1969), ovine (Potts et al, 1970), and rat (Raulias et al, 1976) were all isolated from normal thyroid glands of respective species; salmon (O'Dor et al, 1969; Niall et al, 1969) and eel (Otani et al, 1976; Noda & Narita, 1976; Morikawa et al, 1976) were isolated from ultimobranchial bodies. The co-existence of human and salmon CT-like peptide in man has been suggested (Fischer et al, 1983), but not confirmed. Athough all 32 amino acids are required for its hypocalcaemic activity, some of these amino acids can be substituted, either maintaining or occasionally enhancing its biological activity (Potts et al, 1971; Maier et al, 1974; Rittel et al, 1976).

Biosynthesis of CT

As with most other peptide hormones CT is also produced as a precursor molecule. A number of post-translational modifications occur in CT including cleavage and C-terminal amidation, prior to secretion of the mature form of CT (1-32).

The release of CT from C-cells is stimulated by cations Ca^{++} and Mg^{++} and also by glucagon, dibutyryl cyclic AMP, theophyllin (Bell & Kimble, 1970), gastrin, and cholecystokinin (Cooper et al, 1972). CT causes a dose-dependent elevation of cyclic AMP levels (Nicholson et al, 1986; Ito et al, 1985), and the effects of CT on osteoclasts can be mimicked by dibutyryl cyclic AMP (Chambers & Moore, 1983).

The CT gene is located in the short arm of chromosome 11 (Hoppener et al, 1984; Kittur et al, 1985). Clones representing CT messenger RNA (mRNA) had been characterised both in rat (Amara et al, 1980) and in man (Allison et al, 1981). They have been shown to encode a regulatory peptide precursor with a hydrophobic signal peptide and the CT separated by a paired dibasic amino acid from N- and C-terminal flanking peptides. The mRNA is represented in the

Figure 1

	Man	Rat	S-1	S-2	S-3	Eel	*Chick	Bov	Porc	Ovi	*Man[2]
1	Cys	-	-	-	-	-	-	-	-	-	Tyr
2	Gly	-	Ser	Ser	Ser	Ser	Ala	Ser	Ser	Ser	Ser
3	Asn	-	-	-	-	-	Ser	-	-	-	-
4	Leu	-	-	-	-	-	-	-	-	-	-
5	Ser	-	-	-	-	-	-	-	-	-	-
6	Thr	-	-	-	-	-	-	-	-	-	-
7	Cys	-	-	-	-	-	-	-	-	-	-
8	Met	-	Val	-	Val	Val	Val	Val	Val	Val	Leu
9	Leu	-	-	-	-	-	-	-	-	-	Gln
10	Gly	-	-	-	-	-	-	Ser	Ser	Ser	-
11	Thr	-	Lys	Lys	Lys	Lys	Lys	Ala	Ala	Ala	-
12	Tyr	-	Leu	Leu	Leu	Leu	Leu	-	-	-	-
13	Thr	-	Ser	Ser	Ser	Ser	Ser	Trp	Trp	Trp	Leu
14	Gln	-	-	-	-	-	-	Lys	Arg	Lys	-
15	Asp	-	Glu	-	-	Glu	Glu	-	Asn	-	Tyr
16	Phe	Leu	Leu	Leu	Leu	Leu	Leu	Leu	Leu	Leu	Leu
17	Asn	-	His	His	His	His	His	-	-	-	Lys
18	Lys	-	-	-	-	-	-	Asn	Asn	Asn	Asn
19	Phe	-	Leu	Leu	Leu	Leu	Leu	Tyr	-	Tyr	-
20	His	-	Gln	Gln	Gln	Gln	Gln	-	-	-	-
21	Thr	-	-	-	-	-	-	Arg	Arg	Arg	Met
22	Phe	-	Tyr	-	-	Tyr	Tyr	-	-	Tyr	-
23	Pro	-	-	-	-	-	-	Ser	Ser	Ser	-
24	Gln	-	Arg	Arg	Arg	Arg	Arg	Gly	Gly	Gly	Gly
25	Thr	-	-	-	-	-	-	Met	Met	Met	Ile
26	Ala	Ser	Asn	Asn	Asn	Asp	Asp	Gly	Gly	Gly	Asn
27	Ile	-	Thr	Thr	Thr	Val	Val	Phe	Phe	Phe	Phe
28	Gly	-	-	-	-	-	-	-	-	-	-
29	Val	-	Ser	Ala	Ala	Ala	Ala	Pro	Pro	Pro	Pro
30	Gly	-	-	-	-	-	Glu	Glu	Glu	Glu	Gln
31	Ala	-	Thr	Val	Val	Thr	Thr	Thr	Thr	Thr	Ile
32	Pro	-	-	-	-	-	-	-	-	-	-

Amino acid sequences of the nine fully characterised and two
*predicted calcitonins: The invariant residues are
clustered at the two ends of the molecule.

Abbreviations: S = Salmon, Bov = Bovine, Porc = Porcine, Ovi
= Ovine, Man - predicted.

genome by 4 exons: exon I is non coding, exon II and III
encode the signal peptide and N-terminal flanking peptide,
while exon IV encodes CT. A number of groups have
characterized mRNA encoding for CT precursor in *in vitro*
translational systems (either cell-free translation of
polyadenylated mRNA or translation of unfractionated RNA in
whole cells) (Table 1). These studies mostly utilised mRNA
derived from medullary thyroid carcinoma (MTC) tissue, the
richest source of CT, but in some cases mRNA from normal
thyroid tissue was also used. In the MTC tissues up to 10%
of the total polyadenylated mRNA had been shown to encode
for CT mRNA (Alison et al, 1981). Glycosylation has been
suggested to play a role in determining the specificity of

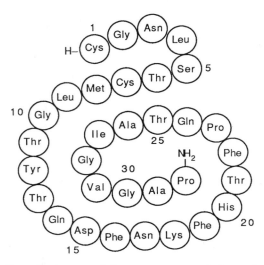

Figure 2.   Amino acid sequence of h-calcitonin

TABLE 1. Summary of studies of *in vitro*   translation of mRNA
coding for calcitonin precursors indicating their
approximate sizes.

Source of Messenger RNA	Translation System	Mr of primary product precipitable by calcitonin antiserum
Human MTC Van der Donk et al (1976)	Xenopus oocyte	65,000
Human MTC, various endocrine tumours Lips et al (1978)	Xenopus oocyte	65,000
Human MTC Goodman et al (1979)	Wheat germ, reticulocyte lysate	15,000 in each case
Codfish ultimobranchial gland, rat MTC. Jacobs et al (1979)	Wheat Germ Reticulocyte lysate	15,000 in each case
Human MTC, normal rat thyroid Desplan et al (1980)	Reticulocyte lysate	14,500 in each case
Rat MTC Amara et al (1980a)	Wheat germ	17,500
Human MTC Allison et al (1981)	Wheat germ	21,000
Rat MTC Jacobs et al (1981a)	Wheat germ	17,000

pre-secretory processing of CT-mRNA. In support of these findings, Baylin et al, 1981, observed that from 5 - 20% of i-CT extracted from human MTC and small cell carcinoma of the lung appeared to be glycosylated. Furthermore, glycosylated CTs of M_r up to 27,000 have been detected in extracts of serially transplanted rat MTC (O'Neil et al, 1981).

During the last 15 years, the development of techniques in recombinant DNA cloning in bacterial plasmids and nucleotide sequence analysis (Maxam & Gilbert, 1977; Sanger et al, 1975) have provided a strong tool to the understanding of eukaryotic genes and their products. Using these techniques further detailed cDNA analysis in rat revealed that the CT gene was more complex, and contained 6 exons. The exon V encodes (sequence of an N-terminal 80 amino acid peptide flanked by a paired dibasic amino acids) a novel 37 amino acid potent vasodilatory peptide (Morris et al, 1984; Brain et al, 1985, 1986) named calcitonin gene-related peptide (CGRP) (Amara et al, 1983; Rosenfeld et al, 1983). A schematic representation of α-CT/CGRP gene, and its transcription and translation are shown in figure 3. A similar peptide was later isolated and sequenced from a MTC in man (Morris et al, 1984). CGRP and its receptors are widely distributed in CNS (Wimalawansa et al, 1987a) and cardiovascular tissues (Wimalawansa et al, 1988b). CGRP is also present in the circulation in the rat (Zaidi et al, 1986; Wimalawansa & MacIntyre, 1988c), in man (Girgis et al, 1985; Wimalawansa, 1989a) and in the cerebrospinal fluid in man (Wimalawansa & MacIntyre, 1987).

The primary nuclear transcript of the α-CT/CGRP gene is processed to give rise to either precursor mRNA for CT and its carboxyl terminal flanking peptide Katacalcin (MacIntyre et al, 1982; Hillyard et al, 1983), or CGRP: CT mRNA is formed from the common intermediate by splicing the third intron and polyadenylating at the end of exon IV. Later studies revealed the existence of another CT/CGRP gene designated beta CT/CGRP gene in man (Hoppener et al, 1985) and in rat (Amara et al, 1985). The cloned beta-gene from rat (Amara et al, 1985) and from man (Hoppener et al, 1985) has been shown to encode a CGRP differing by one amino acid in rat and three in man from the corresponding α-CGRP (Amara et al, 1985; Hoppener et al, 1985). The amino acid sequences of α- and β-hCGRP are shown in Figure 4.

The structure of β-gene is similar to α-gene. However, the amino acid sequence encoded in exon IV has only 67% homology to the corresponding α-CT/CGRP gene (Alevizaki et al, 1986) and this is preceded by a termination codon and expression of this CT-like peptide in man seems unlikely.

Using insitu hybridisation, expressions of both CGRP genes in a variety of neural tissues have been demonstrated (Amara et al, 1985). The existence of the predicted β-hCGRP was proven by isolation and purification of β-CGRP from human spinal cord and its full characterisation by a combination of Fast Atom Bombardment Mass Spectrometry and gas phase sequencing (Wimalawansa et al, 1989a). The expression of both α- and β-CGRP has been demonstrated with indirect immuno-chemical analysis (cleavage of methionine

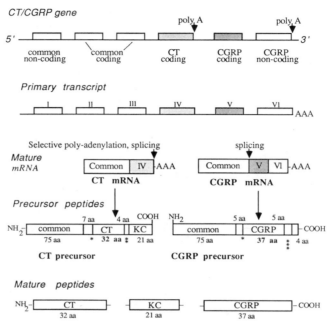

Figure 3. A schematic representation of the structural organisation of the - calcitonin-CGRP gene. Two different mRNA's may
be produced from the alternative processing of same primary transcript and use of two poly-adenylation sites; one coding for the
calcitonin precursor, the other for the calcitonin gene-related
peptide precursor. Post-translational modifications of calcitonin and CGRP includes intra-molecular S-S bridge formation at
the N-terminal region and amidation of the C-terminal amino acid.
acid.

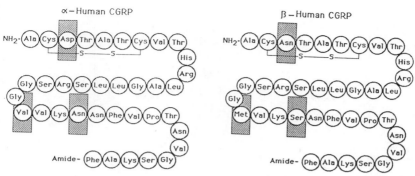

Figure 4. The aminoacid sequences of alpha and beta-calcitonin gene related peptides (Human).

residue with CNBr and by oxidation of methionine to methionine sulphoxide) in plasma and in cerebrospinal fluid in man (Wimalawansa et al, 1989b).

Recently, another peptide (Amylin, DAP, IAAP) with 48% homology to β-hCGRP was isolated from pancreatic amyloid deposit in a type II diabetic and from an Insulinoma (Cooper et al, 1987; Westermark et al, 1986). Comparison of the amino acid sequences of CT gene peptides with amylin is shown in Figure 5. Peptides with reasonable homology to CT, such as calcitonin gene-related peptide (D'Souza et al, 1986; Zaidi et al, 1987b) and amylin (Wimalawansa, Datta, Zaidi & MacIntyre unpublished) are also able to inhibit bone resorption, but at a higher concentration.

Distribution of CT receptors

In addition to osteoclasts (Tashjian et al, 1978; Warshawsky et al, 1980; Marx et al, 1972), CT receptors have been demonstrated in kidney (Marx et al, 1972, 1973; Warshawsky et al, 1980), rat (Fischer et al, 1981a) and human brain (Fischer et al, 1981b; Tschopp et al, 1985; Rizzo et al, 1981), testicular Leidig cells (Chausmer et al, 1982), fish gill (Fouchereau-Peron et al, 1981a), pig lung (Fouchereau-Peron et al, 1981b), lymphoid cell line (Marx et al, 1974), and human breast (Martin et al, 1980; Findlay et al, 1980b; Moseley et al, 1983) and lung cancer cell lines (Findlay et al, 1980a; Martin et al, 1981). CT receptors are rapidly down regulated following exposure to CT (Findlay et al, 1981). Receptors for 1,25 $(OH)_2D_3$ have also been identified on C-cells and on parathyroid cells (Freake & MacIntyre, 1982). Vitamin D has a direct influence on CT synthesis and secretion. This has been confirmed *in vivo* by demonstrating the increase of mRNA for CT following administration of 1,25$(OH)_2D_3$ (Segond et al, 1985). Furthermore, stimulation of CT secretion by 1,25 dihydroxycholecalciferol has also been demonstrated (Care et al, 1982).

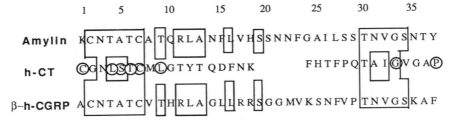

| | 1 | 5 | 10 | 15 | 20 | 25 | 30 | 35 |

Amylin   K C N T A T C A T Q R L A N F L V H S S N N F G A I L S S T N V G S N T Y

h-CT   C G N L S T C M L G T Y T Q D F N K   F H T F P Q T A I G V G A P

β-h-CGRP A C N T A T C V T H R L A G L L R R S G G M V K S N F V P T N V G S K A F

Amylin/CGRP   46% homology   ◯ Represents 8 invarient residues
Amylin/CT   16% homology   in all the calcitonins

Figure 5

Bioactivity of calcitonin

Biological potency of calcitonin is usually assessed by plasma calcium-lowering activity in the rat (Cooper et al, 1967; Kenny, 1971). Thus, salmon calcitonin (sCT) and eel calcitonin (eCT) (CTs of ultimobranchial origin) are the most potent, (Galante et al, 1971; Habener et al, 1971), whereas human (hCT) and porcine calcitonin (pCT) have only 1/50th and 1/30th of the potency of sCT and eCT (Maier, 1977; Findlay et al, 1980). This may be due to the greater affinity of sCT for CT receptor (Marx et al, 1972) or its longer half life in the circulation (Habener et al, 1971). sCT and eCT are more stable than hCT (Otani et al, 1978). Continuous or prolonged administration of CT may result in a loss of potency (Obie & Cooper, 1979): this may be associated with antibody formation (as with non-human CT's) or may be due to increase in the rate of CT catabolism or down-regulation of the CT receptors (Tashjian et al, 1978) or to changes in intracellular biochemical activities (Zanelli et al, 1985). Non-human CTs can be allergenic with roughly 50% of patients developing antibodies within 1 - 3 years. However, actual clinical resistance (neutralising antibodies) will develop in less than a quarter of these patients (Singer et al, 1980). Porcine CT has been shown to be more allergenic than the synthetic salmon and eel CTs. The former is now largely superceded by the latter two and by synthetic hCT. The kidney is the main organ responsible for the metabolism of human and salmon CT, while porcine CT is predominantly degraded in the liver (De Luise et al, 1972).

Assay for CT

Radioimmunoassays (RIA) have been developed for a variety of CTs (MacIntyre et al, 1980, 1984) including porcine, ovine, rat, rabbit, chicken, salmon and human hormones (Heath & Sizemore, 1983). The clinical application of hCT-RIA in measurement of CT in MTC patients has been described (Tashjian et al, 1970). Owing to the lack of immunological cross-reactivity between non-human CT (except rat CT) and human CT, homologous RIA systems are used to quantitate CT in man (Catherwood & Deftos, 1984; Heath et

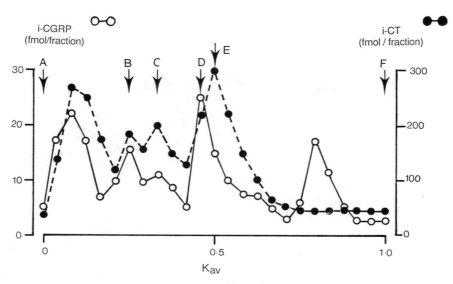

Figure 6. Sephadex G_{50} superfine gel-permeation chromatography of i-CGRP (o-o) and i-CT (●-●) profiles in plasma of medullary thyroid carcinoma patients. The elusion positions of the column calibration markers are: A = void volume (V_0), B = cytochrome C, C = Aprotinin, D = h-CGRP, E = h-CT, F = salt volume (V_t).

al, 1984). International reference preparation of hCT are available for comparative bioassays and also for RIA (Gaines Das & Zanelli, 1980). Multiple immunochemical forms of CT had been shown in MTC (Goltzman & Tischler, 1978; Heath & Sizemore, 1979; Baylin et al, 1981) and in plasma obtained from MTC patients (Singer & Habener, 1974; Deftos et al, 1975; Sizemore & Heath, 1975; Wimalawansa, 1989a) and in lung cancer (Becker et al, 1978). Immunochemical heterogeneity of CT in man and their effects on RIA had been shown previously (Snider et al, 1977; Ziegler & Rane, 1984). Figure 6 shows the gel-permeation chromatographic profile of plasma obtained from MTC patients demonstrating the immuno-chemical heterogeneity of CT in the circulation. A plasma extraction assay has been suggested (instead of neat plasma) in RIA to minimise the effects of these multiple immuno-chemical forms of CT (Body & Heath, 1983). However, this may underestimate the total bioactive CT in plasma, as some of the larger molecular weight forms are also bioactive (Seth, Wimalawansa, Zaidi & MacIntyre, unpublished). During the last few years non-isotopic ligand assays have been developed including fluorescence and enzyme immunoassays (Self et al, 1985; Wimalawansa et al, 1987c; Seth et al, 1987, 1988) improving the detectability of CT. Highly sensitive and specific CT assays have been developed using monoclonal antibodies in two-site (immuno-radiometric or enzyme) assays (Seth et al, 1988). A typical standard curve using such an assay for measurement of i-CT is shown in Figure 7.

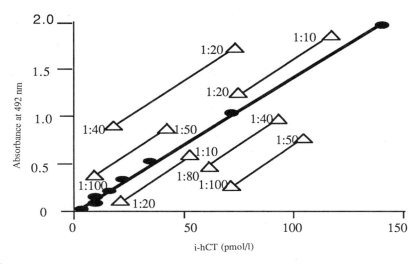

Figure 7. Calibration graph for the measurement of i-hCT (o) in plasma with two site enzyme-immunoassay using monoclonal antibodies. (Δ) indicates the parallel dilutions to the standard curve obtained from plasma of 4 MTC patients. (After Seth et al, 1988).

Physiology

The physiological role of CT is now beginning to emerge and appears to be concerned with maintenance of the skeleton during periods of calcium stress such as growth, pregnancy and lactation (Samaan et al, 1975; Stevenson et al, 1979, 1981; Talmage et al, 1980; MacIntyre & Stevenson, 1986). The role of CT in maintaining the skeleton during lactation is schematically shown in Figure 8. During pregnancy oestrogens, progesterone and androgens all show a gradual increase, but the mean CT levels are similar in each trimester of gestation and it is not clear which hormone "switches on" the CT production and why the levels do not increase further. From these results, it can be seen that CT is important in the protection of the skeleton during pregnancy. Testosterone appears to be a potent stimulus to CT production. High levels of CT are found in women during pregnancy and on oral contraceptives where the i-CT levels may rise to the male range. It is not yet clear which component of the pill is responsible for the raised i-CT levels and further studies with progesterone-only pills are needed to elucidate this point. In addition, at physiological concentrations, circulatory CT may have a tonic effect on osteoclastic activity. CT may not be regarded as a calcium-regulating hormone in the adult, but as the most potent endogenous direct inhibitor of osteoclastic bone resorption.

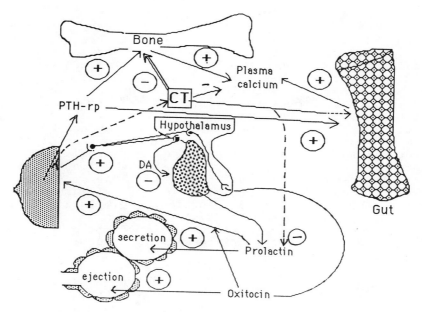

Figure 8. Various hormones involved in lactation and the protective role calcitonin on bone.

It is clear that women have a greater requirement for such a hormone during times of calcium stress such as pregnancy and lactation. At such a time, there might be a retention of calcium by the foetus at the expense of the mother and increased secretion of CT might exert a protectiv effect on the maternal skeleton. In support of this, raised i-CT levels are seen in pregnant women and a failure of CT to rise may well explain the pregnancy-associated osteoporosis. It is surprising that the basal CT levels in women are much lower than those found in men; the reason for these sex differences in circulating CT levels are not yet apparent. It is possible that, at the menopause, the cessation of sex hormone production could cause a further drop in the already low CT levels in the normal female. This might be sufficient to trigger bone resorption, a probable factor in the development of post-menopausal osteoporosis. CT reserves have also been shown to decrease progressively with age in both sexes (Samaan et al, 1975; Deftos et al, 1980). Not only do women have a lower level of plasma i-CT (Heath & Sizemore, 1977; Hillyard et al, 1978; Parthemore & Deftos, 1978), but also a much smaller CT reserve irrespective of age. A circadian variation of plasma CT has been reported, peak values occurring at around midday (Hillyard et al, 1977).

Formation and resorption of bone are tightly coupled. Therefore, any treatment which influences one process will eventually affect the other in the same direction. Thus inhibition of osteoclastic bone resorption by CT will soon be followed by a decrease in bone formation by osteoblasts. When a patient with rapid bone turnover is treated with CT, a rapid decrease in urinary excretion of hydroxyproline/ creatinine (marker of osteoclastic activity) can be observed. This is then followed up with a decrease in plasma bone specific alkaline phosphatase and osteocalcin (marker of osteoblastic activity). Therefore, in many cases of osteoporosis, long term treatment with CT alone may not be satisfactory and the positive effects may not be sustained. It is logical, therefore, to combine CT with perhaps an agent capable of stimulating osteoclasts. Alternatively, osteoporotic patients in whom oestrogens are contra-indicated or unacceptable (first line of therapy), may be treated with CT perhaps in a cyclical fashion. Whatever the therapy, it is beneficial to maintain a calcium intake of around 1 gram per day. The occasional elderly patient presenting with osteomalacia needs to be recognised and treated with an appropriate vitamin D supplement and calcium.

Following natural and artificial menopause, there is a fall in circulating levels of i-CT (Taggart et al, 1982; Stevenson et al, 1982) and deficient CT response to calcium infusion (Taggart et al, 1982). It has been proposed that increased osteoclastic activity associated with oestrogen deficiency following the menopause (and consequently CT deficiency) may in part be responsible for the development of postmenopausal osteoporosis (Milhaud et al, 1978). Furthermore, plasma i-CT levels rise during the follicular phase of the cycle, are maximum just after ovulation and then fall during the luteal phase (Milhaud et al, 1982). Chronic oestrogen administration may increase plasma i-CT levels and its synthesis in C-cells (Stevenson et al, 1981). However, some researchers have found no difference in basal plasma CT levels, but the levels rose significantly in response to calcium infusion (Morimoto et al, 1980).

Calcitonin has been shown to inhibit bone resorption *in vitro* (Reynolds et al, 1968; Chambers et al, 1985a, 1985b) and resorption induced by parathyroid hormone (Aliapoulious et al, 1966; Chambers et al, 1985a), and also steroid induced osteoporosis. Further, CT is able to decrease urinary excretion of hydroxyproline and calcium (Aer, 1968).

Actions of CT in Bone

Soon after its discovery, studies conducted on tissue cultures revealed that CT is a potent inhibitor of bone resorption (Friedman & Raisz, 1965; Foster et al, 1969). In addition to *in vivo* bio-assay in rats using its calcium lowering effects, tissue cultures also have been used as bioassays for measurement of CT activity (Raisz et al, 1967).

CT acts directly on osteoclasts and alters their behaviour (Chambers & Magnus, 1982; Chambers, 1985). CT inhibits osteoclast activity and thus is able to reduce bone resorption (Chambers et al, 1985a). This inhibitory effect of CT on osteoclast activity (Kallio et al, 1972) is the basis of a recently developed, highly sensitive, *in vitro* bioassay (Chambers et al, 1986). However, both *in vivo* and *in vitro* bioassays are tedious and expensive. Therefore, for clinical purposes, plasma i-CT levels are routinely measured with either radioimmunoassay (Hillyard et al, 1977; Heath et al, 1984; MacIntyre et al, 1980, 1984) or by immunometric assays (Seth et al, 1988).

An osteoclast is a large multi nucleated highly motile cell (Figure 9A). Osteoclasts are one of the main target cells for CT and contain large numbers (more than 10^6) of CT receptors (Wong & Cohn, 1975; Nicholson et al, 1986). Within a few minutes of administration of CT, osteoclasts decrease its motility and then start to retract (Chambers & Moore, 1983; Chambers & Dunn, 1983; Chambers et al, 1986) (Figure 9B). CT is also able to diminish the size of the cavities excavated in bone substrate by osteoclastic activity (Chambers et al, 1985; Zaidi et al, 1987b). During excavation of bone, osteoclasts liberate enzymes (e.g. acid phosphatases) and acids which subsequently hydrolyse the bone matrix leaving multiple pits (Figure 10). It has been shown that physiological levels of plasma CT are capable of controlling osteoclasts (Zaidi et al, 1988). Although the site of the target cells is unknown, CT when given over weeks or months causes a decrease in recrusion of osteoclasts from its precursor cells and thereby reduces the osteoclast numbers (Foster et al, 1969). This effect is of great importance in the treatment of Paget's disease and osteoporosis. When CT is injected intravenously into growing rats or into patients with Paget's disease, plasma calcium levels fall significantly (Woodhouse et al, 1970; McCredie et al, 1971). The basis of this plasma calcium lowering action of CT is an acute inhibitory effect on the osteoclasts. However, plasma calcium falls only when the bone turnover is high. Presumably, acute inhibiton of osteoclastic activity diminishes the flow of calcium from bone to blood. A plasma calcium-lowering effect of calcitonin is not seen in normal adults even with large doses because of the 'slow' (normal) rate of bone turnover (MacIntyre et al, 1967; Foster et al 1969; Singer et al, 1969).

Actions of CT in the kidney

Calcitonin has a weak action on the kidney enhancing the excretion of sodium, potassium, phosphate (Robinson et al, 1966), calcium and magnesium (Russell & Fleisch, 1968; MacIntyre et al, 1972; Carney & Thompson, 1981). A second messenger system for CT in the kidney is linked to an adenylate cyclase system (Bell, 1974). Further, in experimental animals CT also enhances the renal production of 1,25 dihydroxyvitamin D_3 (Galante et al, 1972) by selective stimulation of 25-hydroxylase activity in a cyclic AMP-independent pathway in the proximal straight tubule (Kawashima et al, 1981). CT stimulates the production of 1,25-dihydroxyvitamin D_3 in proximal kidney tubules by a cyclic AMP independent pathway (Horiuchi et al, 1979; Kawashima et al, 1981). This may be of physiological importance particularly during childhood and pregnancy.

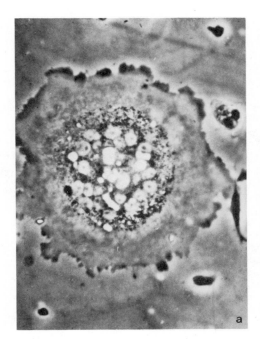 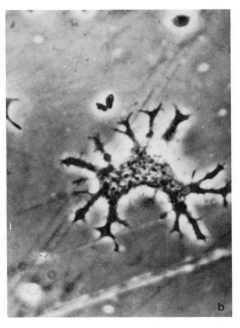

Figure 9. a) Appearence of a motile osteoclast after 2 hour incubation in control medium, showing lobulated peripheri with pseudopodial ruffling activity. Phase contrast X 320. b) Appearence of an osteoclast 30 minutes after addition of salmon calcitonin into the medium. (Courtesy of Professor T.J. Chambers, St. George's Hospital, London).

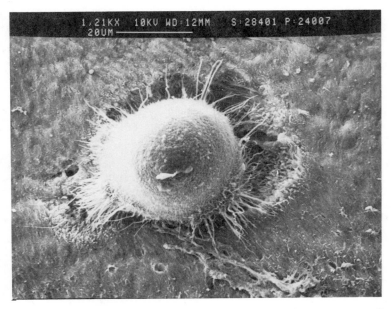

Figure 10. Scanning electron micrograph of an osteoclast after 8 hours incubation on a human cortical bone slice. An area of resorption can be seen where the cell was attached to the bone by osteoclast microvilli (After Chambers et al, 1985a).

Actions of CT in gastrointestinal tract

In addition to its major role of skeletal maintenance, CT also acts on a number of other tissues. In the gastrointestinal tract, it increases the intestinal secretion of sodium, potassium, chloride and water (Gray et al, 1973), and increases the intestinal absorption of calcium (Jaeger et al, 1986) and magnesium (Robinson et al, 1969). CT also inhibits gastric emptying, gastric acid secretion (Levine et al, 1984) and pancreatic functions. It also inhibits the secretion of several gastrointestinal regulatory peptides including gastrin (Fahrenkrug et al, 1975), insulin (Cantalamessa et al, 1978), glucagon, motilin and gastric inhibitory peptide (Stevenson et al, 1985). However, it is unlikely that the actions of CT on the gastrointestinal tract are of major physiological importance.

Besides hypercalcaemia, CT secretion is stimulated by a number of gastrointestinal hormones including gastrin, glucagon, and pancreozymin (Care et al, 1975). It may be speculated that CT also serves as an intestinal calcium conserving hormone; after a meal or ingestion of milk, the circulatory levels of gastro-intestinal hormones increases, which subsequently may increase CT secretion. CT itself delays the process of digestion (Bueno et al, 1983) in order to facilitate the absorption. This may, perhaps diminish the potential loss of calcium via kidneys during the post-prandial phase of hypercalcaemia (Gray & Munson, 1969). CT is able to inhibit gastrin and gastric acid secretion (Levine et al, 1984) in patients with peptic ulcer (Becker et al, 1974). The therapeutic use of CT in gastric ulcers and in pancreatitis is based on the above two hypotheses.

Actions of CT in the central nervous system

A number of studies have suggested that CT may act in the central nervous system (CNS) as a neuro-modulator. The CNS actions of CT have been demonstrated on animal models including analgesia and suppression of feeding (Pecile et al, 1975; Freed et al, 1979) and modification of behaviour (Nicoletti et al, 1982). Reduction in feeding has been observed in man, monkey and in rat, (Perlow et al, 1980) and in diabetic mice (Morley et al, 1982) following injection of CT.

Potent analgesic effects of CT have been reported in man (Fiore et al, 1985), and in animals (Pecile et al, 1975). Intra cerebro-ventricular (ivc) injection of 2 µg of sCT in conscious rabbits has produced an analgesic effect comparable to that resulting from 40 µg of morphine (Pecile et al, 1975). In contrast to the rapidly attenuating actions of morphine, no tachyphylaxis was seen with ivc administration of sCT over several days. Confirming these CNS effects, high affinity specific binding sites for salmon CT have been reported in several regions of the rat brain (Fischer et al, 1981a; Rizzo & Goltzman, 1981), the highest concentration being in the hypothalamus. Inhibitory effects of CT on the secretion of pituitary hormones, including growth hormone (Cantalamessa et al, 1978), thyroid-stimulating hormone (Mitsuma et al, 1984) and luteinizing hormone (Leicht et al, 1974) have been described.

Pathophysiology

CT is a major product of the medullary carcinoma of the thyroid (MTC). Cultures of MTC cells are able to secrete CT (Lichtenberger & Singer, 1975). Furthermore, dense granules and CT-like activity have been shown in MTC (Mayer & Abdel-Bari, 1968). MTC is a malignant neoplasm of the CT secreting C-cells of the thyroid gland (Hazard et al, 1959), and accounts for 6-10% of malignant thyroid tumours (Williams et al, 1966). Although MTC has a relatively undifferentiated appearance, the cells show generally sparse mitoses and the prognosis is better than many other thyroid carcinomas. MTC occurs in both sporadic and familial forms. A tendency is for the disease to be inherited as an autosomal trait. Occurrence of familial forms accounts for 25-50% of all cases reported (Milhaud et al, 1982). It is often associated with other endocrine tumours such as phaeochromocytoma and parathyroid adenoma in the multiple endocrine neoplasia syndrome (Sipple, 1961; Williams, 1965; Steiner et al, 1968). Most MTC produces excessive CT (Melvin & Tashjian, 1969). Very high plasma levels of CT (> 10ng/ml) are pathognomonic of MTC, although other causes of ectopic CT production should be excluded (Liddle et al, 1969; Milhaud et al, 1974; Martin et al, 1981). Nevertheless, i-CT measurements are useful in confirming a clinical diagnosis of MTC and in the early identification of relapses after surgery and determining those members of families affected by familial chromattinomatosis, who may be carrying the gene.

Although it is not always necessary to treat the immediate family members of patients with familial MTC surgically, it is important to know which patients are at risk of developing either MTC or phaeochromocytoma. Such patients can then be monitored regularly. Family history of the disease is an important factor in deciding on the appropriate treatment. A patient with an elevated CT level should be checked for symptoms of phaeochromocytoma: if this tumour is present it must be removed before any other surgery is considered. Patients with MTC may tolerate grossly elevated levels of plasma CT, CGRP and katacalcin (MacIntyre et al, 1982; Hillyard et al, 1983) without exhibiting hypocalcaemia or generalised vasodilation. Possibly, down-regulation of receptor may occur with persistent stimulation by these peptides, in analogy with the *in vitro* 'escape' phenomenon (Raisz et al, 1967; Tashjian et al, 1978) and *in vivo* tachyphylaxis (Obie & Cooper, 1979) observed for CT.

Diagnosis of medullary thyroid carcinoma

Occult MTC or C-cell hyperplasia occurring in asymptomatic members of affected kindreds who have normal basal plasma i-CT levels may be identified by an exaggerated CT response to provocative testing (Melvin et al, 1972; Hennessey et al, 1973, 1974; Jackson et al, 1973; Parthemore et al, 1974; Rude & Singer, 1977; Telenius-Berg et al, 1977). In addition to MTC, a variety of non-thyroidal malignancies have also been known to cause elevated plasma i-CT levels (Silva et al, 1973; Coombes et al, 1974) including breast (Coombes et al, 1975; Hillyard et al, 1976) and lung carcinoma (Ellison et al, 1975; Coombes et al, 1976; Bertagna et al, 1978), and myeloid leukaemic cells (Foa et al, 1982; Oscier et al, 1983).

Measurement of plasma i-CT levels (for hypersecretion) as an index of pre-malignant or malignant C-cell disease is an accepted screening test for the cancer prophylaxis in high risk populations (families of patients with MTC). The originally introduced screening tests measured the hCT response in blood during infusion of cacium, 15 mg/kg body weight over four hours (Melvin et al, 1971). Later the schedule was modified into an infusion of calcium (as chloride) 2-3 mg/kg body weight (Parthemore et al, 1974) and calcium gluconate, 4 mg/kg body weight over 1 - 2 minutes (Rude & Singer, 1977). Glucagon, cholecystokinin and secretin which are CT secretagogues *in vitro* (Telenius-Berg et al, 1977) have largely been discarded due to their unpleasantness and unpredictability (Telenius-Berg et al, 1977). hCT response to oral ethanol has also been used as a screening test (Dymling et al, 1976; Hillyard et al, 1978). Pentagastrin (0.5 mg/kg body weight) administered over 10-15 seconds is a popular screening test as no infusions are involved (Hennessey et al, 1974; Sizemore et al, 1975). Nevertheless, both false postive and false negative results have been reported with all these tests (Hennessey et al, 1974; Telenius-Berg et al, 1977; Rude et al, 1977).

In view of this and the heterogeniety of responses both in normals and in patients with MTC, sequential multiple screening tests have been suggested. Although plasma CGRP is elevated in many patients with MTC, the measurement of plasma i-CGRP by RIA as a screening test for MTC is not as sensitive and specific as i-CT measurements (Girgis et al, 1987). Nevertheless, measurement of receptor-active CGRP by a radioreceptor assay (Wimalawansa, 1989b) can be used successfully in conjunction with i-CT-RIA, during stimulation tests (Wimalawansa & MacIntyre, 1989a, 1989c).

Therapeutic uses of CT

Although CT is a very old hormone in phylogenesis, it is a 'modern' hormone with respect to our knowledge regarding physiological, clinical and therapeutic significance. Indications for CT therapy include Paget's disease of bone, osteoporosis, Sudeck's atrophy, hypercalcaemia and metastatic bone pain. Since CT is a peptide, it is not possible to give orally. However, with research into various delivery systems and chemical modifications of CT molecule, may eventually allow CT to be administered orally or at least by buccal-mucosal route. Presently available CT can be given by intravenous, intramuscular, subcutaneous or by intranasal routes.

Side-effects are greatest with intravenous administration. This route of administration is important in obtaining beneficial central analgesic effects, but intra-thecal administration has been shown to be most effective. Prior administration of an anti-emetic is essential when CT is given intravenously. Side-effects are less with intramuscular and least with intranasal administration and subcutaneous injections. Nausea and

flushing are common but mild, and vomiting is rare. About
30-50% of patients will utter such complaints in the
beginning, but in most cases the severity declines or
disappears upon continued therapy (Ziegler et al, 1976;
Stevenson and Evans, 1981). The prior administration of an
oral anti-emetic is usually helpful to prevent nausea and
vomiting. Other rare side-effects include diarrhoea,
diuresis, and immunological reactions with non-human CT's
(Singer et al, 1972; Dube et al, 1973).

Indications

1. Paget's disease of bone

Calcitonin has been widely used in the treatment of
Paget's disease of bone (Foster et al, 1969; Galante et al,
1973; Woodhouse et al, 1971, 1972; Martin & Woodhouse,
1977; Maier et al, 1977; Singer et al, 1980;   Zanelli et
al, 1985). CT is an ideal treatment for Paget's disease
(which is characterized by very high bone turnover), as it
not only inhibits osteoclast activity, but also prevents
the generation of new osteoclasts. The inhibition of
osteoclastic activity explains the short term (acute)
effects of CT: long term responses are related to the
decrease in the number of osteoclasts. CT is effective in
alleviating pain and improving clinical, biochemical,
radiological and histological features of the disease
(Maier, 1977; Singer et al, 1980; Zanelli et al, 1985).
EHDP (etidronate sodium; ethane-1-hydroxy-1, 1,-
diphosphonate disodium) is an alternative form of therapy
for Paget's disease. However, higher doses (> 15mg kg/body
weight) of EHDP may cause formation of osteoid seams
resembling osteomalacia, and hence is contra-indicated in
osteolytic forms of Paget's disease (Nagant de Deuxchaisnes
et al, 1979). The new generation of diphosphonates does not
seem to have this adverse effect.

The major indication for CT therapy in Paget's disease
is bone pain of Pagetic origin (Evans, 1979). A symptomatic
response rarely starts before two weeks and is usually
apparent only after 6-12 weeks of treatment (Greenberg et
al, 1974). Therapy is usually continued until maximal
symptomatic relief is obtained and for at least a further 6
months. If a patient has radiological evidence of an
osteolytic lesion in a weight-bearing bone (which may
predispose to a fracture), CT should be given (e.g. a dose
of 100 IU daily by subcutaneous injection) until
radiological healing has occurred. This may take 1-2 years.
If relapses occur, repeat courses of CT are indicated and
usually effective. If clinical resistance develops, the
type of CT used should be changed to another immunological
species, preferably human. Alternatively, intravenously
administered newer disphosphonate [e.g. 3-amino-1-
hydroxypropylidene-1,1-biphosphonate (APD), Dimethyl -APD,
clodronate disodium (dichloromethylene diphosphonate,
Cl_2MPD)] can be given successfully. Some improvement of
neurological deficits due to Paget's disease have been
described after CT therapy (Singer et al, 1980). CT is also
useful prior to major orthopaedic surgery of Pagetic bone,
in order to reduce blood flow, facilitating surgery. If a

prosthesis is being set into a Pagetic bone, such treatment should be considered for an indefinite period postoperatively in order to prevent loosening or displacement of the prosthesis (Woodhouse et al, 1971). Furthermore, fracture healing in patients with Paget's disease can also be improved with CT therapy and immobilisation hypercalcaemia in Paget's disease is rapidly corrected with CT.

2.   Osteoporosis

Osteoporosis is a result of imbalance between bone formation and resorption resulting in a net loss of bone (Meunier et al, 1981; Whyte et al, 1982) leading to decrease in bone mass and fractures. Although the ideal treatment for osteoporosis should increase bone mass, an inhibitor of bone resorption (such as CT and diphosphonates) should at least arrest further bone loss. Both Paget's disease and osteoporosis are due to over-activation of osteoclasts. CT has been successfully and widely used in Paget's disease of bone and it is, therefore, logical to use this therapy in both the prevention and treatment of osteoporosis.

In addition to the universal decline in $1,25 (OH)_2D_3$ responsiveness associated with ageing, there seems to be an added abnormality in parathyroid hormone secretory function in osteoporosis (Silverberg et al, 1989). Furthermore, there are CT receptors in parathyroid cells and both the plasma levels of i-CT and the secretory capacity of C-cells has been shown to decrease with age. In addition to $17-\beta-$

oestradiol all three hormones mentioned above may also play a part in postmenopausal osteoporosis.

The positive effects of CT in osteoporosis are now well established (Chesnut et al, 1981; Leggate et al, 1984; MacIntyre et al, 1988). Calcitonin has been shown to be effective in increasing bone mass in osteoporosis (Wallach et al, 1977; Rasmussen et al, 1980; Gruber et al, 1984; Wimalawansa et al, 1987b). It is most likely to be of greatest benefit in types of osteoporosis where increased resorption is a feature, and hence it has been particularly employed in postmenopausal (Chesnut et al, 1981) and steroid-induced osteoporosis. The function of CT as a hormone protecting the skeleton may perhaps be extended to the role of controlling bone ageing. Common dosage used in clinical studies has been 100 IU daily (Wallach et al, 1977; Gruber et al, 1984), but it is likely that lower and less frequent doses may be effective in the prevention of postmenopausal osteoporosis (MacIntyre et al, 1988). The smallest fully active dose of CT should be used, as frequent high doses may impair receptor sensitivity and may lead to a therapeutic escape. Smaller doses, such as 20 IU of human CT thrice weekly, have been shown to be highly effective in preventing postmenopausal bone loss (MacIntyre et al, 1988; Wimalawansa et al, 1987b). Furthermore, the combination of oestrogen and CT may have an additive effect (Wimalawansa et al, 1987b, 1988).

The accepted first line of therapy for postmenopausal osteoporosis is oestrogen replacement therapy (Conference Report, 1987; Wimalawansa, 1988). Plasma 17β-oestradiol levels >60 pg/ml are necessary to maintain the bone mass in postmenopausal women, when oestrogen is administered parenterally (Wimalawansa & MacIntyre, 1988a; MacIntyre & Wimalawansa, 1989). However, CT is a suitable alternative therapy in patients in whom oestrogen is contra-indicated or unacceptable. The availability of a non-injectable form of CT (e.g. intra-nasal preparations) should increase its acceptability. Other second line therapies available for prevention and treatment of osteoporosis include diphosphonate (either on its own or as ADFR regimen), anabolic steroids and sodium fluoride. The concept of stimulating bone turnover (activation) by one means, and inhibiting bone resorption (depression) by another (ADFR regimen) has been tried by many researchers (Rasmussen & Bordier, 1974). Acceptance of this regimen in routine therapy is hindered by its complexity and in some cases its side effects. In many studies, phosphate or PTH was used as an activating agent, and CT or diphosphonates as a depressing agent. In the author's view cyclical therapy with diphosphonates (or perhaps CT) alone (e.g. two weeks therapy in every three months) is likely to be as effective as other, more complicated ADFR regimens.

Rapid bone loss associated with weightlessness is a major medical problem in space travel. This accelerated bone loss may also be arrested with adequate doses of CT given through an appropriate route. Further research is necessary to assess the beneficial effects of CT therapy in space travel.

Immobilization is another condition associated with rapid bone loss. This may be due to the removal of the stimuli provided by physical activity, which may be necessary for normal osteoblast/osteoclast activity. Similar changes in bone to those which were observed during the weightless state have been reported with immobilization.

Increased osteoclastic activity characterised by hypercalcaemia, hypercalciuria and increased excretion of hydroxyproline in urine have been shown within weeks of spinal cord injury resulting in paraplegia (Klein et al, 1966; Chantraine, 1971). This has also been confirmed by quantitative histological methods (Minaire et al, 1974). Longer periods of immobilization carried out on monkeys have shown a substantial loss of trabecular bone with loss of trabecular architecture. More importantly, once re-mobilized, these lost trabecular plates were not replaced and the original bone mass was not recovered. CT seems to be very effective in preventing this rapid bone resorption (Minaire et al, 1986), irrespective of the cause of immobilization. Although most of the bone loss is directly due to immobilization, additional neurological factors have also been suggested (Chantraine et al, 1986). It has been shown that CT could prevent this rapid bone loss (mainly axial trabecular bone) which occurs below the lesion in patients with spinal injury, without substantial inhibition of bone formation. Prevention of bone loss from paraplegic and hemiplegic patients may greatly facilitate their rehabilitation.

In childhood, since the bone turnover is high, rapid loss of trabecular bone can occur during immobilization. CT had been shown to be successful in preventing bone loss distal to fractures of the femoral diaphysis in children (Mallet et al, 1986). Similarly, patients presenting with recent vertebral compression fractures will also benefit by CT therapy. In these patients, in addition to the prevention of further bone loss due to fracture and pain associated immobilization, pain itself may be lessened with daily CT therapy (Levernieux et al, 1986).

3. Hypercalcaemia

Calcitonin produces an acute reduction of plasma calcium in some patients with hypercalcaemia. A fall in plasma calcium of 0.5 to 1.0 mmol per litre may be observed within 24 hours of commencing CT therapy. However, in the absence of additional glucocorticoid therapy, the effect may not be maintained beyond 48 to 72 hours (Mundy & Martin, 1982). Calcitonin is most likely to be effective in cases of hypercalcaemia where a generalised increase in bone resorption is a prominent feature, such as primary hyperparathyroidism and some humoral hypercalcaemia of malignancy. The calciuric effect of CT may also play a role in reducing the raised plasma calcium. Possible sites of actions and the role of CT in tumour associated hypercalcaemia are shown in Figure 11. CT has been successfully used in combination with a new generation of diphosphates (e.g. amino propylidene disphosphonate) for humoral hypercalcaemia of malignancy (Ralston et al, 1986).

4. Metastatic bone pain

Calcitonin has been used for the treatment of bone pain in patients with metastatic malignancy, where an analgesic effect has been observed in three quarters of the patients treated (Fiore et al, 1985). CT has also been used successfully in the treatment of intractable pain from advanced malignancy (Allan, 1983). When injected into the sub-arachnoid space sCT acts as a potent analgesic (Fraioli et al, 1982). It is likely that the main site of action is in the CNS, but the mechanism of its analgesic action is still not understood. The analgesic effects of CT has been postulated to occur through a number of mechanisms. A direct central action (Fabbri et, 1981), and an indirect one through interference with the classical neurotransmitters such as serotonin (Clementi et al, 1984, 1985) and prostaglandin, which is independent of endorphin (Braga et al, 1977, 1978), and a peripheral action mediated via the inhibition of the chemical factors involved in inflammation. Interestingly, bone pain associated with hormone sensitive tumours (e.g. breast, prostate, thyroid) shows a good response together with some lung tumours secreting ectopic hormones.

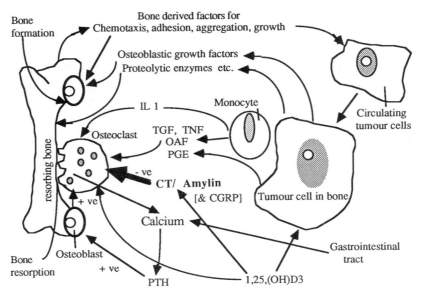

Figure 11. Schematic drawing of possible interactions between various cells, lymphokinines and calcium regulating hormones in bone formation and bone resorption. Calcitonin and amylin are the two most potent peptide hormones capable of directly inhibiting the osteoclast. CGRP at higher concentrations ($>10^3$ molar excess) may have a similar effect.

In addition to the possibility of the effects of CT on β-endophin release, CT may also bind to CGRP receptors in the central nervous system. CGRP distribution in the brain and the dorsal spinal cord (Wimalawansa et al, 1987a) suggests that it may be involved in the processing of pain sensation (Rosenfeld et al, 1983). *In vitro* studies have shown that CT could interact with CGRP binding sites in the kidney (Wohlwend et al, 1985) and in the nervous system (Wimalawansa, 1989b). This suggests that when pharmacological doses of CT are administered it could interact with CGRP receptors in the CNS, which may modulate the sensory neuro-transmission.

SUMMARY

The 32 amino acid polypeptide hormone CT, is a potent inhibitor of the osteoclast. Therapy with CT is particularly effective in controlling osteoclastic bone resorption in disorders characterized by high bone turnover. These disorders include Paget's disease of bone, Osteoporosis, Sudeck's atrophy and hypercalcaemic states.

ACKNOWLEDGEMENTS

The author acknowledges the secretarial assistance of Mrs. Wendy Grant and Mrs. Brenda Salvage, and Professor Timothy Chambers for the pictures of osteoclasts.

REFERENCES

Aer, J., 1968, Effect of thyrocalcitonin on urinary hydroxy-proline and calcium in rats, Endocrinology, 83:379.

Alevizaki, M., Shiraishi, A., Rassool, F.V., Ferrier, G.J.M., MacIntyre, I., and Legon, S., 1986, The calcitonin-like sequence of the β-CGRP gene. FEBS Lett., 206:47-52.

Aliapoulios, M.A., Goldhaber, P., and Munson, P.L., 1966, Thyrocalcitonin inhibition of bone resorption induced by parathyroid hormone in tissue culture, Science, 151:330-332.

Allan, E., 1983, Calcitonin in the treatment of intractable pain from advanced malignancy, Pharmatherapeutica, 3:482-486.

Allison, J., Hall, L., MacIntyre, I., and Craig, R., 1981, The construction and partial characterization of plasmids containing complementary DNA sequences to human calcitonin precursor polyprotein. Biochem J., 199:725-731.

Amara, S.G., David, D.N., Rosenfeld, M.G., Roos, B.A., and Evans, R.M., 1980a, Characterisation of rat calcitonin mRNA, Proc. Natl. Acad. Sci. USA., 77:4444-4448.

Amara, S.G., Arriza, J.L., Leff, S.W., Swanson, L.W., Evans, R.M., and Rosenfeld, M.G., 1985, Expression in brain of a messenger RNA encoding a novel neuropeptide homologous to calcitonin gene-related peptide. Science, 229:1094-1097.

Amara, S.G., Rosenfeld, M.G., Birnbaum, R.S., and Roos, B.A., 1980a, Identification of the putative cell-free translation product of rat calcitonin mRNA. J. Biol Chem, 255:2645-2648.

Baghdiantz, A., Foster, G.V., Edwards, A., Kumar, M.A., Slack, E., Soliman, H.A., and MacIntyre, I., 1964, Extraction and purification of calcitonin, Nature, 203:1027-1028.

Baylin, S.B., Wieman, K.C., O'Neil, J.A., amd Roos, B.A., 1981, Multiple forms of human tumor calcitonin demonstrated by denaturing polyacrylamide gel electrophoresis and lectin affinity chromatography, J. Clin. Endocrinol. Metab., 53:489-497.

Becker, H.D., Reeder, D.D., Scurry, M.T., and Thompson, J.C., 1974, Inhibition of gastrin release and gastric secretion by calcitonin in patients with peptic ulcer, Am. J. Surg., 127:71-75.

Becker, K.L., Snider, R.H., Silva, O.L., and Moore, C.F., 1978, Calcitonin heterogeneity in lung cancer and medullary thyroid cancer, Acta Endocrinol., 89:89-99.

Becker, K.L., Monaghan, K.G., and Silva, O.L., 1980, Immunocytochemical localisation of calcitonin in Kulchitsky cells of human lung, Arch. Pathol. Lab. Med., 104:196-198.

Becker, K.L., Silva, O.G., Post, R.M., Ballenger, J.C., Carmen, J.S., Snider, R.H., and Moore, C.F., 1980, Immunoreactive calcitonin in cerebrospinal fluid of man, Brain Res., 194:598-602.

Bell, N.H., 1974, Evidence for a separate adenylate cyclase system responsive to beta-adrenergic stimulation in the renal cortex of the rat, Acta Endocrinol., 77:604-611.

Bell, N.H., and Kimble, J.B., 1970, Effects of glucagon, dibutyryl cyclic 3',5'-adenosine monophosphate, and theophylline on calcitonin secretion in vitro, J. Clin. Invest., 49:1368-1373.

Bertagna, X.Y., Nicholson, W.E., Pettengill, O.S., Sorenson, G.D., Mount, C.D., and Orth, D.N., 1978, Ectopic production of high molecular weight calcitonin and corticotropin by human small cell carcinoma cells in tissue culture: evidence for separate precursors, J. Clin. Endocrinol. Metab., 47:1390-1393.

Body, J-J, and Heath, H. III., 1983, Estimates ofcirculating monomeric calcitonin: physiological studies in normal and thyroidectomised man, J. Clin. Endocrinol. Metab., 57:897-903.

Braga, P.G., Ferri, S., Olgiati, V.R., and Pecile, A., 1977, Caratterizzazione farmacologica dell'analgesia indotta da Calcitonina. Atti Simp. Int. Appl. Ter. della Calcitonina, Capri, 17-18 maggio, p.185.

Braga, P., Ferri, S., Santagostino, A., Oligiati, V.R., and Pecile, A., 1978, Lack of opiate receptor involvement in centrally induced calcitonin analgesia, Life Sci., 22:971.

Brain, S.D., MacIntyre, I., and Williams, T.J., 1986, A second form of calcitonin gene-related peptide which is a potent vasodilator. Eur. J. Pharmacol., 124:349-352.

Brain, S.D., Williams, T.J., Tippins, J.R., Morris, H.R., and MacIntyre, I., 1985, Cacitonin gene-related peptide (CGRP) is a potent vasodilator. Nature, 313:54-56.

Brewer, H.B., and Ronan, R., 1969, Amino acid sequence of bovine thyrocalcitonin, Proc. Natl. Acad. Sci. USA., 63:940-947.

Bueno, L., Fioramonti, J., and Ferre, J.P., 1983, Calcitonin-CNS action to control the pattern of intestinal motility in rats, Peptides, 4:63-65.

Bussolatti, G., and Pearse, A.G.E., 1967, Immunofluorescent localisation of calcitonin in C-cells of the pig and dog thyroid, J. Endocrinol., 37:205-209.

Cantalamessa, L., Catania, A., Roschini, E., and Peracchi, M., 1978, Inhibitory effect of calcitonin on growth hormone and insulin secretion in man, Metabolism, 27:987-992.

Care, A.D., Bates, R.F.L., Swaminathan, R., Scanes, C.G., Peacock, M., Mawer, E.B., Taylor, C.M., De Luca, H.F., Tomlinson, S., and O'Riordan, J.L.H., 1975, The control of parathyroid hormone and calcitonin secretion and their interaction with other endocrine systems, in: "Calcium Regulating Hormones", Proc. Vth Parathyroid Conference, Oxford, 1974, R.V. von Talmage., M. Owan, and I.A. Parson, eds., Excerpta Med. ICS, 346.

Care, A.D., Ross, R., Pickard, D.W., and Cooper, C.W., 1982, Stimulation of secretion of calcitonin by 1,25 dihydroxycholecalciferol, in: "Vitamin D, Chemical, Biochemical and Clinical Endocrinology of Calcium Metabolism", A.W. Norman, K. Schaefer, Dv. Herrath, and H.G. Grigoleit, eds., New York, Walter de Gruyter, pp.575-577.

Carney, S., and Thompson, L., 1981, Acute effect of calcitonin on rat renal electrolyte transport, Am. J. Physiol., 240:F12.

Catherwood, B.D., and Deftos, L.J., 1984, General
    principles, problems and interpretation in the
    radioimmunoassay of calcitonin, Biomed. Pharmacother.,
    38:235-241.
Chambers, T.J., 1985, The pathobiology of the osteoclast, J.
    Clin. Path., 38:241-245.
Chambers, T.J., and Magnus, C.J., 1982, Calcitonin alters
    behaviour of isolated osteoclasts, J. Pathol., 136:27-
    36.
Chambers, T.J., and Dunn, C.J., 1983, Pharmacological
    control of osteoclastic motility, Calcif. Tiss.
    Internat., 35:566-570.
Chambers, T.J. and Moore, A., 1983, The sensitivity of
    isolated osteoclasts to morphological transformation by
    calcitonin, J. Clin. Endocrinol. Metab., 57:819-824.
Chambers, T.J., Fuller, K., McSheehy, P.M.J., and Pringle,
    J.A.S., 1985a, The effects of calcium regulating
    hormones on bone resorption by isolated human
    osteoclastoma cells, J. Pathol., 145:297-305.
Chambers, T.J., McSheehy, P.M.J., Thompson, B.M., and
    Fuller, K, 1985b, The effect of calcium regulating
    hormones and prostaglandins on bone resorption by
    osteoclasts disaggregated from rabbit long bones,
    Endocrinol., 116:234-239.
Chambers, T.J., Chambers, J.C., Symonds, J., and Darby,
    J.A., 1986, The effect of human calcitonin on the
    cytoplasmic spreading of rat osteoclasts, J. Clin.
    Endocrinol. Metab., 63:1080-1085.
Chantraine, A., 1971, Clinical investigation of bone
    metabolism in spinal cord lesions, Paraplegia, 8:253-
    259.
Chantraine, A., Nusgens, B., and Lapiere, C.M., 1986, Bone
    remodeling during the development of osteoporosis in
    paraplegia, Calcif. Tissue Int., 38:323-327.
Chausmer, A., Stevens, M.D., and Severn, C., 1982,
    Autoradiographic evidence for a calcitonin receptor on
    testicular Leidig cells, Science, 216:735-736.
Chesnut, C.H. III., Baylink, D.J., Roos, B.A., Gruber, H.E.,
    Ivey, J.L., Matthews, M., Nelp, W.B. and Sisom, K.,
    1981, Calcitonin and postmenopausal osteoporosis, in:
    "Calcitonin 1980", A. Pecile, Excerpta Medica,
    Amsterdam, pp.247-255.
Clementi, G., Prato, A., Confroto, G., and Scapagnini, U.,
    1984, Role of serotonin in the analgesic activity of
    calcitonin, Eur. J. Pharmacol., 98:449-452.
Clementi, G., Amico Roxas, M. de., Rapisarda, E., Caruso,
    A., Prato, A., Thormbadore, S., Priolo, G., and
    Scapagnini, U., 1985, The analgesic activity of
    calcitonin and the central serotonergic system, Eur. J.
    Pharmacol., 108:71-73.
Conference Report. 1987, Prophylaxis and treatment of
    osteoporosis. Consensus Development Conference:
    Aalborg, Denmark, Br. Med. J., 295:914-915.
Coombes, R.C., Hillyard, C.J., Greenberg, P.B., and
    MacIntyre, I., 1974, Plasma immunoreactive calcitonin
    in patients with non-thyroid tumours, Lancet, i:1080-
    1083.
Coombes, R.C., Easty, G.C., Detre, S.I., Hillyard, C.J.,
    Stevens, U., Girgis, S.I., Galante, L.S., Heywood, L.,

MacIntyre, I., and Neville, A.M., 1975, Secretion of immunoreactive calcitonin by human breast carcinomas, Br. Med. J., 4:197-199.

Coombes, R.C., Ellison, M.L., Easty, G.C., Hillyard, C.J., James, R., Galante, L., Girgis, S., Heywood, L., MacIntyre, I., and Neville, A.M., 1976, The ectopic secretion of calcitonin by lung and breast carcinomas, Clin. Endocrinol., 5, Suppl:387s-396s.

Cooper, C.W., Hirsch, P.F., Toverud, S.V., and Munson, P.L., 1967, An improved method for the biological assay of calcitonin, Endocrinol., 81:610-612.

Cooper, C.W., Schlesinger, W.H., and Mahgoub, A.M., 1972, Calcium, Parathyroid Hormone and the Calcitonins, Excerpta Medica, Amsterdam, p.128.

Cooper, G.J.S., Willis, A.C., Clark, A., Turner, R.C., Sim, R.B., and Reid, K.B.M., 1987, Purification and characterization of a peptide from amyloid-rich pancreases of type 2 diabetic patients, Proc. Natl. Acad. Sci. USA., 84:8628-8632.

Copp, D.H., Cameron, E.C., Cheney, B.A., Davidson, R.G.F., and Henze, K.G., 1962, Evidence for calcitonin - a new hormone from the parathyroid that lowers blood calcium, Endocrinology, 70:638-649.

Copp, D.H., and Henze, K.G., 1964, Parathyroid origin of calcitonin - evidence from perfusion of sheep glands, Endocrinology, 75:49-51.

Copp, D.H., Cockcroft, D.W., and Kueh, Y., 1967, Calcitonin from the ultimobranchial glands of dogfish and chickens, Science, 158:924-925.

Craig, R.K., Hall, L., Edbrooke, M.R., Allison, J., and MacIntyre, I., 1982, Partial nucleotide sequence of human calcitonin precursor mRNA identifies flanking cryptic peptides, Nature, 295:345-347.

Culter, G.B. Jr., Habener, J.F., and Potts, J.T. Jr., 1977, Biosynthesis and secretion of calcitonin by avian ultimobranchial glands, Endocrinology, 100:537-540.

Deftos, L.J., Roos, B.A., Bronzert, B., Parthemore, J.G., 1975, Immunochemical heterogeneity of calcitonin in plasma, J. Clin. Endocrinol. Metab., 40:407-412.

Deftos, L.J., Burton, D., Catherwood, B.D., Bone, H.G., Parthemore, J.G., Guillemin, R., Watkins, W.B., and Moore, R.Y., 1978a, Demonstration by immunoperoxidase histochemistry of calcitonin in the anterior lobe of the rat pituitary, J. Clin. Endocrinol. Metab., 47:457-460.

Deftos, L.J., Burton, D., Bone, H.G., CXatherwood, R.B., Parthemore, J.,G., Moore, R.Y., Minic, S., and Guillemin, R., 1978b, Immunoreactive calcitonin in the intermediate lobe of the pituitary gland, Life Sci., 23:743-748.

Deftos, L.H., Weisman, M.H., Williams, G.W., Karpf, D.B., Frumar, A.M., Davidson, B.J., Parthemore, J.G., and Judd, H.L., 1980, Influence of sex and age on plasma calcitonin in human beings, N. Engl. J. Med., 302:1351-1353.

De Luise, M., Martin, T.J., Greenberg, P.B., and Michaelangeli, V., 1972, Metabolism of porcine, human and salmon calcitonin in the rat, J. Endocrinol., 53:475-482.

Desplan, C., Benicourt, C., Julienne, A., Segond, N., Calmettes, C., Moukhar, M.S., and Milhaud, G., 1980, Cell-free translation of mRNA coding for human and murine calcitonin, FEBS Lett., 117:89-92.

D'Souza, S.M., MacIntyre, I., Girgis, S.I., and Mundy, G.R., 1986, Human synthetic calcitonin gene-related peptide inhibits bone resorption in vitro, Endocrinology, 119: 58-61.

Dubé, W.J., Goldsmith, R.S., Arnaud, S.B., and Arnaud, C.D., 1973, Development of antibodies to porcine calcitonin during treatment of Paget's disease of bone, Mayo Clin. Proc., 48: 43-48.

Dymling, J.F., Ljungberg, O., Hillyard, C.J., Greenberg, P.B., Evans, I.M.A., and MacIntyre, I., 1976, Whisky: a new provocative test for calcitonin secretion, Acta Endocrinol., 82:500-509.

Ellison, M., Woodhouse, D., Hillyard, C., Dowsett, M., Coombes, R.C., Gilbey, E.D., Greenberg, P.B., and Neville, A.M., 1975, Immunoreactive calcitonin production by human lung carcinoma cells in culture, Br. J. Cancer, 32:373-379.

Evans, I.M.A., 1979, Human calcitonin in the treatment of Paget's disease: long-term trials, in: "Human Calcitonin and Paget's Disease", I. MacIntyre, ed., Hans Huber, Bern, pp.111-121.

Fabbri, A., Santoro, G., Moretti, C., Cappa, M., Fraioli, F., Di Julio, C.G., Galluzzi, T., and Lamanna, V., 1981, The analgesic effect of calcitonin in humans: studies on the role of opioid peptides, Int. J. Clin. Pharm. Ther. Tossic., 19:509.

Fahrenkrieg, J., Hornum, I., Rehfeld, J.F., 1975, Effect of calcitonin on serum gastrin concentration and component pattern in man, J. Clin. Endocrinol. Metab., 41:149-152.

Findlay, D.M., deLuise, M., Michaelangeli, V.P., Ellison, M., and Martin, T.J., 1980a, Properties of a calcitonin receptor and adenylate cyclase in BEN cells, a human cancer cell line, Cancer Res., 40:1311-1315.

Findlay, D.M., Michaelangeli, V.P., Eisman, J.A., Frampton, R.J., Moseley, J.M., MacIntyre, I., Whitehead, R., and Martin, T.J., 1980b, Calcitonin and 1,25-dihydroxyvitamin D_3 receptors in human breast cancer cell lines, Cancer Res., 40:4762-4767.

Findlay, D.M., deLuise, M., Michaelangeli, V.P., and Martin, T.J., 1981, Independent down regulation of insulin and calcitonin receptors in human tumour cell line, J. Endocrinol., 88:271.

Findlay, D.M. Michaelangeli, V.P., Orlowski, R.C., and Martin, T.J., 1984, Biological activities and receptor interactions of des-Leu-16-salmon and des-phe-16-human calcitonin, Endocrinol., 112:1288-1291.

Fiore, C.E., Castorina, F., Malatino, L.S., and Petralito, A., 1985, Calcitonin and cancer pain: comparison of effects of different calcitonins and routes of administration, in: "Calcitonin 1984. Chemistry, Physiology, Pharmacology and Clinical Aspects", A. Pecile, ed.

Fischer, J.A., Sagar, S.M., and Martin, J.B., 1981a, Characterisation and regional distribution of calcitonin binding sites in the rat brain, Life Sci., 29:663-666.

Fischer, J.A., Tobler, P.H., Kauffmann, M., Born, W., Henke, H., Cooper, P.E., Sagar, S., and Martin, J.B., 1981b, Calcitonin: regional distribution of the hormone and its binding sites in the human brain and pituitary, Proc. Natl. Acad. Sci. USA., 78:7801-7805.

Fischer, J.A., Tobler, P.H., Henke, H., and Tschopp, F.A., 1983, Salmon and human calcitonin-like peptides coexist in the human thyroid and brain, J. Clin. Endocrinol. Metab., 57: 1314-1316.

Flynn, J.J., Margules, D.L., and Cooper, C.W., 1981, Presence of immunoreactive calcitonin in the hypothalamus and the pituitary lobes of rat, Brain Res. Bull., 6:547-549.

Foa, R., Oscier, D.G., Hillyard, C.J., Incarbone, E., MacIntyre, I., and Goldman, J.M., 1982, Production of immunoreactive calcitonin by myeloid leukaemic cells, Br. J. Haematol., 50:215-223.

Foster, G.V., Baghdiantz, A., Kumar, M.A., Slack, E., Soliman, H.A., and MacIntyre, I., 1964a, Thyroid origin of calcitonin, Nature, 202:1303-1305.

Foster, G.V., MacIntyre, I., and Pearse, A.G.E., 1964b, Calcitonin production and the mitochondrion-rich cells of the dog thyroid, Nature, 203:1029-1030.

Foster, G.V., Doyle, F.H., Bordier, P., and Matrajt, H., 1969, In vivo effect of hypocalcitonin on bone. in: Les Tissus Calcifies, ve Symposium Europeen. Paris, Societe d'Edition d'Enseignement Superieur, 173-177.

Foster, G.V., Joplin, G.F., MacIntyre, I., Melvin, K.E.W., and Slack, E., 1969, Effect of thyrocalcitonin in man, Lancet, i:107-109.

Fouchereau-Peron, M., Moukhtar, M.S., Benson, A.,A., and Milhaud, G., 1981a, Demonstration of specific receptors for calcitonin in isolated trout gill cells, Comp. Biochem. Physiol., 68a:417.

Fouchereau-Peron, M., Moukhtar, M.S., Benson, A.A., and Milhaud, G., 1981b, Characterisation for specific receptors for calcitonin in porcine lung, Proc. Natl. Acad. Sci. USA., 78:3973-3975.

Fraioli, F., Fabbri, A., Gnessi, L., Moretti, C., Santore, C., and Feleci, M., 1982, Subarachnoid injection of salmon calcitonin induces analgesia in man, Eur. J. Pharmacol., 78:381-383.

Freake, H.C., and MacIntyre, I., 1982, Specific binding of 1,25 dihydroxycholecalciferol in human medullary thyroid carcinoma, Biochem. J., 206:181-182.

Freed, W.J., Perlow, M.J., and Wyatt, R.J., 1979, Calcitonin: inhibitory effect of eating in rats, Science, 206:850-852.

Friedman, J., and Raisz, L.G., 1965, Thyrocalcitonin: inhibitor of bone resorption in tissue culture, Science, 150:1465-1467.

Fritsch, H.A.R., Van Noorden, S., and Pearse, A.G.E., 1979, Localisation of somatostatin, substance P and calcitonin-like immunoreactivity in neural ganglia of Ciona intestinalis, Cell Tiss. Res., 202:263-274.

Fritsch, H.A.R., Van Noorden, S., and Pearse, A.G.E., 1980, Calcitonin-like immunochemical staining in the alimentary tract of Ciona intestinalis, Cell Tiss. Res., 205:439-444.

Fritsch, H.A.R., Van Noorden, S., Pearse, A.G.E., 1982, Gastrointestinal and neurohormonal peptides in the alimentary tract and cerebral complex of Ciona intestinalis (Ascidiaceae), Cell Tiss. Res., 223:369.

Gaines Das, R.E., and Zanelli, J.M., 1980, International Reference Preparation of calcitonin, human, for bioassay: assessment of material and definition of the International Unit, Acta Endocrinol., 93:37-42.

Galan Galan, F., Rogers, R.M., Girgis, S.I., and MacIntyre, I., 1981, Immunoreactive calcitonin in the central nervous system of the pigeon, Brain Res., 212:59-63.

Galante, L.S., Colston, K.W., MacAuley, S.J., and MacIntyre, I., 1972, Effect of calcitonin on vitamin D metabolism, Nature, 288:271-273.

Galante, L., Horton, R., Joplin, G.F., Woodhouse, N.J.Y., and MacIntyre, I., 1971, Comparison of human, porcine and salmon synthetic calcitonins in man and in the rat, Clin. Sci., 40:9P.

Girgis, S.I., Galan Galan, F., Arnett, T.R., Rogers, R.M., Bone, Q., Ravazzola, M., and MacIntyre, I., 1980, Immunoreactive human calcitonin-like molecule in the nervous systems of protochordates and a cyclostome, Myxine, J. Endocrinol., 87:375-382.

Girgis, S.I., Macdonald, D.W.R., Stevenson, J.C., Bevis, P.J.R., Lynch, C., Wimalawansa, S.J., Self, C.H., Morris, H.R., and MacIntyre, I., 1985, Calcitonin gene-related peptide: potent vasodilator and major product of the calcitonin gene, Lancet, ii:14-16.

Girgis, S.I., Lynch, C., Hillyard, C.J., Stevenson, J.C., Hill, P.A., Macdonald, D.W.R., and MacIntyre, I., 1987, Calcitonin gene-related peptide: the diagnostic value of measurements in medullary thyroid carcinoma, Henry Ford Hosp. Med. J., 35:118-119.

Goltzman, D., and Tischler, A.S., 1978, Characterization of the immunochemical forms of calcitonin released by a medullary thyroid carcinoma in tissue culture, J. Clin. Invest., 61:449-458.

Goodman, R.H., Jacobs, J.W., and Habener, J.F., 1979, Cell-free translation of mRNA coding for a precursor of human calcitonin, Biochem Biophys Res Comm., 91:932-938.

Gray, T.K., and Munson, P.L., 1969, Thyrocalcitonin: evidence for physiological function, Science, 166:512-513.

Gray, T.K., Bieberdorf, F.A., and Fordtran, J.S., 1973, Thyrocalcitonin and the jejunal absorption of calcium, water and electrolytes in normal subjects, J. Clin. Invest., 52:3084-3088.

Greenberg, P.B., Doyle, F.H., Fisher, M.T., Hillyard, C.J., Joplin, G.F., Pennock, J., and MacIntyre, I., 1974, Treatment of Paget's disease of bone with synthetic human calcitonin, Am. J. Med., 56:867-870.

Gruber, H.E., Ivey, J.L., and Baylink, D.J., 1984, Long-term calcitonin therapy in postmenopausal osteoporosis, Metabolism, 33:295-303.

Habener, J.F., Singer, F.R., Deftos, L.J., Neer, R.M., and Potts, J.T. Jr., 1971, Explanation for the unusual potency of salmon calcitonin, Nature New Biol., 232:91-92

Hazard, J.B., Hawk, W.A., Crile, G., 1959, Medullary (solid) carcinoma of the thyroid. A clinicopathological entity, J. Clin. Endocrinol. Metab., 19:152-161.

Heath, H. III., and Sizemore, G.W., 1979, Immunochemical heterogeneity of calcitonin in tumour, tumour venous effluent and peripheral blood of patients with medullary thyroid carcinoma, J. Lab. Clin. Med., 93:390-394.

Heath, H. III., and Sizemore, G.W., 1983, Radioimmunoassay for calcitonin, in: "Assay of Calcium Regulating Hormones", D.D. Bilke, eds., Springer Verlag, Berlin, pp.229-244.

Heath, H. III., Body, J.J., and Fox, J., 1984, Radioimmunoassay of calcitonin in normal human plasma: problems, perspectives and prospects, Biomed. Pharmacother., 38:241-246.

Heath, H. III., and Sizemore, G.W., 1977, Plasma calcitonin in normal man. Difference between men and women, J. Clin. Invest., 60:1135-1140.

Heersche, J.N.M., Marcus, R., and Aurbach, G.D., 1974, Calcitonin and the formation of 3',5'-AMP in bone and kidney, Endocrinology, 94:241-247.

Hennessy, J.F., Gray, T.K., Cooper, C.W., and Ontjes, D.A., 1973, Stimulation of thyrocalcitonin secretion by pentagastrin and calcium in 2 patients with medullary carcinoma of the thyroid, J. Clin. Endocrinol. Metab., 36:200-203.

Hennessy, J.F., Wells, S.A. Jr., Ontjes, D.A., and Cooper, C.W., 1974, A comparison of pentagastrin injection and calcium infusion as provocative agents for detection of medullary thyroid carcinoma, J. Clin. Endocrinol. Metab., 39:487-495.

Hillyard, C.J., Coombes, R.C., Greenberg, P.B., Galante, L.S., and MacIntyre, I., 1976, Calcitonin in breast and lung cancer, Clin. Endocrinol., 5:1-8.

Hillyard, C.J., Cooke, T.J.C., Coombes, R.C., Evans, I.M.A., and MacIntyre, I., 1977, Normal plasma calcitonin: circadian variation and response to stimuli, Clin. Endocrinol., 6:291-298.

Hillyard, C.J., Stevenson, J.C., and MacIntyre, I., 1978, Relative deficiency of plasma calcitonin in normal women, Lancet, i:961-962.

Hillyard, C.J., Myers, C.M., Abeyasekera, G., Stevenson, J.C., Craig, R.K., and MacIntyre, 1983, Katacalcin: a new plasma calcium lowering hormone, Lancet, i:846-848.

Hoppener, J.W.M., Steenbergh, P.H., Bakker, E., Pearson, P.L., Geurts van Kessel, A.H.M., Jansz, H.S., and Lips, C.J.M., 1984, Localization of the polymorphic human calcitonin gene on chromosome 11, Hum. Genet., 66:309-312.

Hoppener, J.W.M., Steenbergh, P.H. Zandberg, J., Geurts Van Kessel, A.H.M., Baylin, S.B., Nelkin, B.D., Jansz, H.S., and Lips, C.J.M., 1985, The second human calcitonin/CGRP gene is located on chromosome 11, Hum. Genet., 70:259-263.

Horiuchi, N., Takahashi, M., Matsumoto, T., Takahashi, N., Simazawa, E., Suda, T., and Ogata, E., 1979, Salmon calcitonin-induced stimulation of 1,25 dihydroxyvitamin D_3 in rats involving a mechanism independent of adenosine 3'-5'-cyclic monophosphate, Biochem. J., 184:269-271.

Jacobs, J.W., Goltzman, D., and Habener, J.F., 1982, Absence of detectable calcitonin synthesis in the pituitary using cloned complementary deoxyribonucleic acid probes, Endocrinology, 111:2014-2019.

Jacobs, J.W., Lund, P.K., Potts, J.T. Jr., Bell, N.H., and

Habener, J.F., 1981a, Procalcitonin is a glycoprotein, J. Biol. Chem., 256:2803-2807.

Jacobs, J.W., Potts, J.T. Jr., Bell, N.H., and Habener, J.F., 1979, Calcitonin precursor identified by cell-free translation of mRNA, J. Biol. Chem., 254:10600-10603.

Jaeger, P., Jones, W., Clemens, T.L., and Hayslett, J.P., 1986 Evidence that calcitonin stimulates 1,25-dihydroxy-vitamin D production and intestinal absorption of calcium, in vivo J. Clin. Invest., 78:456.

Kallio, D.M., Garant, P.R., and Minkin, C., 1972, Ultrastructural effects of calcitonin on osteoclasts in tissue culture, J. Ultrastruct. Res., 39:205-216.

Kawashima, H., Torikai, S., and Kurokawa, K., 1981, Selective stimulation of 25-hydroxyvitamin D^3-1 -hydroxylase by calcitonin in the proximal straight tubule of the rat kidney, Nature, 291:327-329.

Kenny, A.D., 1971, Determination of calcitonin in plasma by bioassay, Endocrinology, 89:1005-1009.

Klein, L., van de Noort, S., and Dejak, J.J., 1966, Sequential studies of urinary hydroxyproline and serum alkaline phosphatase in acute paraplegia, Med. Serv. J. Can., 22:524-533.

Kittur, S.D., Hoppener, J.W.M., Antonaratis, S.E., Daniels, J.D.J., Mayers, D.A., Maestri, N.E., Jansen, M., Kormeulk R.G., Neltin, B.D., and Kazazian, H.H., 1985, Linkage map, of the short arm of human chromosome 11: location of the genes for catalase and insulin-like gorwth factor II., Proc. Natl. Acad. Sci., 82:5064-5066.

Le Douarin, N., and Le Leivre, C., 1970, Demonstration de l'origine neurale des cellules a calcitonine du corps ultimobranchial chez l'embryon de poulet, C. R. Acad. Sci., 270:2857-2859.

Leggate, J., Farish, E., Fletcher, C.D., McIntosh, W., Hart, D.M., and Sommerville, J.M., 1984, Calcitonin and post-menopausal osteoporosis, Clin. Endocrinol., 20:85-92.

Levernieux, J., Julien, D., and Caulin, F., 1986, The effect of calcitonin on bone pain and acute resorption related to recent osteoporotic crush-fractures - result of a double blind and an open study, in: "Calciotropic Hormones and Calcium Metabolism", M. Cecchettin, and G. Segre, eds., Elsevier, Amsterdam, pp.171-178.

Levine, A.S., Hughes, J.J., Morley, J.E., Gosnell, B.A., and Silvis, S.E., 1984, Calcitonin as a regulator of gastric acid secretion, Psychopharmacol. Bull., 20:459-462.

Lichtenberger, L.M., and Singer, F.R., 1975, Release of calcitonin by cultures of medullary carcinoma of the thyroid, Endocr. Res. Comm., 2:527-536.

Liddle, G.W., Nicholson, W.E., Island, D.P., Orth, D.N., Abe, K., and Lowder, S.C., 1969, Clinical and laboratory studies of ectopic humoral syndromes, Recent Progr. Horm. Res., 25:283-314.

Lips, C.G.M., Van der Sluys Veer, J., Van der Donk, J.A., Van Dam, R.H., and Hackeng, W.H.L., 1978, Common precursor molecule as origin for the ectopic-hormone producing tumour syndrome, Lancet, i:16-18.

MacIntyre, I., 1972, Calcitonin, in: "Proc. Internat. Symp. Metab. Water Electrolytes,", Siena, pp.311-318.

MacIntyre, I., and Stevenson, J.C., 1980a, Chemistry, physiology and therapeutic applications of calcitonin, Arth. Rheum., 23:1139-1147.

MacIntyre, I., and Stevenson, J., 1980b, Calcitonin: a modern
    view of its physiological role and interrelation with
    other hormones, in: "Calcitonin 1980: Chemistry,
    Physiology, Pharmacology and Clinical Aspects", A.
    Pecile, ed., Excerpta Medica, Amsterdam, pp.1-10.
MacIntyre, I., Parsons, J.A., and Robinson, C.J., 1967, The
    effect of thyrocalcitonin on blood-bone calcium
    equilibrium in the perfused tibia of the cat, J.
    Physiol., 191:393-405.
MacIntyre, I., Galante, L.S., and Hillyard, C.J., 1980, Radio-
    immunoassay and bioassay of calcitonin, in: "Handbuch de
    Inneren Medizin Vol 6/Ia, F. Kuhlencordt, and H.
    Bartelheimer, eds., Springer Verlag, Berlin, pp.623-634.
MacIntyre, I., Hillyard, C.J., Murphy, P.K., Reynolds, J.J.,
    Gaines Das, R.E., and Craig, R.K., 1982, A second plasma
    calcium lowering peptide from the human calcitonin
    precursor, Nature, 300:460-462.
MacIntyre, I., Girgis, S.I., and Hillyard, C.J., 1984,
    Essential steps in measurement of normal circulating
    levels of calcitonin, Biomed. Pharmacother., 38:230-234.
MacIntyre, I., Stevenson, J.C., Whitehead, M.I., Wimalawansa,
    S.J., Banks, L.M., and Healy, M.J.R., 1988, Calcitonin
    for prevention of postmenopausal bone loss, Lancet,
    i:900-902.
MacIntyre, I., and Wimalawansa, S.J., 1989, Positive
    relationship of plasma 17 -oestradiol with prevention of
    post-menopausal bone loss, ASBMR/ICCRA First Joint
    Meeting, Quebec, Canada, (Abstr).
Maier, R., 1977, Pharmacology of human calcitonin, in:
    "Human Calcitonin and Paget's Disease", I. MacIntyre,
    ed., Hans Huber, Bern, pp.66-77.
Maier, R., Riniker, B., and Rittel, W., 1974, Analogues of
    human calcitonin. I. Influence of modifications of
    aminoacid positions 29 and 31 on hypocalcaemic
    activities in the rat, FEBS Letts., 48:68-71.
Mallet, E., Lefort, J., and Caulin, F., 1986, Prevention of
    trabecular bone loss in children's femoral fracture:
    effects of treatment with calcitonin, Clin. Sci, 70
    (suppl. 13):82P.
Martin, T.J., Woodhouse, N.J.Y., 1977, Calcitonin in the
    treatment of Paget's disease, in: "Bone Disease and
    Calcitonin", J. Kanis, ed., Armour Pharmaceuticals
    Ltd., Eastbourne, pp.11-24.
Martin, T.J., Findlay, D.M., MacIntyre, I., Eisman, J.A.,
    Michaelangeli, V.P., Moseley, J.M., and Partridge,
    M.C., 1980, Calcitonin receptors in a cloned human
    breast cancer cel line (MCF7), Biochem. Biophys. Res.
    Commun., 96:150-154.
Martin, T.J., Moseley, J.M., Findlay, D.M., and
    Michaelangeli, V.P., 1981, Calcitonin production and
    calcitonin receptors in human cancers, in: "Hormones in
    Normal and Abnormal Human Tissues", New York, Walter de
    Gruyter, pp.429-457.
Marx, S.J., Woodward, C.J., and Aurbach, G.D., 1972,
    Calcitonin receptors of the kidney and bone, Science,
    178:998-1001.
Marx, S.J., Woodward, C.J., Aurbach, G.D., Glassman, H., and
    Keutmann, H.J., 1973, Renal receptors for calcitonin,
    Binding and degradation of hormone, J. Biol. Chem.,
    248:4797-4802.

Marx, S.J., Aurbach, G.D., Gavin, J.R., and Buell, J.W., 1974, Calcitonin receptors on cultured human lymphocytes, J. Biol. Chem., 249:6812.

Maxam, A.M., and Gilbert, W., 1977, A new method for sequencing DNA, Proc. Natl. Acad. Sci. USA., 74:560:564.

McCredie, D.A., Dixon, S.R., Martin, T.J., Melick, R.A., Rotenberg, E., and Shipman, R., 1971, The effects of calcitonin in children in health and disease, in: "Proc. XIII Internat. Congr. Paediatrics, Verlag der Weiner Medizinischen Akademie, Vienna, p.155-161.

Melvin, K.E.W., and Tashjian, A.H. Jr., 1969, The syndrome of excessive thyrocalcitonin produced by medullary carcinoma of the thyroid, Proc. Natl. Acad. Sci. USA, 59:1216-1222.

Melvin, K.E.W., Tashjian, A.H., and Miller, H.H., 1972, Studies in familial (medullary) thyroid carcinoma, Recent Prog. Horm. Res., 28:399-470.

Meunier, P.J., Sellami, S., Brancon, D., and Edouard, C., 1981, Histological heterogeneity of apparently idiopathic osteoporosis, in: "Osteoporosis. Recent Advances in Pathogenesis and Treatment", H.F. DeLuca, H.M. Frost, W.S.S. Jee, et al, eds., University Park Press, Baltimore, pp.293-301.

Meyer, J.S., and Abdel-Bari, W., 1968, Granules and thyrocalcitonin-like activity in medullary carcinoma of the thyroid gland, New Engl. J. Med., 278:523-529.

Milhaud, G., Calmette, C., Taboulet, J., Julienne, A., and Moukhtar, M.S., 1974, Hypersecretion of calcitonin inneoplastic conditions, Lancet, i:462-463.

Milhaud, G., Benezech-Lefevre, M., and Moukhtar, M.S., 1978, Deficiency of calcitonin in age related osteoporosis, Biomedicine, 28:272-276.

Milhaud, G., 1982, Immunoassay of human calcitonin, in: Proc. Internat. Workshop on Human Calcitonin, A. Caniggia, ed., pp.29-47.

Minaire, P., Meunier, P., and Edouard, C., 1974, Quantitative histological data on disuse osteoporosis, Calcif. Tissue Res., 17:57-73.

Minaire, P., Meunier, P., and Depassio, J., 1986, Treatment of active osteoporosis with calcitonin, in: "Osteoporosis", C. Christiansen, C.D. Arnaud, B.E.C. Nordin, et al, eds., Glostrup Hospital, Copenhagen, pp.613-615.

Mitsuma, T., Nogimori, T., and Chaya, M., 1984, Peripheral administration of eel calcitonin inhibits thyrotropin secretion in rats, Eur. J. Pharmacol., 102:123-126.

Morley, J.E., Levine, A.S., Brown, D.M., and Hand, B.S., 1982, The effect of calcitonin on food intake in diabetic mice, Peptides, 3:17-20.

Morikawa, T., Munekata, E., Sakakibara, S., Noda, T., and Otani, M., 1976, Synthesis of eel-calcitonin and Asu^{1,7}-eel-calcitonin: contribution of the disulphide bond to the hormonal activity, Experientia, 32:1104-1106.

Morimoto, S., Tsuji, M., Okada, Y., Onishi, T., and Kumahara, Y., 1980, The effect of oestrogens on human calcitonin secretion after calcium infusion in elderly female subjects, Clin. Endocrinol.,13:135-143.

Morris, H.R., Panico, M., Etienne, T, Tippins, J., Girgis, S.I., and MacIntyre, I., 1984, Isolation and characterization of human calcitonin gene-related peptide, Nature, 308:746-748.

Moseley, J.M., Findlay, D.M., Gorman, J.J., Michaelangeli, V.P., and Martin, T.J., 1983, The calcitonin receptor on T47D breast cancer cells. Evidence for glycosylation, Biochem J., 212:609-611.

Mundy, G.R., and Martin, T.J., 1982, The hypercalcaemia of malignancy: pathogenesis and management, Metabolism, 31:1247-1277.

Nagant de Deuxchaisnes, C., Rombouts-Lindemans, C., Huaux, J.P., Devogelaer, J.P., Malghem, J., and Maldague, B., 1979, Roentgenologic evaluation of the action of the diphosphonate EHDP and of combined therapy (EHDP and calcitonin) in Paget's disease of bone, in: "Molecular Endocrinology", I. MacIntyre and M. Szelke, eds., Elsevier/North Holland, Amsterdam, pp.405-433.

Neher, R., Riniker, B., Maier, R., Byfield, P.G.H., Gudmundsson, T.V., and MacIntyre, I., 1986, Human calcitonin, Nature, 220:984-986.

Niall, H.D., Keutmann, H.T., Copp, D.H., and Potts, J.T. Jr., 1969, The amino acid sequence of salmon ultimobranchial calcitonin, Proc. Natl. Acad. Sci. USA., 64:771-778.

Nicholson, G.C., Moseley, J.M., Sexton, P.M., Mendelsohn, F.A.O., and Martin, T.J., 1986, Abundant calcitonin receptors in isolated rat osteoclasts. Biochemical and autoradiographic characterisation, J. Clin. Invest., 78:355-360.

Nicoletti, F., Clementi, G., Patti, F., Canonico, P.L., diGiorgio, R.M., Matera, M., Pennsei, G., Angelussi, L., and Sapagnini, U., 1982, Effects of calcitonin on rat extrapyramidal motor system: behavioural and biochemical data, Brain Res., 250:381.

Noda, T., and Narita, K., 1976, Amino acid sequence of eel calcitonin, J. Biochem. (Tokyo), 79:353;359.

Obie, J.F., and Cooper, C.W., 1979, Loss of calcemic effects of calcitonin and parathyroid hormone infused continuously into rats using the Alzet osmotic minipump, J. Pharmacol. Exp. Ther., 209:422-428.

O'Dor, R.K., Parkes, C.D., and Copp, D.H., 1969, The amino acid composition of salmon calcitonin, Canad. J. Biol., 47:873-875.

Oscier, D.G., Hillyard, C.J., Arnett, T.R., MacIntyre, I., and Goldman, J.M., 1983, Immunoreactive calcitonin production by a human promyelocytic cell line HL60, Blood, 61:61-65.

Otani, M., Yamauchi, H., Meguro, T., Kitazawa, S., Watanabe, S., and Orimo, H., 1976, Isolation and characterisation of calcitonin from pericardium and esophagus of eel, J. Biochem. (Tokyo), 79:345-352.

Otani, M., Kitazawa, S., Yamaguchi, H., Meguro, T., and Orimo, H., 1978, Stability and biological activity of eel calcitonin in rats, Horm. Met. Res., 10::252-256.

Parthemore, J.C., Bronzert, D., Roberts, G. and Deftos, L.J., 1974, A short calcium infusion in the diagnosis of medullary thyroid carcinoma, J. Clin. Endocrinol. Metab., 39:101-111.

Parthemore, J.G., and Deftos, L.J., 1978, Calcitonin secretion in normal human subjects, J. Clin. Endocrinol. Metab., 47:184-188.

Pearse, A.G.E., 1966, The cytochemistry of the thyroid C-cells and their relationship to calcitonin, Proc. Roy. Soc. Lond., 164:478-487.

Pearse, A.G.E., and Carvalheira, A.F., 1967, Cytochemical evidence for an ultimobranchial origin of rodent thyroid C-cells, Nature, 214:929-930.

Pearse, A.G.E., and Polak, J.M., 1971, Cytochemical evidence for the neural crest origin of mammalian ultimobranchial C-cells, Histochemie, 27:96-102.

Pecile, A., Ferri, S., Braga, P.C., and Olgiati, V.R., 1975, Effects of intracerebroventricular calcitonin in the conscious rabbit, Experientia, 31:332-333.

Perez Cano, R., Galan Galan, F., Girgis, S.I., Arnett, T.R., and MacIntyre, I., 1981, A human calcitonin-like molecule in the ultimobranchial body of the amphibian (Rana pipiens), Experientia, 37:1116-1117,

Perez Cano, R., Girgis, S.I., Galan Galan, F., and MacIntyre, I., 1982a, Identification of both human and salmon calcitonin-like molecules in birds, suggesting the existence of two calcitonin genes, J. Endocrinol., 92:351-355.

Perez Cano, R., Girgis, S.I., and MacIntyre, I., 1982b, Further evidence for calcitonin gene duplication: the identification of two different calcitonins in a fish, a reptile and two mammals, Acta Endocrinol., 100:256-261.

Perlow, M.J., Freed, W.J., Carman, J.S., and Wyatt, R.J., 1980, Calcitonin reduces feeding in man, monkey and rat, Biochem. Behav., 12:609-614.

Potts, J.T. Jr., Niall, H.D., Keutman, H.T., Brewer, H.B. Jr., and Deftos, L.J., 1968, The amino acid sequence of porcine calcitonin, Proc. Natl. Acad. Sci. USA., 59:1321-1328.

Potts, J.T. Jr., Niall, H.D., Keutmann, H.T., Deftos, L.J., and Parsons, J.A., 1970, Calcitonin: recent chemical and immuological studies, in: "Calcitonin 1969, Proc. 2nd Int. Symp..", S.F. Taylor, ed., Heinemann Medical Books, London, pp.56-73.

Potts, J.T. Jr., Keutmann, H.T., Niall, H.D., and Tregear, G.W., 1971, The chemistry of parathyroid hormone and the calcitonins, Vitam. Horm., 29:41-93.

Queener, S.F., and Bell, N.H., 1975, Calcitonin: a general survey, Metabolism, 24:555-567.

Raisz, L.G., Au, W.Y.W., Friedman, J., and Neimann, I., 1967, Thyrocalcitonin and bone resorption - studies employing a tissue culture bioassay, Am. J. Med., 43:684-689.

Ralston, S.H., Alzaidi, A.A., Gardner, M.D., and Boyle, I.T., 1986, Treatment of cancer-associated hyper-calcaemia with combined aminopropylidene diphosphonate and calcitonin, Br. Med. J., 292:1549-1550.

Rasmussen, H., Bordier, P., 1974, "The Physiological and Cellular Basis of Metabolic Bone Disease", Williams and Wilkins, Baltimore.

Rasmussen, H., Bordier, P., Marie, D., Anquier, K., Eisinger, J.R., Kuntz, D., Caulin, F., Argemi, B., Gueris, J., and Julien, A., 1980, Effect of combined therapy with phosphate and calcitonin on bone volume in osteoporosis, Metab. Bone Dis. Rel. Res., 2:107-111.

Raulias, D., Hagaman, J., Ontjes, D.A., Lundblad, R.L., and Kingdon, H.S., 1976, The complete amino acid sequence of rat thyrocalcitonin, Eur. J. Biochem., 64:607-611.

Ravazzola, M., Orci, L., Girgis, S.I., Galan Galan, F., and MacIntyre, I., 1981, The lung is the major source of calcitonin in the lizard, Cell Biol. Int. Rep., 5:937-944.

Reynolds, J.J., Dingle, J.T., Gudmundsson, T.V., and
    MacIntyre, I., 1968, Bone resorption in vitro and its
    inhibition by calcitonin, in: "Calcitonin, Proceedings of
    the Internat. Symp. on Thyrocalcitonin and the C-cells",
    S.F. Taylor, eds., Heinemann Medical Books, London,
    pp.223-229.
Rittel, W., Maier, R., Brugger, M., Kamber, B., Riniker, B.,
    and Sieber, P., 1976, Structure-activity relationship of
    human calcitonin. III. Biological activity of synthetic
    analogues with shortened or terminally modified peptide
    chains, Experientia, 32:246-248.
Rizzo, A.J., and Goltzman, D., 1981, Calcitonin receptors in
    the central nervous system of the rat, Endocrinology,
    108:1672-1677.
Robinson, C.J., Martin, T.J., and MacIntyre, I., 1966,
    Phosphaturic effect of thyrocalcitonin, Lancet, ii:83-84.
Robinson, C.J., Matthews, E.W., and MacIntyre, I. 1969, The
    effect of parathyroid hormone and thyrocalcitonin on the
    intestinal absorption of calcium and magnesium, in: "Les
    Tissues Calcifies: Proc. Vth Europ. Symp.", G. Milhaud,
    eds., Paris, S.E.D.E.S., pp.279-282.
Rosenfeld, M.G., Mermod, J-J., Amara, S.G., Swanson, L.W.,
    Sawchenko, P.E., Rivier, J., Vale, W.W., and Evans, R.M.,
    1983, Production of a novel neuropeptide encoded by the
    calcitonin gene via tissue specific RNA processing,
    Nature, 304:129-135.
Rude, R.K., and Singer, F.R., 1977, Comparison of serum
    calcitonin levels after a 1-minute calcium injection and
    after pentagastrin injection in the diagnosis of medullary
    thyroid carcinoma, J. Clin. Endocrinol. Metab., 44:980-
    983.
Russell, R.G.G., and Fleisch, H., 1968, The renal effects of
    thyrocalcitonin in the pig and dog, in; "Calcitonin,
    Proceedings of the Internat. Symp. on Thyrocalcitonin
    and the C-cells", S. Taylor, eds., Heinemann Medical
    Books, London, pp. 297-305.
Samaan, N.A., Anderson, G.D., and Adam-Mayne, M.E., 1975,
    Immunoreactive calcitonin in the mother, neonate, child
    and adult, Am. J. Obstet. Gynecol., 121:622-625.
Sanger, F., Nicklen, S., and Coulson, A.R., 1975, DNA
    sequencing with chain-terminating inhibitors, Proc. Natl.
    Acad. Sci. USA., 74:5463-5467.
Segond, N., Legendre, B., Tahri, E.H., Besnard, P., Julienne,
    A., Moukhtar, M.S., Garel, J.M., 1985, Increased level of
    calcitonin mRNA after 1,25-dihydroxyvitamin D_3 injection
    in the rat, FEBS Letts., 184:2-5.
Seiber, P., Brugger, M., Kamber, B., Riniker, B., and Rittel,
    W., 1968, Mensliches calcitonin III. Die synthesis von
    calcitonin M, Helv. Chim. Acta, 51:2057-2061.
Self, C.H., Wimalawansa, S.J., Johannsson, A., Bates, D.,
    Girgis, S.I., and MacIntyre, I., 1985, A new sensitive
    and fast peptide immunoassay based on enzyme
    amplification: used in the determination of CGRP and the
    demonstration of its presence in the thyroid, Peptides,
    6:627-630.
Seth, R., Kehely, A., Wimalawansa, S.J., Self, C.H., Motté,
    P., Bonnay, M., Bellet, D., and MacIntyre, I., 1987,
    The development of a two-site enzyme-immunometric assay
    for calcitonin and its application in the measurement
    of the hormone in normal subjects, MTC patients and

post-menopausal women, in: "Proc. Mtg. on Multiple Endocrine Neoplasia, type 2, Heidelberg, West Germany".

Seth, R., Motté, P., Kehely, A., Wimalawansa, S.J., Self, C., Bellet, D., Bohuon, C., and MacIntyre, I., 1988, A sensitive and specific enzyme-immunometric assay for human calcitonin using monoclonal antibodies. J. Endocrinol., 119:351-357.

Silva, O.L., Becker, K.L., Primack, A., Doppman, J., and Snider, R.H., 1973, Ectopic production of calcitonin, Lancet, ii:317-319.

Silverberg, S.J., Shane, E., de la Cruz, L., Segre, G.V., Clemens, T.L., and Bilezikian, J.P., 1989, Abnormalities in parathyroid hormone secretion and 1,25-dihydroxyvitamin D_3 formation in women with osteoporosis, New Engl. J. Med., 320:277-281.

Singer, F.R., Alfred, J.P., Neer, R.M., Krane, S.M., Potts, J.T. Jr., and Bloch, K.J., 1972, An evaluation of antibodies and clinical resistance to salmon calcitonin, J. Clin. Invest., 51:2331-2336.

Singer, F.R., Fredericks, R.S., and Minkin, C., 1980, Salmon calcitonin therapy for Paget's disease of bone: the problem of acquired clinical resistance, Arth. Rheum., 23:1148-1154.

Singer, F.R., Woodhouse, N.J.Y., Parkinson, D.K., and Joplin, G.F., 1969, Some acute effects of administered porcine calcitonin in man, Clin. Sci., 37:181-190.

Singer, F.R., and Habener, J.F., 1974, Multiple immunoreactive forms of calcitonin in human plasma, Biochem. Biophys. Res. Commun., 61:710-716.

Sipple, J.H., 1961, The association of phaeochromocytoma with carcinoma of the thyroid gland, Am. J. Med., 31:163-166.

Sizemore, G.W., and Heath, H. III., 1975, Immunochemical heterogeneity of calcitonin in plasma of patients with medullary thyroid carcinoma, J. Clin. Invest, 55:1111-1118.

Snider, R.H., Silva, O.L., Moore, C.F., and Becker, K.L., 1977, Immunochemical heterogeneity of calcitonin in man: effect on radioimmunoassay, Clin. Chim. Acta, 76:1-14.

Steiner, A.L., Goodman, A.D., and Powers, S.R., 1968, Study of a kindred with phaeochromocytoma, medullary thyroid carcinoma, hyperparathyroidism and Cushing's disease: multiple endocrine neoplasia type II, Medicine, 47:371-409.

Stevenson, JC., Hillyard, C.J., MacIntyre, I., Cooper, H., and Whitehead, M.I., 1979, A physiological role for calcitonin: protection of the maternal skeleton, Lancet, 2:769-770.

Stevenson J.C., Abeyasekera, G., Hillyard, C.J., Phang, K.G., MacIntyre, I., Campbell, S., Townsend, P.T., Young, O., and Whitehead, M.I., 1981, Calcitonin and the calcium-regulating hormones in post menopausal women: effect of oestrogens, Lancet, i:693-695.

Stevenson, J.C., and Evans, I.M.A., 1981, Pharmacology and therapeutic use of calcitonin, Drugs, 21:257-262.

Stevenson, J.C., White, M.C., Joplin, G.F., and MacIntyre, I., 1982, Osteoporosis and calcitonin deficiency, Br. Med. J., 285:1010-1011.

Stevenson, J.C., Adrian, T.E., Christofides, N.D., and Bloom, S.R., 1985, Effect of calcitonin on gastro-

—intestinal regulatory peptides in man, Clin. Endocrinol., 22:655-660.

Taggart, H.McAS., Chesnut, C.H. III., Ivey, J.L., Baylink, D.J., Sisom, K., Huber, M.B., and Roos, B.A., 1982, Deficient calcitonin response to calcium stimulation in postmenopausal osteoporosis?, Lancet, i:475-478.

Talmage, R.V.,Grubb, S.A., Norimatsu, H., and Vanderwiel, C.J., 1980, Evidence for an important physiological role for calcitonin, Proc. Natl. Acad. Sci. USA., 77:609-613.

Tashjian, A.H. Jr., Wright, D.R., Ivey, J.L., and Pont, A., 1978, Calcitonin binding sites in bone: relationships to biological response adn 'escape', Recent Progr. Horm. Res., 34:285-334.

Tashjian, A.H., Jr., Howland, B.G., Melvin, K.E.W., and Hill, C.S. Jr., 1970, Immunoassay of human calcitonin: clinical measurement, relation to serum calcium and studies in patients with medullary thyroid carcinoma, New Engl. J. Med., 283:890-895.

Tauber, S.D., 1967, The ultimobranchial oreigin of calcitonin, Proc. Natl. Acad. Sci. USA., 58:1684-1687.

Telenius-Berg, M., Almquist, S., Hedner, P., Ingemansson, S., Tibblin, S., and Wasthed, B., 1975, Screening for medullary carcinoma of the thyroid, Lancet, i:390.

Tschopp, F.A., Henke, H., Petermann, J.B., Tobler, P.H., Janzer, R., Hokfelt, T., Lundberg, J.M., Cuello, C., and Fischer, J.A., 1985, Calcitonin gene-related peptide and its binding sites in the human central nervous system and pituitary, Proc. Natl. Acad. Sci. USA., 82:248-252.

Van der Donk, J.A., Van Dam, R.H., Goudswaard, J., Hackeng, W.H.L., and Lips, C.J.M., 1976, Precursor molecule for calcitonin, Lancet, ii: 1133.

Wallach, S., Cohn, S.H., Atkins, H.L., Ellis, K.J., Kohberger, R., Aloia, J.F., and Zanzi, I., 1977, Effect of salmon calcitonin on skeletal mass in osteoporosis, Curr. Ther. Res., 22:556-572.

Warshawsky, F., Goltzman, D., Rouleau, M.F., and Bergeron, J.M., 1980, Direct in vivo demonstration by radioautography of specific binding sites for calcitonin in skeletal and renal tissues of rat, J. Cell Biol., 88:682-694.

Westermark, P., Wernstedt, C., Wilander, E., and Sletten, K., 1986, A novel peptide in the calcitonin gene-related peptide family as an amyloid fibril protein in the endocrine pancreas, Biochem. Biophys. Res. Commun., 140:826-831.

Whyte, M.P., Bergeld, M.A., and Murphy, W.A., 1982, Postmenopausal osteoporosis. A heterogeneous disorder as assessed by histomorphometric analysis of iliac crest bone from untreated patients, Am. J. Med., 72 193-202.

Williams, E.D., 1965, A review of 17 cases of carcinoma of the thyroid and phaeochromocytoma, J. Clin. Path., 18:288-292.

Williams, E.D., Brown, C.L., and Donach, I., 1966, Pathological and clinical findings in a series of 67 cases of medullary carcinoma of the thyroid, J. Clin. Path., 19:103-113.

Wimalawansa, S.J., 1988, Osteoporosis: a preventable disease, Bone, 5:4.

Wimalawansa, S.J., 1989a, Immunochemical heterogeneity, and
    the effect of a meal and pentagastrin stimulation on
    different molecular weight forms of calcitonin gene-
    related peptide and calcitonin in man, Submitted to
    Journal of Endocrinology.
Wimalawansa, S.J., 1989b, Sensitive and specific radio-
    receptor assay for calcitonin gene-related peptide, J.
    Neuroendocrinol., 1:15-19.
Wimalawansa, S.J., and MacIntyre, I. 1987, Demonstration of
    calcitonin gene-related peptide in the human
    cerebrospinal fluid, Brain, 110:1647-1655.
Wimalawansa, S.J. and MacIntyre, I., 1988a, Can we determine
    the lowest dose of oestradiol still active on bone?,
    in: "Recent Research on Gynecological Endocrinology,
    vol. 2", A.R. Genazzani, F. Petraglia, and A. Volpe,
    eds., Parthenon Publishing Group, U.K., pp.314-316.
Wimalawansa, S.J., and MacIntyre, I., 1988b, Calcitonin
    gene-related peptide and its specific binding sites in
    the cardiovascular system of the rat, Int. J. Cardiol.,
    20:29-37.
Wimalawansa, S.J., and MacIntyre, I., 1988c, Heterogeneity
    of plasma calcitonin gene-related peptide: partial
    characterisation of immunoreactive forms, Peptides, in
    press.
Wimalawansa, S.J., and MacIntyre, I., 1989a, The value of
    CGRP radioreceptor assay for the detection of medullary
    thyroid carcinoma, CRC Medullary Thyroid Group
    Newsletter, MEN, type 2, in press.
Wimalawansa, S.J., and MacIntyre, I., 1989b, Calcitonin, in:
    "Therapeutic Drugs: A Clinical Pharmacopia", C.T.
    Dollery, ed., Churchill Livingstone, Edinburgh, in
    press.
Wimalawansa, S.J., and MacIntyre, I., 1989c, Application of a
    novel radio-receptor assay for CGRP, ASBMR/ICCRA First
    Joint Meeting, Quebec, Canada, (Abstr.).
Wimalawansa, S.J., Emson, P.C., and MacIntyre, I., 1987a,
    Regional distribution of calcitonin gene-relatedpeptide
    and its specific binding sites in the rat, with
    particular reference to the nervous system,
    Neuroendocrinology, 46:131-136.
Wimalawansa, S.J., Kehely, A., Banks, L.M., Stevenson, J.C.,
    Endacott, J., Whitehead, M.I., and MacIntyre, I.,
    1987b, The effects of percutaneous oestradiol and low
    dose human calcitonin on postmenopausal vertebral bone
    loss, in: "Osteoporosis 1987", C. Christiansen, J.S.
    Johansen, and B.J. Riis, eds., Norhaven A/S, Viborg,
    pp.528-532.

Wimalawansa, S.J., Stevenson J.C., Kehely, A., Banks, L.M.,
    and MacIntyre, I., 1988, The minimal doses of
    calcitonin and 17 -oestradiol necessary for maintenance
    of skeleton in postmenopausal women, in: "Recent
    Research on Gynecological Endocrinology, vol. 2", A.R.
    Genazzani, F. Petraglia, and A. Volpe, eds., Parthenon
    Publishing Group, U.K., pp.239-244.
Wimalawansa, S.J., Morris, H.R., Panico, M., Etiner, A.,
    Blench, I., and MacIntyre, 1989a, Isolation,
    purification and characterisation of -hCGRP from human
    spinal cord, submitted to J. Biol. Chem.

Wimalawansa, S.J., Morris, H.R., and MacIntyre, I., 1989b, Both - and -calcitonin gene-related peptides are present in plasma cerebrospinal fluid and spinal cord in man, submitted to J. Mol. Endocrinol.

Wimalawansa, S.J., Seth, R., and MacIntyre, I., 1987c, Novel non-radioisotopic assay for calcitonin, for diagnosis and management of medullary thyroid carcinoma, CRC Medullary Thyroid Group, CRC, London.

Wohlwend, A., Malmstrom, K., Henke, H., Murer, H., Vassali, J.D., and Fischer, J.A., 1985, Calcitonin and calcitonin gene-related peptide interact with the same receptor in cultured LLC-PK$_1$ kidney cells, Biochem. Biophys. Res. Commun., 131:537-542.

Wong, G.L., and Cohn, D.V., 1975, Target cells in bone for parathormone and calcitonin are different: enrichment for each cell type by sequential digestion of mouse calvaria and selective adhesion to polymeric surfaces, Proc. Natl. Acad. Sci. USA., 72:3167-3171.

Woodhouse, N.J.Y., Bordier, P., Fisher, M., Joplin, G.F., Reiner, M., Kalu, D.N., Foster, G.V., and MacIntyre, I., 1971, Human calcitonin in the treatment of Paget's bone disease, Lancet, i:1139-1143.

Woodhouse, N.J.Y., Joplin, G.F., MacIntyre, I., and Doyle, F.H., 1972, Radiological regression in Paget's disease treated by human calcitonin, Lancet, ii:992-994.

Woodhouse, N.J.Y., Reinter, M., Kalu, D.N., Galante, L., Leese, B., Foster, G.V., Joplin, G.F., and MacIntyre, I., 1970, Some effects of acute and chronic calcitonin M administration in man, in: "Calcitonin 1969, Proceedings of the Second International Symposium", S. Taylor, ed., Heinemann, London, pp.504-513.

Zaidi, M., Bevis, P.J.R., Abeyasekera, G., Girgis, S.I., Wimalawansa, S.J., Morris, H.R., and MacIntyre, I., 1986, The origin of circulating calcitonin gene-related peptide in the rat. J. Endocrinol., 110:185.

Zaidi, M., Breimer, L.H., and MacIntyre, I., 1987a, The biology of the peptides from the calcitonin genes, Quart. J. Exp. Physiol., 72:371-408.

Zaidi, M., Fuller, K., Bevis, P.J.R., Gaines Das, R.E., Chambers, T.J., and MacIntyre, I., 1987b, Calcitonin gene-related peptide inhibits osteoclastic bone resorption: a comparative study, Calcif. Tissue Int., 40:149-154.

Zanelli, J.M., Salmon, D.M., Azria, M., and Zanelli, G.D., 1985, A rat model for clinical resistance to chronic treatment with salmon calcitonin; application of quantitative cytochemistry, in: "Calcitonin 1984. Chemistry, Physiology, Pharmacology and Clinical Aspects", A. Pecile, ed., Excerpta Medica, Amsterdam, pp.223-230.

Ziegler, R., Holz, G., Raue, H., Minne, H., and Delling, G., 1976, Therapeutic studies with human calcitonin, in: "Human Calcitonin and Paget's Disease, Proceedings of the International Workshop, London", I. MacIntyre, ed., Huber, Vienna, p.167.

Ziegler, R., and Raue, F., 1984, Variations in plasma calcitonin levels measured by radioimmunoassay systems for human calcitonin, Biomed. Pharmacother., 38:245-256.

OSTEOGENIN: ROLE IN BONE INDUCTION AND REPAIR

A.H. Reddi and S. Ma

Bone Cell Biology Section
National Institute of Dental Research
National Institutes of Health
Bethesda, MD 20892   U.S.A.

INTRODUCTION

     Bone has considerable potential for repair and regeneration. The
aim of this article is to provide a concise review of bone induction. It
presents the hypothesis that endogenous growth and differentiation factors
isolated from bone matrix in conjunction with exogenous growth factors
isolated from elsewhere will initiate and promote cartilage and bone repair.
The potential for regeneration and repair of skeletal tissue is well known
from the days of Hippocrates in ancient Greece. Almost a century ago Senn
(1) described the utility of decalcified bone implants in the care of osteo-
myelitis. Pierre Lacroix (2), a Belgian orthopaedic surgeon proposed that
bone may contain a substance christened "osteogenin" which may initiate
bone growth. Marshall Urist (3) made the key discovery that demineralized,
lyophilized bone matrix induced bone formation. Bone induction by
demineralized bone matrix recapitulates the stages of long bone development
(4-7).

BONE FORMATION AND REPAIR: A CASCADE

     Bone formation in the developing embryo is evident in the epiphysis
of long bones and is a developmental cascade (4). The growth and
differentiation of mesenchymal cells into cartilage and bone during
endochondral ossification is a continuum and is confined to the epiphyseal
growth plate. The changes during the repair of bone following fracture
consists of a sequential response that recapitulates the major steps in
bone development in the embryo. In addition, the bone induction elicited
by implantation of demineralized bone matrix powder is reminiscent of
embryonic endochondral bone differentiation and fracture repair (5-8).
The major phases of the cellular response to demineralized diaphyseal bone
matrix include chemotaxis and attachment of progenitor cells, mitosis of
responding cells and differentiation into cartilage and finally bone and
marrow (Table I).

     Chemotaxis and Cell Attachment   Chemotaxis may be defined as the
directed migration of cells in response to a chemical gradient.
Implantation of demineralized bone matrix promotes the chemotaxis of cells
into the interior of the implant. In less than a day the implant forms a
plano-convex conglomerate of particles of implanted bone matrix, an

TABLE I
Bone Induction: Cellular and Biochemical Changes

Time after Implantation	Cellular Changes	Biochemical Changes
1 min	Blood clot formation. Platelet release.	Fibrin network formation. Release of platelet-derived growth factors. Binding of plasma fibronectin to implanted matrix.
3–18 h	Accumulation of PMN. Adhesion of cells.	Limited proteolysis and release of chemotactic peptides for fibroblasts.
day 1	Chemotaxis for fibroblasts and cell attachment to the implanted extracellular matrix.	Release of peptides of fibronectin. Increased cell motility.
day 3	Cell proliferation. Release of growth factors.	^{3}H–Thymidine incorporation into DNA. Type III collagen synthesis.
day 5	Differentiation of chondroblasts.	Increase in $^{35}SO_4$ incorporation into proteoglycans.
day 7	Synthesis and secretion of cartilage matrix.	Type I collagen synthesis, cartilage-specific proteoglycans.
day 9	Hypertrophy of chondrocytes. Calcification of cartilage matrix. Vascular invasion. Endothelial cell proliferation.	Increase in ^{45}Ca incorporation and alkaline phosphatase activity. Type IV collagen, Laminin and Factor VIII in blood vessels.
days 10–12	Osteoblasts. Bone formation and mineralization. Chondrolysis.	Type I collagen synthesis. Bone proteoglycan synthesis. Peak in ^{45}Ca incorporation and alkaline phosphatase activity.
days 12–18	Osteoclast differentiation. Bone remodeling and dissolution of the implanted matrix.	Increase in lysosomal enzymes. Release of collagenases and proteases.
day 21	Bone marrow differentiation.	Increase in ^{59}Fe incorporation into heme. Accumulation of lysozyme. Type III collagen.

irregular meshwork of fibrin and polymorphonuclear leukocytes (PMNs). Chemotaxis for fibroblast-like mesenchymal cells continues for the next 2-3 days. Plasma fibronectin binds to the implanted collagenous bone matrix (9, 10). Mesenchymal cells migrate and attach to the matrix. The cellular fibronectin has also been implicated in cell attachment. Fibronectin is a protein with a molecular mass of 450 kDa and has affinity for collagen, fibrin, and heparin, the major constituents in the site of any musculo-skeletal trauma. It is well known that peptides derived from fibronectin are chemotactic and possibly mitogenic for mesenchymal cells.

Partially purified proteins from the solubilized demineralized bone matrix possess chemotactic activity for osteoblast-like cells and muscle-derived mesenchymal cells (11,12). In addition to proteins released from the demineralized bone matrix local release of platelet-derived growth factor (PDGF) may play a role in chemotaxis of mesenchymal cells (13,14) and may be involved in the initial attraction and assembly of progenitor cells in the bone and cartilage fracture site.

Mitosis and Growth Factors   The newly attached mesenchymal cells undergo proliferation. The implanted collagenous bone matrix is a local mitogen (15). The mitogenic activity was quantitated using radioautography and tritiated thymidine incorporation. Growth factors with potential to increase cell number in tissue culture were isolated from demineralized rat bone matrix (16). The response to the partially purified growth factor is concentration-dependent. A skeletal growth factor was isolated from human bone matrix (17) with an apparent molecular weight of 60 to 85 kDa. The human skeletal growth factor has been identified as Insulin-like growth factor II (IGF-II) based on amino acid sequence homology (18). Bone cells appear to elaborate growth factors that regulate their own growth (autocrine factors) as demonstrated by Canalis and colleagues (19). A bone derived growth factor (BDGF) of 11 kDa molecullar mass was purified and identified as Beta-2 microglobulin (20). More recently Hauschka (21) has isolated a variety of growth factors from bovine bone by heparin affinity chromato-graphy that includes acidic and basic fibroblast growth factors (22) and PDGF-like factors (23).

Differentiation of Cartilage and Bone   The proliferation of the mesenchymal progenitor cells is followed by differentiation of chondrocytes. Hyaline cartilage with abundant chondrocytes are evident on days 7-8. On day 9 there is angiogenesis and calcification of the hypertrophic cartilage matrix . In close proximity to the invading capillaries monocytes, macrophages and multinucleated chondroclasts are observed in local areas of chondrolysis. Thereafter on days 10-11 with increasing vascularization numerous osteoprogenitor cells and osteoblasts are seen adjacent to the pericytes of the invading blood vessels. New bone matrix is deposited by osteoblasts on the surface of calcified cartilage matrix and on the particles of implanted demineralized matrix. The newly formed bone is remodeled by osteoclasts on days 12-18. By day 21 the remodeled ossicle is replete with hematopoietic marrow (Table I).

The emergence of cartilage and bone in a heterotopic extraskeletal site permits an unambiguous analysis of the de novo osteogenic response. The subcutaneous site allows the study of the developing stages of endochondral bone at discrete time points and the assessment of the various biochemical and endocrine parameters. Incorporation of radioactive ^{35}S-sulfate into proteoglycans is maximal on day 7. Mineralization of cartilage and bone matrix was monitored by ^{45}Ca incorporation into the acid soluble mineral phase and was high on days 11-14 (4,5). This increase in mineralization is preceded by alkaline phosphatase activity, an enzyme known to be intimately involved in ossification (5). Erythropoiesis in the marrow elements was monitored by ^{59}Fe incorporation into heme (Table I). These various biochemical assays provide a foundation for further quest in the isolation of osteogenic and bone morphogenetic proteins (8).

ISOLATION OF OSTEOGENIN

Progress in the isolation of osteogenins has been difficult and slow due to the fact that bone matrix is in the solid state. We have shown that the osteogenic activity of bone matrix can be dissociatively extracted by 4.0 M guanidine, 8 M urea or 1% sodium dodecyl sulfate at pH 7.4 (24). The extracted proteins can be reconstituted with inactive collagenous bone matrix residue to restore bone induction (24). This important advance provided a method for assay of soluble components for induction of bone differentiation in vivo and permitted further purification. The putative differentiation factors have a molecular mass of less than 50,000 daltons and appear to be homologous in several mammals (25). These factors have the potential to transform muscle-derived mesenchymal cells into chondrocytes (26) and stimulate chick limb bud chondrogenesis (27). The osteogenic potential of demineralized bone matrix was inhibited by pretreatment with heparin (28). In view of this we explored the utility of heparin affinity columns to purify the osteogenic protein(s) termed collectively as "osteogenins". Recent work demonstrated that osteogenins bind to heparin affinity columns and are eluted by 0.5 M NaCl (29). The osteogenins were further purified by hydroxyapatite, high performance liquid chromatography (HPLC) on molecular sieve columns and reverse-phase HPLC. Active fractions were further purified by sodium dodecly sulfate gel electrophoresis. Osteogenin activity was localized in a zone between 30 and 40 kDa. The amino acid sequence of a number of tryptic peptides of the gel eluted material were determined (30). Recently the amino acid sequences of four bone morphogenetic proteins (BMPs) were reported (31). The amino acid sequence of osteogenin shows considerable homology to BMP-3. However, unlike recombinant BMP-3 which only induces cartilage, purified osteogenin from bovine bone initiated both cartilage and bone formation.

The osteogenic response elicited by osteogenin is rather specific. Several homogeneous growth factors including platelet-derived growth factor (PDGF), epidermal growth factor (EGF), transforming growth factor Beta (TGF), fibroblast growth factor (FGF), insulin, growth hormone, and insulin-like growth factor I were inactive in the in vivo osteogenic bioassay. However, it is possible that these factors may promote bone formation initiated by osteogenin.

PROMOTION OF BONE FORMATION BY GROWTH FACTORS

The possible role of growth factors to promote bone formation during fracture healing was explored by using the bone-matrix induced endochondral bone formation model. A systematic study of the effects of PDGF, FGF, EGF, and TGF on cartilage and bone formation was performed. PDGF is stored in platelets and is also produced by macrophages (23). PDGF has the characteristic of a wound hormone whose main function is to increase the migration and mitosis of mesenchymal cells in the wound prior to the reparative response. PDGF is released locally to promote chemotaxis and recruitment of cells. At higher concentrations PDGF is a mitogen for mesenchymal cells. In view of this the effect of PDGF and other growth factors on cartilage and bone formation was examined. Cartilage formation was quantitated by type II collagen messenger RNA levels and bone formation by alkaline phosphatase activity and calcium content. PDGF supplement increased cartilage and bone formation in older rats but not in young animals. The PDGF response is age-dependent. It is likely that the rate of bone formation is already maximal in young rats and therefore PDGF does not exhibit any additional stimulatory effect. On the other hand, the bone formation is submaximal in older rats and is enhanced by PDGF. These effects of PDGF were not observed with EGF,

FGF, and TGF Beta (32). TGF Beta was recently isolated from bovine bone matrix (33) and is known to increase synthesis of cartilage proteoglycans and type II collagen by muscle derived mesenchymal cells in vitro. However, in vivo this growth factor did not induce new bone or cartilage (29). Future experiments should explore combinations of growth factors for synergistic effects. The increasing availability of growth and differentiation factors engineered by recombinant DNA technology will result in a new generation of prostheses for bone repair in the near future.

SUMMARY

The developmental cascade in response to demineralized bone matrix implantation includes: binding of fibronectin to the implanted matrix, chemotaxis of cells, mitosis of progenitor cells, differentiation into chondroblasts and osteoblasts and marrow. The bone matrix is a repository of growth and differentiation factors that govern the major phases of the repair cascade. Osteogenin, a bone inductive protein was isolated by heparin affinity chromatography and the amino acid sequence determined. Osteogenin in conjunction with collagenous matrix initiated new bone formation locally. Growth factors present endogenously in bone can be supplemented with exogenous growth factors and formulated in an optimal collagen-based delivery system to obtain a predictable and rapid repair of bone.

REFERENCES

1. N. Senn, On the healing of aseptic bone cavities by implantation of antiseptic decalcified bone. Am. J. Med. Sci. 98:219 (1889).
2. P. Lacroix, Recent investigations on the growth of bone. Nature 156:576 (1945).
3. M. Urist, Bone formation by autoinduction. Science 150:893 (1965).
4. A.H. Reddi, Cell biology and biochemistry of endochondral bone development. Collagen Rel. Res. 1:209 (1981).
5. A.H. Reddi and C.B. Huggins, Biochemical sequences in the transformation of normal fibroblasts in adolescent rats. Proc. Natl. Acad. Sci. USA 69:1601 (1972).
6. A.H. Reddi and W.A. Anderson, Collagenous bone matrix-induced endochondral ossification and hemopoiesis. J. Cell Biology 69:557 (1976).
7. A.H. Reddi, Extracellular matrix and development, in "Extracellular Matrix Biochemistry," K.A. Piez and A.H. Reddi, eds., Elsevier, New York (1984).
8. M.R. Urist, R.J. Delange and G.A.M. Finerman, Bone cell differentiation and growth factors. Science 220:680 (1983).
9. R.E. Weiss and A.H. Reddi, Synthesis and localization of fibronectin during collagenous matrix-mesenchymal cell interaction and differentiation of cartilage and bone in vivo. Proc. Natl. Acad. Sci. USA 77:2074 (1980).
10. R.E. Weiss and A.H. Reddi, Role of fibronectin in collagenous matrix-induced mesenchymal cell proliferation and differentiation in vivo. Exp. Cell Res. 133:247 (1981).
11. M. Somerman, A.T. Hewitt, H.H. Varner, E. Schiffman, J.D. Termine, and A.H. Reddi, Identification of a bone matrix-derived chemotactic factor. Calcif. Tiss. Int. 35:481 (1983).
12. R. Landesman and A.H. Reddi, Chemotaxis of muscle-derived mesenchymal cells to bone-inductive proteins of rat. Calcif. Tiss. Int. 39:259 (1986).
13. V. Gauss-Miller, H.K. Kleinman, G.R. Martin and E. Schiffman, Role of attachment factors and attractants in fibroblast chemotaxis. J. Lab. Clin. Med. 96:1071 (1980).

14. H. Seppa, G. Grotendorst, S. Seppa, E. Schiffman and G.R. Martin, Platelet-derived growth factor is chemotactic for fibroblasts. J. Cell Biol. 92:584 (1980).
15. N.C. Rath and A.H. Reddi, Collagenous bone matrix is a local mitogen. Nature 278:855 (1979).
16. T.K. Sampath, D.P. DeSimone and A.H. Reddi, Extracellular bone matrix-derived growth factor. Exp. Cell Res. 142:460 (1982).
17. J.R. Farley and D.J. Baylink, Purification of a skeletal growth factor from human bone. Biochemistry 21:3502 (1982).
18. S. Mohan, J.C. Jennings, T.A. Linkhart, J.F. Wergedal and D.J. Baylink, Primary structure of human skeletal growth factor (SGF): Homology with IGF-II. J. Bone Mineral Res. 3:S218 (1988).
19. E. Canalis, W.A. Peck and L.G. Raisz, Stimulation of DNA and collagen synthesis by autologous growth factor in cultured fetal rat calvaria. Science 200:1021 (1980).
20. E. Canalis, T. McCarthy and M. Centrella, A bone-derived growth factor isolated from rat calvariae is Beta-2 microglobulin. Endocrinology 121:1198 (1987).
21. P.V. Hauschka, A.E. Mavrakos, M.D. Iafrati, S.E. Doleman and M. Klagsbrun, Growth factors in bone matrix: isolation of multiple types by affinity chromatography on heparin-Sepharose. J. Biol. Chem. 261: 12665 (1986).
22. D. Gospodarowicz, G. Neufeld and L. Schweigerer, Fibroblast growth factor: structural and biological properties. J. Cell Physiol. Suppl. 5:15 (1987).
23. R. Ross, E.W. Raines and D.F. Bowen-Pope, The biology of platelet-derived growth factor. Cell 46:155 (1986).
24. T.K. Sampath and A.H. Reddi, Dissociative extraction and reconstitution of bone matrix components involved in local bone differentiation. Proc. Nanl. Acad. Sci. USA 78:7599 (1981).
25. T.K. Sampath and A.H. Reddi, Homology of bone inductive proteins from human, monkey, bovine and rat extracellular matrix. Proc. Natl. Acad. Sci. USA 80:6591 (1983).
26. T.K. Sampath, M. Nathanson and A.H. Reddi, In vitro trasformation of mesenchymal cells derived from embryonic muscle into cartilage in response to extracellular matrix components of bone. Proc. Natl. Acad. Sci. USA 81:3419 (1984).
27. G.T. Syftestad, J.T. Triffit, M.R. Urist and A.I. Caplan, An osteo-inductive bone matrix extract stimulates the conversion of mesenchyme into chondrocytes. Calcif. Tiss. Int. 36:625 (1984).
28. A.H. Reddi, Collagenous bone matrix and gene expression in fibroblasts. in: Extracellular Matrix Influences on Gene Expression. H.C. Slavkin and R.C. Greulich, eds., Academic Press, New York (1975).
29. T.K. Sampath, N. Muthukumaran and A.H. Reddi, Isolation of osteogenin, an extracellular matrix-associated bone inductive protein by heparin affinity chromatography. Proc. Natl. Acad. Sci. USA 84:7109 (1987).
30. F.P. Luyten, N.S. Cunningham, S. Ma, N. Muthukumaran, R.G. Hammonds, W.B. Nevins, W.I. Wood and A.H. Reddi, Purification and partial amino acid sequence of osteogenin, a protein initiating bone differentiation. J. Biol. Chem. 264:13377 (1989).
31. J.M. Wozney, V. Rosen, A.J. Celeste, L.M. Mitsock, M.J. Whitters, R.W. Kriz, R.M. Hewick and E.A.Wang, Novel regulators of bone formation: Molecular clones and activities. Science 242;1528 (1988).
32. R. Howes, J.M. Bowness, G.R. Grotendorst, G.R. Martin and A.H. Reddi, Platelet-derived growth factor enhances demineralized bone matrix-induced cartilage and bone formation. Calcif. Tiss. Int. 42:34 (1987).
33. S.M. Seyedin, P. Segarini, D.M. Rosen, A.Y. Thompson, H. Bentz and J. Graycar, Cartilage-inducing factor B is a unique protein structurally and functionally related to transforming growth factor Beta. J. Biol. Chem. 262:1946 (1987).

APPROACHES TO THE STUDY OF THE FUNCTION AND ACTIVITY OF BONE REGULATORY FACTORS: ESTABLISHED AND POTENTIAL METHODS

Joan M Zanelli and Nigel Loveridge

National Institute for Biological Standards and Control, Blanche Lane, South Mimms, Potters Bar, EN6 3QG (JMZ)[*] and Bone Growth and Metabolism Unit, Rowett Research Institute, Aberdeen, AB2 9SB (NL), UK.

I. INTRODUCTION

The aim of this paper is to review methodological approaches which can either be used to *explore* the biological activities of bone regulatory factors or be used to *measure* the amount of a particular factor. The discrimination between *explore* and *measure* needs to be made at the outset because practical and scientific considerations for each of these aspects can, at times, appear to be mutually exclusive. This is not intended to be a comprehensive review of methodologies and we do not propose to compare and contrast individual methods for individual substances; instead, we aim to review the rationale of choosing, or developing, appropriate laboratory techniques. We will also propose potential methods, based on in situ biochemistry, which are expected to make a major research contribution to the study of bone regulatory factors. Selection of the most appropriate methodologies requires an objective assessment of the scientific questions to be asked and the relevance of the experimental answers likely to be obtained.

The term "bone regulatory factors" is a general one which includes endocrine substances, which are transported from the site of production to the site of action through the blood circulation; paracrine substances where the site of production and site of action is localised within a tissue and autocrine substances where the site of production and site of action is within the same class of cell. Examples of bone regulatory factors are given in Table I but it should be stressed that this is by no means an exclusive list.

Endocrine factors, by definition are transported through the circulation and thus are likely to have a biological effect on more than one target tissue. Classic examples of endocrine bone regulatory factors are parathyroid hormone (PTH), calcitonin (CT) and vitamin D metabolites. The effects of PTH on bone have been reviewed elsewhere in these proceedings but the basic spectrum of in vivo and in vitro

---

[*]Present address: Bone Disease Research Group, Clinical Research Centre, Harrow, HA1 3UJ

techniques for exploring the biological activities of PTH or for measuring the potency of preparations of PTH or the concentrations of PTH in biological fluids or tissues are similar to those for most hormones and are represented in Figure 1. Before dealing with the types of approaches available to assay bone regulatory factors the question of bioassays as opposed to immunoassays and the need for biological standards will be dealt with.

TABLE I. SOME OF THE MAJOR SYSTEMIC AND LOCAL FACTORS INVOLVED IN THE REGULATION OF BONE GROWTH AND METABOLISM

SYSTEMIC FACTORS

    CALCIOTROPIC HORMONES:

PARATHYROID HORMONE	(PTH)
CALCITONIN	(CT)
VITAMIN D METABOLITES	
PARATHYROID HORMONE-RELATED PEPTIDE	(PTHrP)

    GROWTH PROMOTERS:

GROWTH HORMONE	(GH)
INSULIN-LIKE GROWTH FACTORS	(IGF-I, IGF-II)

    OTHERS:

ESTRADIOL	(E_2)
THYROID HORMONES	(T_3, T_4)
VITAMIN A	
INTERLEUKINS	

AUTOCRINE/PARACRINE FACTORS

    GROWTH PROMOTERS/DIFFERENTIATORS:

TRANSFORMING GROWTH FACTORS	$(TGF\alpha, TGF)$
OSTEOCLAST GROWTH FACTOR	(OGF)
FIBROBLAST GROWTH FACTORS	(aFGF, bFGF)
INSULIN-LIKE GROWTH FACTOR-I	(IGF-I)
SKELETAL GROWTH FACTOR/INSULIN LIKE GROWTH FACTOR-II	(SGF/IGF-II))
INTERLEUKINS	
EPIDERMAL GROWTH FACTOR	(EGF)

    OTHERS:

PROSTAGLANDINS	(PG's)

II. BIOASSAYS AND IMMUNOASSAYS

With the universal application of immunoassays it may seem that bioassays, with all their attendent problems are an irrelevance. However it has become increasingly obvious that while immunoassays are indeed almost universally applicable, there are situations where the hormone concentration as measured by immunoassay does not reflect the clinical condition (for review see Robertson et al 1987). Broadly speaking biological assays are based on the quantification of a specific biochemical response of an organism, target organ, cells or parts of cells to a particular agent. In contrast immunoassays are based on the presence of antigenic determinants on the agent, which may or may not be the same as those determinants responsible for biological activity. Thus in summary, bioassays reflect the functional activity, which may be mimicked by other factors which have the same biological effect, while immunoassays reflect the analytical approach which will be specific for an amino acid sequence, but not necessarily reflect the bioactivity of a molecule containing that sequence. It is obvious therefore that these types of approaches are complementary to each other.

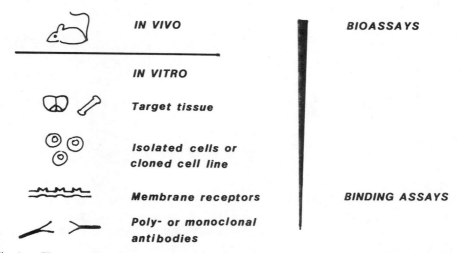

Fig 1   The basic spectrum of techniques available for the assessment of bone regulatory factors.

As far as bone regulatory factors are concerned, the discrepancy between bioactivity and immunoreactivity occurs mainly with the polypeptide hormones. For instance oxidation of parathyroid hormone (eg the 1-34 fragment of hPTH) can lead to a marked loss of biological activity but this has no effect on immunoreactivity (Fig 2). Similarly the removal of the first two amino acids of the 1-34 molecule to leave the 3-34 molecule results in the production of an in vitro inhibitor of PTH bioactivity (Rosenblatt et al 1977). Lastly, the presence in the circulation of a molecule with PTH-like bioactivity which was not reflected by equivalent levels of PTH immunoreactivity was reported in patients with humoral hypercalcaemia of malignancy (Goltzman et al 1981). This factor now generally called PTH-related peptide (PTHrP) has been identified (Moseley et al 1987;Burtis et al 1987; Strewler et al 1987) and it shares a certain degree of sequence homology with PTH in the 1-16 portion of PTH, which is thought to contain the determinants for biological activity.

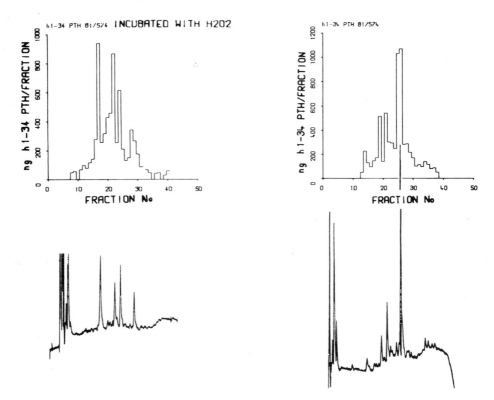

Fig 2   HPLC (lower panels) and immunoreactivity (upper panels) profiles for synthetic human PTH 1-34 peptide. Following incubation with hydrogen peroxide which reduces the biological activity of the peptide, the HPLC profile shows three oxidation products (methionine sulphoxides and sulphone) in addition to a small residues of unoxidised peptide. All components appear to have equal immunoreactivity (left side panels). The untreated peptide showing the position of the major components together with small proportions of the characteristic oxidation products (resulting from processing and freeze-drying procedures) is shown for comparison (right side panels).

As far as other bone regulatory factors are concerned bioassays are important because some of these factors are found in a latent state, while others have binding proteins which appear to affect their biological activity. For instance, transforming growth factor ß (TGFß) is generally found in a latent state, bound to a large molecule. Biological activity is only disclosed when acidification of this precursor releases the biologically active TGFß (see Sporn et al 1987). Interestingly, isolated osteoclasts because of their ability to acidify their local enviroment are also capable of releasing TGFß from its precursor (Orrefo et al 1989). Both growth hormone (GH) and insulin-like growth factor I (IGF-I) are found in the circulation attached to binding proteins but their effects are different. In the case of GH, the binding protein prevents proteolytic degradation so prolonging the half-life of the hormone and increasing its total biological effect (Baumann et al 1987). In the case of IGF-I, a number of binding proteins have been isolated, most of which are inhibitory to the action of this growth factor (eg Zapf et al 1979; Knauer & Smith 1980; Drop et al 1979), although recently a stimulatory binding protein has been reported (Cornell et al 1987).

III. STANDARDISATION AND UNITAGE OF BIOLOGICAL PREPARATIONS

The historical in vivo method for detecting biological activity was by injection of a tissue extract into an animal and observing or analysing for a particular response. Some 65 years ago the first crude extracts of bovine parathyroid glands were tested by injection into dogs to determine whether or not the extracts had hypercalcaemic activity indicating the presence of the active factor, PTH. The dog test provided the basis for the first quantitative estimates of the biological potency, measured in dog units, of various extracts. These units were "animal" units with variability from dog to dog, laboratory to laboratory and time to time. Nevertheless the dog hypercalcaemia unit provided the basis for the USP (United States Pharmacopaeia) unit used for many years for calibrating the Parathyroid Extract (Lilly) manufactured by the Eli Lilly Company for clinical administration in the Ellsworth Howard diagnostic provocation test. The USP unit for bovine PTH was defined as " one hundredth of the amount required to raise the calcium content of 100 ml of the serum of normal dogs 1mg within 16-18 hours after administration". In 1967 the first reference preparation of bovine parathyroid extract was ampouled by the Division of Biological Standards at the Medical Research Council's National Institute for Medical Research, London so that laboratories around the world could thus have access to ampoules of a single standardised stable research standard for comparative testing of their laboratory preparations. The assignment of potency to the reference ampoule was based on an international collaborative study and preserved continuity with the USP unit. As the unit (subsequently established by the World Health Organisation as the International Unit) was subsequently defined by an ampouled reference standard it became possible to develop biological assays in different species of animals and to develop in vitro systems (see review by Zanelli and Parsons 1980). It should be noted that in 1976, the National Institute for Biological Standards and Control (designated as a WHO International Laboratory for Biological Standards) was established, funded through the UK Department of Health, and replaced the MRC Division of Biological Standards.

A similar history underlies the biological standardisations of the calcitonins (CT's). The International Units assigned to the ampouled WHO international standards for porcine, salmon and human CT's derive from and maintain continuity with the rat hypocalcaemia units originally used to assess the potency of extracts of porcine thyroid tissue, human medullary thyroid carcinomas and salmon ultimobranchial glands. In cases of licensed products (porcine and salmon but not human CT) manufactured for the treatment of certain metabolic bone diseases, most national regulatory specifications require that the biological potency of each batch be measured in International Units, relative to the relevant international standard, to a defined degree of statistical precision using the rat 60 minute hypocalcaemia bioassy described in the appropriate pharmacopaeia.

IV. IN VIVO METHODS FOR ASSESSMENT OF THE BIOLOGICAL ACTIVITIES OF BONE REGULATORY FACTORS

In order to evaluate the biological activities of PTH, designed synthetic PTH analogues and inhibitors and PTHrP, Horiuchi and Rosenblatt (1987) described a complex animal model involving rats kept on a vitamin D deficient diet for 7 weeks, followed by surgical procedures to thyroparathyroidectomize the rats and insert cannulae into the right and left femoral veins and into the bladder. The animals, restrained individually in holders at controlled temperature and humidity, are infused with a maintenance solution containing calcium, magnesium, sodium and potassium chlorides in glucose for up to 25h and test substances given by infusion for various periods. This model, carried out on 10-20 rats at a time is a multiparameter biological evaluation system which can provide dose and time dependent stimulus induced responses by analysis of blood and urine samples for calcium, inorganic phosphate, cAMP, 1,25 dihydroxychole-calciferol and creatinine etc. However it depends upon specialised facilities and expertise and would not be a practical in vivo evaluation method for many laboratories to undertake. It is not suitable for precise quantitative measurement of biological activities.

Most bioassays for PTH are based on a hypercalcaemic response either in the parathyroidectomised rat, five hours after a subcutaneous injection (Munson 1961) or in the intact young chick (Parsons et al 1973) or Japanese quail (Dacke & Kenny 1973) at 60 minutes after the subcutaneous or intravenous injection. The comparison of the responses to usually three doses of a test preparation of PTH relative to three doses of the appropriate standard preparation is the basis of the design of the classical parallel line bioassay (Finney 1953, Gaines Das and Tydeman 1982). The chick hypercalcaemia assay, believed to represent a bone response to PTH, has been exploited, in conjunction with in vitro assays , in structure- function studies on synthetic fragments and analogues, of PTH (Parsons et al 1975). More recently (Lane & Zanelli 1988) it has been used as a relatively simple in vivo test for hypercalcaemic activity of synthetic fragments of parathyroid hormone related peptide (PTHrP; see Smith, these proceedings), the humoral factor believed to cause the hypercalcaemia associated with malignancy (Moseley et al 1987; Burtis et al 1987; Strewler et al 1987). Suitably optimised to take account of the short time course of acute hypercalcaemia induced by PTHrP, the chick system also appears suitable for quantitative assays of PTHrP preparations. Certainly an acute hypercalcaemic effect in intact chicks has practical advantages over the infused parathyroidectomized rat model developed by Horiuchi and Rosenblatt 1987, although the latter may be a more appropriate model for the study of the actions of PTHrP in causing the sustained hypercalcaemia which is a feature of the clinical condition and which is likely to be a composite rather than a bone specific effect.

An alternative in vivo system which is tissue (bone or kidney) specific has been developed, based on the PTH-induced stimulation of adenylate cyclase and the tissue accumulation of cAMP. This effect in mouse calvaria and kidney is very rapid, occurring within two minutes of intravenous injection of PTH and a "heat fixation" step, using microwave irradiation, is needed to ensure that the heat-stable cAMP is not degraded by phosphodiesterases in the tissue before it can be removed from the animal and the cAMP extracted and analysed (Zanelli et al 1985a). However, whereas the renal response does not appear to discriminate markedly between the bovine intact (1-84) PTH and the synthetic bovine and human 1-34 fragments, the bone cAMP response does give obvious discrimination between intact PTH and the 1-34 fragments.

The classical in vivo bioassays for the CT's, as described in the national pharmacopaeas, are based on the hypocalcaemic response in young rats, 60 minutes after intravenous or subcutaneous injection of test and standard preparations of CT (Kumar et al 1965).

Other in vivo biological tests include tissue localisation studies whereby a radiolabelled factor is injected into an animal followed by whole body autoradiography (Ullberg 1977) or specific tissue radiography (Bergeron et al 1981). Such in vivo whole body autoradiographic studies have been widely used in pharmacology (reviewed by Rico et al 1980) but cannot give detailed information on cellular, or sub-cellular localisation. The application of high resolution autoradiographic localisation of binding sites in skeletal cells for PTH and CT after in vivo injection at both the light and electron microscope level, has been reported by Warshowsky et al (1980) and Rouleau et al (1986;1988).

Although these techniques have provided valuable information on the biological interaction between a biological factor and its target cell they are not suitable for quantitative estimates of potency of the injected substance. Autoradiographic studies can also be used for in vitro demonstrations of binding sites in specific tissues as described by Pecile in these proceedings (see also Clark & Hall 1986).

It can be argued that in vivo systems should be the methods of choice for evaluating the overall biological activities of endocrine bone regulatory factors, particularly those which may be used clinically. There is also the counter argument that laboratory animals are not necessarily an appropriate model for man. In many countries, it is now becoming socially unacceptable to use animals for experimental research although reference to in vivo bioassays are likely to remain in the pharmacopaeias for some years yet. There has been a steady trend towards the development of in vitro systems for defining and measuring biological effects of endocrine substances and it is likely that in vitro techniques already long-established for the study of endocrine bone regulatory factors will be the first generation of techniques for the study of the increasing number of paracrine and autocrine bone regulatory factors.

V. IN VITRO METHODS FOR ASSESSING THE BIOLOGICAL ACTIVITIES OF BONE REGULATORY FACTORS

In the previous section we have outlined in vivo methods for the investigation of the activities of the endocrine bone regulatory factors such as PTH. With the need to move away from the use of large numbers of experimental animals several in vitro methods have been developed. In addition, this type of assay provides a means of isolating the response of one target tissue or cell under controlled conditions. These methods can be broadly divided into four separate categories, each of which have particular advantages and disadvantages.

EXPLANTS

Bone explants of either fetal (Gaillard 1955, 1961) or neonatal (Goldhaber 1958; 1961) rat and mouse tissues were first used to analyse the effects of PTH. Since that time the use of explants has become one of the most widely used methods for investigating the response to bone regulatory factors. The means of measuring that response are numerous and range from histological changes to collagen production or alkaline phosphatase activity. A marker for the resorptive effect of bone regulatory factors is calcium release, either as ^{45}Ca from bones prelabelled in utero (Raisz 1963;1965) or postnatally (Reynolds and Dingle 1970). In post-natal bones it is possible to measure calcium release without the use of isotopes (Zanelli et al 1969). More recently, these types of explant techniques have been applied to the study of the effects of different growth factors on bone (Tashjian and Levine 1978; Tashjian et al 1982,1987; Canalis and Raisz 1980; Canalis 1980; Ibbotson et al 1985). For example, Canalis et al (1988) have investigated the effect of basic fibroblast growth factor (bFGF) on DNA synthesis (by ^{3}H thymidine incorporation) and collagen and non-collagenous protein production in fetal calvaria.

The two most common techniques are based on fetal rat long bones or neonatal mouse calvaria. While most factors that affect bone resorption in one system do so in the other there are occasional differences. For instance, TGFß was shown to stimulate bone resorption in calvaria by stimulating the production of prostaglandins (Tashjian et al 1985). However, in long bone cultures, TGFß did not induce bone resorption and inhibited the resorption caused by interleukin I (IL-I) or $1,25(OH)_2D_3$ (Pfeilschifter et al 1988). It should be noted that these differences could be due to the types of bone being used, intramembranous or endochondrial, species differences or differences in responses between fetal and neonatal tissue and highlights the possible discrepancies between the various explant systems.

Another more recent use of the explant system, has been to study the proliferation and differentiation of osteoclasts (Scheven et al 1986a). By starting with long bones at an age when they do not contain osteoclasts it is possible, not only to determine the source of the osteoclast precursors (Scheven et al 1986b) but also to study the effects of bone regulatory factors on osteoclast formation (Scheven and Hamilton 1990). Lastly this system, along with the bone marrow system mentioned below has been used to characterise a novel factor which is released by osteoblasts and stimulates the production, but not the activity, of osteoclasts (Dickson and Scheven 1989).

The advantage of the explant method is that it gives an integrated response of whole bone to particular stimuli. It is also suitable for both exploration and for measurement of biological activities of bone regulatory factors. The major disadvantages are the relatively poor sensitivity, at least to calciotropic hormones, and the fact that it is not possible to ascribe responses to particular cell types within the explant culture.

FRESHLY ISOLATED CELLS

Because it has become clear that some bone regulatory factors act primarily on one of the cell types within bone, it has become necessary to develop methods for the preparation of isolated osteoclasts or osteoblasts.

Isolated osteoclasts

There are three basic methods for the preparation of isolated osteoclasts. The first method is dependent on the sequential release of bone cell types from collagenase treated calvaria (Wong & Cohn 1974;1975). In this method the cells released first are of the osteoclastic lineage, while those released after longer treatment with collagenase are more osteoblastic in nature (see Heersche, these proceedings). A variation of this involves the use of Percoll gradients to fractionate collagenase digests of bone, usually fetal calvaria (Braidman et al 1983;1986). The second method uses femurs and tibias from neonatal rats The bones are split, curretted and the released osteoclasts are cultured in the presence or absence of the regulatory factor under test (Chambers and Magnus 1982). Lastly the culture of bone marrow cells to study the osteoclast has become quite common (Testa et al 1981;Ibbotson et al 1984; van de Wijngaert et al 1987; MacDonald et al 1987).

There are a number of ways of quantifying the number and activity of isolated osteoclasts. Histological methods include the presence of multinuclearity and/or acid phosphatase activity. Although the latter is present in many tissues it is particularly prominent in the osteoclasts (Wergedal and Baylink 1969). There is also a substantial body of evidence which suggests that this or similar enzymes are involved in osteoclast responses to bone regulatory factors (Vaes 1968; Eilon and Raisz 1978; Miller 1985; Braidman et al 1986; Chambers et al 1987). The addition of tartrate to the reaction medium results in inhibition of acid phosphatase activity in all cells with the exception of osteoclasts (Hammerstein et al 1971; Minkin et al 1982). Therefore tartrate resistant acid phosphatase (TRAP) has been used as a histochemical marker for the estimation of osteoclast numbers both in sections (Mostafa et al 1982; Chappard et al 1983; Scheven et al 1986a) and in bone marrow preparations (Ibbotson et al 1984; Pharoah and Heersche 1985; MacDonald et al 1987;Dickson and Scheven 1989). However, in sections at least, some doubt has recently been recorded both as to the degree of tartrate resistance (Webber et al 1989) and TRAP activity has been shown to be present in osteoblasts and osteocytes as well as osteoclasts (Bianco et al 1988; Lundy et al 1988; see also Bonucci, these proceedings). Because of this and the fact that bone resorbing cells are not necessarily multinucleate (Fuller & Chambers 1987), Chambers and colleagues have questioned whether or not multinuclearity and TRAP activity are good markers for osteoclast proliferation and differentiation (Hattersley & Chambers 1989).

Other methods for identifying the number and activity of osteoclasts are available. The changes in cell shape have been used as a basis of an assay for responses to calcitonin (Magnus and Chambers 1982; Chambers et al 1986; see also Wimalawansa, these proceedings). Another method involves the activity of osteoclasts seeded on to bone chips. In this situation, the osteoclasts excavate bone leaving a number of resorption pits which can be quantified using a scanning electron microscope (Chambers et al 1985; Jones et al 1986). This quantification can involve not only number but also the volume of each pit. Lastly the expression of osteoclast cell surface antigens, as determined by monoclonal antibodies, has been used as a means of identifying osteoclasts and their precursors (Horton et al 1985; Nijweide et al 1985; Oursler et al 1985; Athanasou et al 1988).

Isolated Osteoblasts

Isolated osteoblasts are prepared in a number of ways. Firstly, the simple outgrowth of cells from trabecular bone (MacDonald et al 1984, 1986; Beresford et al 1986; Lomri & Marie 1988), secondly by the sequential digestion of calvaria and the culturing of particular fractions (Wong and Cohn 1974; Luben et al 1976; see also Heerche these proceedings) and lastly by using the osteogenic cells from bone marrow preparations (Freidenstein 1980; Owen 1985).

The methods of measuring responses are varied and include collagen production, alkaline phosphatase release osteocalcin production and cAMP release and/or production. In some cases (see Heersche) the cells are cultured under conditions which induce bone nodule formation. Using these preparations responses to a number of growth factors such as TGFß have been reported as have responses to PTH and vitamin D metabolites.

The advantage of isolated cells is that they can be relatively sensitive (in particular the osteoclastic responses to calcitonin) and it is possible to define the dominant cell type with which you are dealing. These systems can also be used as the basis of bioassays but have not been widely applied for this purpose. The major disadvantage of isolated cells is that none of the methods guarantees a pure population of a particular cell type and therefore it is conceivable that some of the responses are being mediated through contact with or factors produced by other cell types in the same culture.

CLONAL CELL LINES

Because of the problems associated with freshly isolated cells, many groups have turned to the use of clonal cell lines. Most clonal cell lines currently in use are derived from either rat (ROS: Majeska et al 1978;1980; UMR: Martin 1976; Partridge et al 1980;1981) or human (SaOS-2, Boland et al 1986:MG-63, Franceschi et al 1988) osteosarcomas. Other cell line includes MC3T3-E1 (Sudo et al 1983) derived from mouse calvaria, and the OK cell line (Teitelbaum & Strewler 1984) derived from the opossum kidney. There is no osteoclastic-like cell line currently available. Most of the osteoblastic cell lines express the characteristics of the osteoblastic phenotype such as high alkaline phosphatase activity, synthesis of type I collagen (Aubin et al 1982), osteocalcin (Nishimoto and Price 1980) and have receptors for PTH (see review by Rodan & Rodan 1984). An in vitro bioassay for PTH, based on the accumulation of cAMP in rat osteosarcoma cells has been described (Lindall et al 1983) but it is not sufficiently sensitive for clinical purposes using unextracted serum.

The major advantage of the use of clonal cell lines is the fact that these are a single cell type of a defined phenotype. They are reasonably sensitive to bone regulatory factors and there is in theory at least an unlimited supply. As noted for freshly isolated cells, these systems can be used as the basis of bioassays but have not been widely applied for this purpose. The major disadvantage is that these transformed cells have an inherent growth potential which may be of importance of assessing the effects of growth factors on these cells and in making the assumption that what happens in say an osteosarcoma cell is the same as that which occurs in a natural

TABLE II. OUTLINE OF THE ADVANTAGES AND DISADVANTAGES OF THE ESTABLISHED TECHNIQUES FOR THE ANALYSIS AND MEASUREMENT OF BONE REGULATORY FACTORS

TECHNIQUE	ADVANTAGES	DISADVANTAGES
1 EXPLANTS	* Cell-cell & cell-matrix interactions maintained	* Relatively insensitive
	* Whole bone response	* Cannot ascribe response to particular cell type.
2 FRESHLY ISOLATED CELLS	* Natural cell type	* Cell-cell contact lost
	* Can be very sensitive	* Purity of the cell population
	* Ascribe response to particular cell type	* Stability of the cell population
3 CLONAL CELLS	* Excellent for assay	* Cell-cell contact lost
	* Sensitive	* Not necessarily similar to native cell type.
	* Ascribe response to particular cell type	* No osteoclast cell line
4 MEMBRANE PREPARATIONS	* Sensitive	* Variabilty between preparations
	* Specificity can be a problem	* Limited application

osteoblast. For instance it has been reported that TGFß stimulates alkaline phosphatase activity in osteosarcoma cells (Pfeilschifter et al 1987; Noda and Rodan 1986a) but inhibits activity in the clonal mouse osteoblastic MC3T3-E1 cells (Noda and Rodan 1986b) and in freshly isolated osteoblasts (Rosen et al 1988). Doubts have also been raised about the stability of the phenotype through successive generations (eg Cole et al 1989).

MEMBRANE PREPARATIONS

A well established method for assaying the biological activity of bone regulatory factors such as PTH, its fragments and analogues, is the use of membrane preparations in which the receptor is coupled to adenylate cyclase. Nissenson et al (1981) used preparations of renal membranes from the dog and a non-hydrolysable analogue of GTP which enhances the cAMP response to PTH (Goltzman et al 1978), as the basis for a sensitive bioassay for PTH. Other groups have used human renal membranes (Neipel et al 1983) or chicks (Seshadri et al 1985a). However, problems have arisen with this type of assay system which have led to the need to either extract PTH from the plasma (Hsu et al 1983) or use specific inhibitory analogues of PTH as a means of ensuring the specificity of the response (Seshadri et al 1985b). To the best of our knowledge, bone cell membranes have not been developed for structure-function studies or bioassays.

It should be pointed out that simple measurement of the binding of a ligand to its cell surface receptor is not per se an indication of biological activity but radio-receptor assays can provide a practical approach to structure function studies when used in combination with other techniques (Kremer et al 1982). Generally speaking the domains for hormone binding are distinct from those for activation of the second messenger systems and thus receptor binding studies are more akin to immunoassays than to bioassays.

VI. IN SITU BIOCHEMISTRY: A POTENTIAL APPROACH FOR THE ASSESSMENT OF THE BIOLOGICAL ACTIVITY OF BONE REGULATORY FACTORS

The methods discussed above are all well established. However, as we have outlined each of these methods has various advantages and disadvantages. The main disadvantage of the explant method is its lack of sensitivity and although the isolated cell methods can be very sensitive, cell to cell and cell to matrix contacts are lost. Over recent years it has become apparent that not only are the activities of osteoblasts and osteoclasts coupled (Rodan & Martin 1981; Wong 1984; McSheehy & Chambers 1986) but that the surrounding tissue matrix can affect the state of cell differentiation (Gibson et al 1982; Benya and Shaffer 1982; Kleinman et al 1987).

Theoretically, a possible way around these problems would be to measure biochemical responses to hormones and growth factors in individual cells maintained in situ in their tissue enviroment. Up till the late 1970's, while this approach was feasible for soft tissues, as evidenced by the work of Chayen and colleagues (Chayen 1984), similar techniques were not available for bone. This was due to the fact that it was not possible to prepare sections of bone without prior fixation and or decalcification. It is well known that fixation can result in substantial inhibition or loss of certain enzyme activity (see Chayen et al 1973; Pearse 1980) and alter matrix components, while decalcification can have much the same effect. With the development of suitable cryostats and the use of tungsten tipped knives these problems were overcome and this led to early studies on the changes in enzyme activity in defined cell types within the fracture callus (Dunham et al 1983) and the effect of vitamin deficiency (Dodds et al 1984; 1986). Recent studies on bone from osteoporotic subjects (Kent et al 1983; Dodds et al 1989) and studies on changes in bone biochemistry during loading (Skerry et al 1988) have been reported and indicate the versatility of this type of approach to the biochemistry of bone. Studies on the relationship between bone formation as evidenced by fluorochrome labelling and osteoblastic alkaline phosphatase activity are also in progress (Bradbeer and Reeve 1987).

These techniques involve the use of cryostat sections for analysis of enzymatic activity which leads to the precipitation of a chromogenic reaction product. The amount of chromophore is stoicheiometrically related to the level of enzyme activity and can be measured in discreet cell types by microdensitometry. This relies on the optical isolation of the cell or cells of interest which are then scanned by a flying spot of light at the absorption maximum of the chromophore and the degree of absorption is quantified by a photomultiplier (Chayen 1984; Chayen and Denby 1968; Loveridge 1983).

The most well known of the in situ biochemical techniques are those used in the cytochemical bioassay (CBA) of polypeptide hormones (Chayen et al 1976). The original CBA for PTH (Chambers et al 1978; Goltzman et al 1980) was based on changes in enzyme activity in distinct regions of the nephron. When first reported this assay was the most sensitive of any of the available methods for assaying PTH. At that time it confirmed the suggestion made by Parsons et al (1975) that the circulating level of bioactive PTH in normal subjects was in the region of 10pg/ml. The new two site immunoassays for PTH have recently achieved sufficient sensitivity (eg Brown et al 1987) and the commercially available "Allegro" assay from Nichols Laboratories, USA, although there is still a slight discrepancy between immunoreactive PTH (iPTH) levels and bioPTH levels (Davies et al 1988). Although the CBA has a low throughput, it has been used in a number of clinical situations where there is a possibility of dissociation between serum iPTH levels and the clinical syndrome or immunoassays are not sufficiently sensitive to detect the level of PTH in the circulation. Examples of these are the work on osteoporosis (Saphier et al 1987, Stamp et al 1988), familial hypercalciuric hypercalcaemia (Allgrove et al 1984; Davies et al 1984), the measurement of changes in PTH-like bioactivity during egg-shell formation in birds (van de Velde et al 1984); the pharmacokinetics of PTH bioactivity as compared to immunoreactivity (Kent et al 1985) and a comparison of PTH bioactivity and immunoreactivity in human and fetal blood at delivery (Allgrove et al 1985).

Perhaps the two most important uses of the renal CBA have been in the study of pseudohypoparathyroidism type I (PSPI) and in humoral hypercalcaemia of malignancy (HHM). In the former, the assay has been used to demonstrate that the aetiology of the disease may not be solely due to a defect at the level of the 'G' protein (see Smith, these proceedings) but also involves the presence in the circulation of an inhibitor of PTH bioactivity (Nagant de Deuxchaisnes et al 1981: Loveridge et al 1982; 1986a,b). In HHM the CBA was used to demonstrate the presence of circulating PTH-like bioactivity in the absence of PTH immunoreactivity (Goltzman et al 1981) and the presence of PTH-like bioactivity in tumours (Stewart et al 1983; Loveridge et al 1985). As mentioned earlier, PTHrP has now been identified not only as a tumour product, but also in non-malignant cells (Theide and Rodan 1988). There is now interesting evidence, confirmed by the use of the CBA, that suggests that PTHrP is present in the circulation and parathyroid glands of fetal sheep (Loveridge et al 1988).

PTH is known to act on two major target organs. There is some controversy over whether or not the carboxyl-terminal regions of intact PTH 1-84 are necessary for action on bone (Goltzman 1978; Martin et al 1979; Zanelli et al 1985a). There is recent evidence to suggest that the contribution of the middle and carboxy terminal portions to PTH binding may vary between renal and osseous receptors (Demay et al 1985; Rao & Murray 1985; McKee & Murray 1985; Murray et al 1989). Additionally in certain conditions such as PSPI the renal and skeletal responses to circulating PTH may be different (Dabbagh et al 1984; Kidd et al 1980). Because of this a bioassay based on the skeletal responses to PTH has recently been developed (Bradbeer et al 1988a). This assay is based on changes in enzyme activity in the hypertrophic zone of the growth plate of rat metatarsals. The assay is as sensitive as the renal CBA and has been used to show that the PTH-like bioactivity in the plasma of PSPI patients is more active on the skeleton than on the kidney (Bradbeer et al 1988a). One intriguing aspect of this assay system is that PTH has a similar effect on osteoblasts lining the metaphyseal trabeculae, a lesser effect on the proliferating chondrocytes and no effect on the periosteum or articular chondrocytes. The differing responses to PTH in the growth plate is in agreement with cAMP responses to PTH which, according to the opinion of de Bernard (these proceedings), are lower in the resting chondrocytes than in the deeper layers.

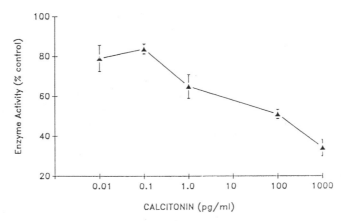

Fig 3.   Inhibition of osteoclastic succinate dehydrogenase activity by calcitonin.

Although to date the in situ methodology described above has mainly been used as the basis of an assay for PTH it has great potential as a means of assessing the actions and interactions of growth factors and calciotropic hormones on bone metabolism. For instance preliminary work suggests that calcitonin inhibits succinate dehydrogenase activity in osteoclasts (fig 3); IGF-I stimulates cell proliferation in chondrocytes as determined by the uptake of 5-bromo-deoxyuridine and TGFß inhibits alkaline and acid phosphatase activity in chondrocytes, osteoblasts and osteoclasts respectively (Loveridge and Farquharson 1989). Another application of this methodology has been to investigate the interactions between vitamin D metabolites and the skeletal response to PTH. Both $1,25(OH)_2D_3$ and $25(OH)D_3$ potentiate the response to PTH (Bradbeer et al 1988b). As this effect occurs after only 8 minutes exposure to PTH it would seem that the vitamin D metabolites must be acting through a non-genomic mechanism similar to that reported for other actions of vitamin D metabolites (Nemere et al 1984). Similarly, in situ biochemistry has shown that alkaline phosphatase activity is elevated in the rat duodenum within 10 minutes of $1,25(OH)_2D_3$ administration (Nasr et al 1988). These techniques have also been used for the analysis of the renal and skeletal responses to exogenous administration of calcitonin to rats by Zanelli and colleagues (Zanelli et al 1985b; Salmon et al 1983) who reported changes in alkaline phosphatase and Ca^{2+}-ATPase activity in the rat.

Like the other methods for analysis of the actions and activities of bone regulatory factors the use of in situ biochemistry does have a number of advantages and disadvantages (TABLE III). Briefly, although these techniques have great potential as a highly sensitive method for investigating the actions of bone regulatory factors they are technically demanding and because of the specialist equipment currently necessary are probably limited to certain laboratories.

TABLE III.   THE ADVANTAGES AND DISADVANTAGES OF IN SITU
              BIOCHEMISTRY

ADVANTAGES	DISADVANTAGES
* Cell-cell & cell-matrix contact maintained	* Technically demanding
* Responses can be measured in discreet cell types	* May be limited to laboratories with specialised equipment
* Highly sensitive	* Too few biochemical methods currently available

VII. SUMMARY

We hope that this chapter has outlined the in vivo and in vitro experimental approaches currently available for the study of the biological activity of bone regulatory factors. Inevitably much of the published work reviewed relates to the endocrine peptide PTH as this is the factor which has been studied extensively by a spectrum of in vivo and in vitro techniques over the last three decades. We have highlighted the differences between biological activity (bioactivity) and binding and immunoreactivity. We have also pointed out the essential role of internationally available reference standards for biological substances which can not be fully characterized by physico-chemical techniques.

The choice of particular methods for the study of the function and activity of bone regulatory factors is a balance dependent on a number of scientific and practical aspects (fig 4) and it should be emphasised that no single method is capable of giving a complete answer as to an assessment of the biological activity of a particular bone regulatory factor.

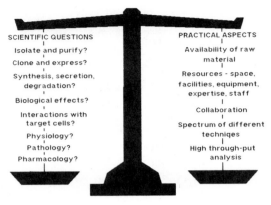

Fig 4.

REFERENCES

Allgrove J, Sangal AK, Low DC, Weller PH, Loveridge N 1984. Biologically active parathyroid hormone in familial hypocalciuric hypercalcaemia. Clin Endocrinol 21:293-298.

Allgrove J, Adami S, Manning RM Chayen J, O'Riordan JLH 1985. Cytochemical bioassay of parathyroid hormone in maternal and cord blood. Arch Dis Chilhood 60:110-115.

Athanasou NA, Quinn J, McGee J O'D 1988. Immunocytochemical analysis of the human osteoclast: phenotypic relationship to other marrow-derived cells. Bone and Mineral 3:317-333.

Aubin JE, Heersche JN, Merrilees MJ, Sodek J 1982. Isolation of bone cell clones with differences in growth, hormone responses and extracellular matrix production. J Cell Biol 92:452-461.

Baumann G, Amburn KD, Buchanan TA. The effect of circulating growth hormone-binding protein on metabolic clearance, distribution and degradation of human growth hormone. J Clin Endocrinol Metab 64:657-660.

Beresford JN, Gallagher JA, Russell RGG 1986. 1,25 dihydroxyvitamin D_3 and human bone derived cells in vitro: effects on alkaline phosphatase type I collagen and proliferation. Endocrinol 119:1776-1785.

Bergeron JJM, Tchervenkov S, Rouleau MF, Rosenblatt M, Goltzman D 1981. in vivo demonstration of receptors in rat liver to the amino terminal region of parathyroid hormone. Endocrinology 109:1552-1559.

Benya PD, Shaffer JD 1982. Dedifferentiated chondrocytes reexpress the differentiated collagen phenotype when cultured in agarose gels. Cell 30:215-224.

Bianco P, Ballanti P, Bonucci E 1988. Tartrate-resistant acid phosphatase activity in rat osteoblasts and osteocytes. Calcif Tiss Int 43:167-171.

Boland CJ, Fried RM, Tashjian AH Jr 1986. Measurement of cytosolic free Ca^{2+} concentration in human and rat osteosarcoma cells: actions of bone resorption-stimulating hormones. Endocrinol 118:980-989.

Bradbeer JN, Dunham J, Fischer JA, Nagant de Deuxchaisnes C, Loveridge N 1988a. The metatarsal cytochemical bioassay of parathyroid hormone: Validation, specificity and application to the study of pseudohyparathyroidism type I. J   Clin Endocrinol Metab, 67: 1237-1243.

Bradbeer JN, Mehdizadeh S, Fraher LJ, Loveridge N 1988b. Certain vitamin D metabolites potentiate the expression of parathyroid hormone bioactivity J Bone Min Res 3:47-52.

Bradbeer JN, Reeve J 1987. In situ measurement of osteoblastic alkaline phosphatase activity in relation to the stages of bone formation. Calcif Tiss Int 41(suppl 2):P95   (abstract).

Braidman IP, Anderson DC, Jones CJP, Weiss JB 1983. Separation of two bone cell populations from fetal rat calvaria and a study of their responses to   parathyroid hormone and calcitonin. J Endocrinol 99:387-399.

Braidman IP, St John JG, Anderson DC, Robertson WR 1986. Effects of physiological concentrations of parathyroid hormone on acid phophatase activity in cultured rat bone cells. J Endocrinol 111:17-26.

Brown RC, Aston JP, Weeks I, Woodhead JS 1987. Circulating intact parathyroid hormone measured by a two-site immunochemiluminometric assay. J Clin Endocrinol Metab 65:407-414.

Burtis WJ, Wu T, Bunch C, Wysolmerski JJ, Insogna KL, Weir EC, Broadus AE Stewart AF 1987. Identification of a novel 17,000 dalton PTH-like adenylate cyclase-stimulating protein from a tumour associated with humoral hypercalcaemia of malignancy. J Biol Chem 262:7151-715.

Canalis E 1980. Effect of insulin-like growth factor I on DNA and protein synthesis in cultured rat calvaria. J Clin Invest 66:709-719.

Canalis E, Raisz LG 1980. Effect of fibroblast growth factor on cultured fetal rat calvaria. Metab Clin Exp 29:108-114.

Canalis E, Centrella M, McCarthy T 1988. Effects of basic fibroblast growth   factor in bone formation in vitro. J Clin Invest 81:1572-1577.

Chambers DJ, Dunham J, Zanelli JM, Parsons JA, Bitensky L, Chayen J 1978. A sensitive bioassay of parathyroid hormone in plasma. Clin Endocrinol 9:375-379.

Chambers TJ, Magnus CJ 1982. Calcitonin alters the behaviour of isolated osteoclasts. J Pathol 136:27-39.

Chambers TJ, McSheehy PMJ, Thompson BM, Fuller K 1985. The effect of calcium regulating hormones and prostaglandins on bone resorption by osteoclasts disaggregated from neonatal rabbit bones. Endocrinol 116:234-239.

Chambers TJ, Chambers JC, Symonds J, Darby JA 1986. The effect of human calcitonin on the cytoplasmic spreading of rat osteoclasts. J Clin Endocrinol Metab 63:1080-1085.

Chambers TJ, Fuller KA, Darby JA 1987. Hormonal regulation of acid phosphatase release by osteoclasts disaggregated from noenatal rat bone. J Cell Physiol 132:90-96.

Chappard D, Alexandre C, Riffat G 1983. Histochemical identification of osteoclasts. Review of current methods and appraisal of a simple procedure for routine diagnosis on undecalcified human iliac bone. Bas Appl Histochem 27:75-85.

Chayen J 1984. Quantitative cytochemistry: a precise form of cellular biochemistry. Biochem Soc Trans 12:887-893.

Chayen J, Denby EF 1968. Biophysical Technique as Applied to Cell Biology Methuen, London.

Chayen J, Bitensky L, Butcher RG 1973. Practical Histochemistry. John Wiley, London, pp 234-246.

Chayen J, Daly JR, Loveridge N, Bitensky L 1976. The cytochemical bioassay of hormones. Rec Prog Horm Res 32:33-79.

Clark CR, Hall MD 1986. Hormone receptor autoradiography: recent developments. Trends Biochem Sci 11:195-199.

Cole JA, Forte LR, Krause WJ, Thorne PK 1989. Clonal sublines that are morphologically and functionally distinct from parental OK cells. Am J Physiol 256:F672-F679.

Cornell HJ, Enberg G, Herington AC 1987. Preferential association of the insulin-like growth factors I and II with metabolically inactive and active carrier bound complexed in serum. Biochem J 241:745-750.

Dabbagh S, Chesney RW, Langer LO, DeLuca HD, Gilbert EF, DeWeerd JH Jr 1984. Renal-nonresponsive, bone responsive pseudohyparathyroidism. Am J Dis Childhood 138:1030-1033.

Dacke CD, Kenny AD 1973. Avian bioassay method for parathyroid hormone. Endocrinol 92:463-470.

Davies M, Adams PH, Lumb GA, Berry JL, Loveridge N 1984. Familial hypocalciuric hypercalcaemia: evidence for continued enhanced tubular reabsorption of calcium following total parathyroidectomy. Acta Endocrinologica 106:499-504.

Davies OK, Hawkins DS, Rubin LP, Posillico JT, Brown EM, Schiff I 1988. Serum parathyroid hormone (PTH) in pregnant women determined by an immunoradiometric assay for intact PTH. J Clin Endocrinol Metab 67:850-852

Demay E, Mitchell J, Goltzman D 1985. Comparison of renal and osseous binding of parathyroid hormone and hormonal fragments. Am J Med 249:E437-445

Dickson IR, Scheven BAA 1989. Regulation of new osteoclast formation by a bone cell-derived macromolecular factor. Biochem Biophys Res Comm 159:1383-1390.

Dodds RA, Catterall A, Bitensky L, Chayen J 1984. Effects on fracture healing of an antagonist of the vitamin K cycle. Calcif Tiss Int 36:233-238.

Dodds RA, Catterall A, Bitensky L, Chayen J 1986. Abnormalities in fracture healing induced by vitamin B6-deficiency in rats. Bone 7:489-495

Dodds RA, Emery RJH, Klenerman L, Bitensky L, Chayen J 1989. Selective depression of particular metabolic activities in cortical osteoblasts at the site of femoral neck fractures. Calcif Tiss Int 44 (suppl): S38 (abstract).

Dunham J, Catterall A, Bitensky L, Chayen J 1983. Metabolic changes in the cells of the callus during fracture healing in the rat. Calcif Tiss Int 35:56-61.

Drop SLS, Valiquette G, Guyda HJ, Corvol MT, Posner BI 1979. Partial purification and characterisation of a binding protein for insulin-like activity (ILAs) in human amniotic fluid: a possible inhibitor of insulin-like activity. Acta Endocr (Copenh) 90:505-518.

Eilon B, Raisz LG 1978. Comparison of the effects of stimulators and inhibitors of resorption on the release of lysosomal enzymes and radioactive calcium from fetal bone in culture. Endocrinol 103:1969-1975.

Finney DJ 1978. Statistical Method in Biological Assay. 3rd Edition. Charles Griffin & Co.

Fuller K, Chambers TJ 1987. Generation of osteoclasts in cultures of rabbit bone marrow and spleen cells. J Cell Physiol 132:441-452.

Franceschi RT, Romano PR, Park K-Y 1988. Regulation of type I collagen synthesis by 1,25-dihydroxyvitamin D_3 in human osteosarcoma cells. J Biol Chem 263:18938-18945.

Friedenstein A 1980. Stromal mechanisms of bone marrow: cloning in vitro and retransplantation in vivo In: Immunobiology of Bone Marrow (Thierenfelder S Ed), Springer Verlag, Berlin pp 19-29.

Gaillard PJ 1955. Parathyroid gland tissue and bone in vitro. Exp Cell Res (Suppl) 3:154-169.

Gaillard PJ 1961. Parathyroid and bone tissue in culture. In: The Parathyroids (eds Greep RO, Talmage RV), Charles C Thomas, Springfield Illinois, pp 20-48.

Gaines-Das RE, Tydeman MS 1978. Interative weighted regression analysis of logit responses. A computer program for analysis of bioassays and immunoassays. Computer Programs in Biomedicine 15:13-22.

Gibson GJ, Schor SL, Grant ME 1982. Effects of matrix macromolecules on chondrocyte gene expression: synthesis of a low molecular weight collagen species by cells cultured within collagen gels. J Cell Biol 93:767-774.

Goldhaber P 1958. The effect of hyperoxia on bone resorption in tissue culture. A M A Arch Pathol 66:635-641.

Goldhaber P 1961. Oxygen dependent bone resorption in tissue culture. In: The Parathyroids (eds Greep RO, Talmage RV), Charles C Thomas, Springfield Illinois, pp 243-254.

Goltzman D 1978. Examination of the requirement for metabolism of PTH in skeletal tissue before biological action. Endocrinol 102:1555-1559.

Goltzman D, Callahan EN, Trgear GW, Potts JT Jr 1978. Influence of guanyl nucleotides on parathyroid hormone-stimulated adenylyl cyclase activity in renal cortical membranes. Endocrinol 103:1352-1360.

Goltzman D, Henderson B, Loveridge N 1980. Cytochemical bioassay of parathyroid hormone: Characteristics of the assay and analysis of circulating hormonal forms. J Clin Invest 65:1309-1317.

Goltzman D, Stewart AF, Broadus AE 1981. Malignancy associated hypercalcaemia: evaluation with a cytochemical bioassay for parathyroid hormone. J Clin Endocrinol Metab 53:899-904.

Hammerstrom LE, Hanker JS, Toverud SU 1971. Cellular differences in acid phosphatase isoenzymes in bone and teeth. Clin Orthop 68:151-167.

Hattersley G, Chambers TJ 1989. Generation of osteoclastic function in mouse bone marrow cultures: Multinuclearity and tartrate-resistant acid phosphatase are unreliable markers for osteoclastic differentiation. Endocrinol 124:1689-1696.

Horiuchi N, Rosenblatt M 1987. Evaluation of a parathyroid hormone antagonist in an in vivo multiparameter bioassay. Am J Physiol 253:E187-E192.

Horton MA, Rimmer EF, Moore A, Chambers TJ 1985. On the origin of the osteoclast: the cell surface phenotype of rodent osteoclasts. Calcif Tiss Int 37:46-50.

Hsu FSF, Pua KH, Nissenson RA 1983. Bioassay of human serum parathyroid hormone using solid phase immunoextraction. Calcif Tiss Int 35:683-689.

Ibbotson KJ, Roodman GD, McManus LM, Mundy GR 1984. Identification and characterization of osteoclast-like cells and their progenitors in culture of feline marrow mononuclear cells. J Cell Biol 99;471-480.

Ibbotson KJ, Twardzik DR, D'Souza SM, Hargreaves WR, Todaro GJ, Mundy GR 1985. Stimulation of bone resorption in vitro by synthetic transforming growth factor-alpha. Science 228:1007-1009.

Jones SJ, Boyde A Ali NN Maconnachie E 1986. Variation in the sizes of resorption lacunae made in vitro. Scanning Electron Microsc 4:1571-1574.

Kent GN, Dodds RA, Bitensky L, Chayen J, Klenerman L, Watts RWE 1983.

Changes in crystal size and orientation of acidic glycosaminoglycans at the fracture site in fractured necks of femur. J Bone Joint Surg (Br) 65:188-194.

Kent GN, Loveridge N, Reeve J, Zanelli JM 1985. Pharmacokinetics of synthetic parathyroid hormone 1-34 in man measured by cytochemical bioassay and radioimmunoassay. Clin Sci 68:171-177.

Kidd GS, Schaaf M, Adler RA, Lassman MN, Wray HL 1980. Skeletal responsiveness in pseudohypoparathyroidism: A spectrum of clinical disease. Am J Med 68:72-77.

Kleinman HK, Luckenbill-Edds L, Cannon FW, Sephel GC 1987. Use of extracellular matrix components for cell culture. Anal Biochem 166:1-13.

Knauer DJ, Smith GL 1980. Inhibition of biological activity of multiplication stimulating activity by binding to its carrier protein. Proc Natl Acad Sci USA 77:7252-7256.

Kumar MA, Slack E, Edwards A, Soliman HA, Baghdiantz A, Foster GV, McIntyre I 1965. A biological assay for calcitonin. J Endocrinol 33:469-475.

Kremer R, Bennet HPJ, Mitchell J, Goltzman D 1982. Characterisation of rabbit renal receptor for native parathyroid hormone employing a radioligand purified by reverse phase liquid chromatography. J Biol Chem 257:14048-14054.

Lane EA, Zanelli JM 1988. Tumour factors associated with the humoral hypercalcaemia of malignancy - acute hypercalcaemic activity of synthetic fragments of parathyroid hormone related peptide. J Endocrinol 119 (suppl) 149 (abstract).

Lindahl AW, Elting J, Elks J, Roos BA 1983. Estimation of biologically active intact parathyroid hormone in normal and hyperparathyroid sera by sequential N-terminal immunoextraction and mid-region immunoassay. J Clin Endocrinol Metab 57:1007-1014.

Lomri A, Marie PJ 1988. Effect of parathyroid hormone and forskolin on cytoskeletal protein synthesis in cultured mouse osteoblastic cells. Biochim Biophys Acta 970:333-342.

Loveridge N 1983. The technique of cytochemical bioassay. In: Cytochemical Bioassays: Techniques and Clinical Applications. (eds Chayen J, Bitensky L), Marcel Dekker, New York pp 45-82.

Loveridge N, Farquharson C 1989. A novel approach to the assay of the skeletal activities of growth factors and calciotropic hormones. J Bone Min Res in press (abstract).

Loveridge N, Fischer JA, Nagant de Deuxchaisnes C, Dambacher MA, Werder E, Devogelaer J-P, De Meyer R, Bitensky L, Chayen J 1982. Inhibition of cytochemical bioactivity of parathyroid hormone by plasma in pseudohypoparathyroidism type I. J Clin Endocrinol Metab 54:1274-1275.

Loveridge N, Kent GN, Heath DA, Jones EL 1985. Parathyroid hormone-like bioactivity in a patient with severe osteitis fibrosa cystica due to malignancy: renotropic actions of a tumour extract as assessed by cytochemical bioassay. Clin Endocrinol 22:135-146.

Loveridge N, Tschopp F, Born W, Devogelaer J-P, Nagant de Deuxchaisnes C, Fischer JA 1986a. Separation of inhibitory activity from biologically active parathyroid hormone in patients with pseudohypoparathyroidism type I. Biochim Biophys Acta, 889:117-122.

Loveridge N, Fischer JA, Devogelaer J-P, Nagant de Deuxchaisnes C 1986b. Suppression of parathyroid hormone inhibitory activity of plasma in pseudohyoparathyroidism type I by IV calcium. Clin Endocrinol 24:549-554.

Loveridge N, Caple IW, Rodda C, Martin TJ, Care AD 1988. Further evidence for a parathyroid hormone-related protein in fetal parathyroid glands of sheep. Quart J Exp Physiol 73: 781-784.

Luben RA, Wong GL, Cohn DV 1976. Biochemical characterization with parathormone and calcitonin of isolated bone cells: provisional identification of osteoclasts and osteoblasts. Endocrinol 99:526-534.

Lundy MW, Lau K-HW, Blair HC, Baylink DJ 1988. Chick osteoblasts contain fluoride sensitive acid phosphatase activity. J Histochem Cytochem 36:1175-1180.

MacDonald BR, Gallagher JA, Anfelt-Ronne I, Beresford JN, Gowen M, Russell RGG 1984. Effects of bovine parathyroid hormone and 1,25 dihydroxyvitamin D_3 on the production of prostaglandins by cells derived from human bone. FEBS Letts 169:49-52.

MacDonald BR, Gallagher JA, Russell RGG 1986. Parathyroid hormone stimulates the proliferation of cells derived from human bone. Endocrinol 118:2445-2449.

MacDonald BR, Takahashi N, McManus LM, Holahan J, Mundy GR, Roodman GD 1987. Formation of multinucleated cells that respond to osteotropic hormones in long term human bone marrow cultures. Endocrinol 120:2326-2333.

Majeska RJ, Rodan SB, Rodan GA 1980. Parathyroid hormone responsive clonal cell line from rat osteosarcoma. Endocrinol 107:1494-1503.

Martin KJ, Hruska KA, Freitag JJ, Klahr S, Slatopolsky E 1979. The peripheral metabolism of parathyroid hormone. N Eng J Med 301:1092-1095.

Martin TJ, Ingelton PM, Underwood JCE, Michelangeli VP, Henk NH, Melick RA 1976. Nature 260:436-438.

McKee MD, Murray TM 1985. Binding of intact parathyroid hormone to chicken renal membranes: evidence for a second binding site with carboxy-terminal specificity. Endocrinol 117:1930-1939.

McSheehy PMJ, Chambers TJ 1986. Osteoblastic cells mediate osteoclastic responsiveness to parathyroid hormone. Endocrinol 118:824-828.

Miller SC 1985. The rapid appearance of acid phosphatase activity at the developing ruffled border of parathyroid hormone activated medullary bone osteoclasts. Calcif Tiss Int 37:526-529.

Minkin C 1982. Bone acid phosphatase: tartrate resistant acid phosphatase as a marker for of osteoclast function. Calcif Tiss Int 34:285-290.

Moseley JM, Kubota M, Diefenbach-Jagger H, Wettenhal REH, Kemp BE, Suva LJ, Rodda CP, Ebeling PR, Hudson PJ, Zajac JD, Martin TJ 1987. Parathyroid hormone-related protein purified from a human lung cancer cell line. Proc Acad Sci USA 84:5048-5052.

Mostafa YA, Meyer RA, Latorraca R 1982. A simple and rapid method for osteoclast indentification using a histochemical method for acid phosphatase. Histochem J 14:409-413.

Munson PL 1961. Biological assay of parathyroid hormone. In: The Parathyroids, (eds Greep RO, Talmage RV), Charles C Thomas, Springfield, Illinois. pp94-113.

Murray TM, Rao LG, Muzaffar SA, Ly H 1989. Human parathyroid hormone carboxylterminal peptide (53-84) stimulates alkaline phosphatase activity in dexamethasone-treated rat osteosarcoma cells in vitro. Endocrinol 124:1097-1099.

Nagant de Deuxchaisnes C, Fischer JA, Dambacher MA, Devogelaer J-P, Arber CE, Zanelli JM, Parsons JA, Loveridge N, Bitensky L, Chayen J 1981. Dissociation of parathyroid hormone bioactivity and immunoreactivity in pseudohypoparathyroidism type I. J Clin Endocrinol Metab 53:1105-1109

Nasr LB, Monet J-D, Lucas PA 1988. Rapid (10 minute) stimulation of rat duodenal alkaline phosphatase activity by 1,25-dihydroxyvitamin D_3. Endocrinol 123:1778-1782.

Nemere I, Yoshimoto Y, Norman AW 1984. Calcium transport in perfused duodena from normal chicks: Enhancement within fourteen minutes of exposure to 1,25-dihydroxy-vitamin D_3. Endocrinol 115:1476-1483.

Niepel B, Radeke H, Atkinson MJ, Juppner H, Hesch RD 1983. A homologous biological assay for parathyroid hormone in human serum. J Immunoassay 4:21-47.

Nijweide PJ, Vrijheid-Lammers T, Mulder RJP, Blok J 1985. Cell surface antigens on osteoclasts and related cells in the quail studied with monoclonal antibodies. Histochemistry 83:315-324.

Nishimoto SK, Price PA 1980. Secretion of the vitamin K dependent protein of bone by rat osteosarcoma cells: evidence for an intracellular precursor. J Biol Chem 255:6579-6583.

Nissenson RA, Abbot SR, Teitelbaum AP, Clark OH, Arnaud CD 1981. Endogenous biologically active human parathyroid hormone: measurement by a guanyl nucleotide-amplified adenylate cyclase assay. J Clin Endocrinol Metab 46:604-612.

Noda M, Rodan GA 1986a. Type ß transforming growth factor inhibits proliferation and expression of alkaline phosphatase in murine osteoblast-like cells. Biochem Biophys Res Commun 140:56-65.

Noda M, Rodan GA 1986b. Type-beta transforming growth factor (TGF-beta) regulation of alkaline phosphatase expression and other phenotype-related messenger RNA's in osteoblastic rat osteosarcoma cells. J Cell Physiol 133:426-437.

Orrefo ROC, Mundy GR, Seyedin SM, Bonewald LF 1989. Activation of the bone-derived latent TGF-ß complex by isolated osteoclasts. Biochem Biophys Res Commun 158:817-824.

Oursler MJ, Bern LV, Clevinger B, Osdoby P 1985. Identification of osteoclast-specific monoclonal antibodies. J Cell Biol 100:1592-1600.

Owen M 1985. Lineage of osteogenic cells and their relationship to the stromal system. In: Bone and Mineral Research Ann Vol 3 (Peck W ed), Excerpta Medica, Amsterdam pp 1-25.

Parsons JA, Reit B, Robinson CJ 1973. A bioassay for parathyroid hormone using chicks. Endocrinol 92:454-462.

Parsons JA, Rafferty B, Gray D, Reit B, Zanelli JM, Keutman HT, Tregear GW, Callahan EN, Potts JT Jr 1975. Pharmacology of parathyroid hormone and some of its fragments and analogues. In: Calcium Regulating Hormones (eds Talmage RV, Owen M, Parsons JA), Excerpta Medica, Amsterdam, pp33-39.

Partridge NC, Frampton RJ, Eisman JA, Michelangeli VP, Elms E, Bradley TR, Martin TJ 1980. Receptors for 1,25(OH)$_2$ vitamin D_3 enriched in clonal osteoblast-like rat osteogenic osteosarcoma cells. FEBS Letts 115:139-142.

Partridge NC, Alcorn D, Michelangeli VP, Kemp BE, Ryan GB, Martin TJ 1981. Functional properties of hormonally responsive cultured normal and malignant rat osteoblastic cells Enodocrinol 108:213-219.

Pearse AGE 1980. Histochemistry: Theorectical and Applied, Vol 1, 4th edition, Churchill-Livingstone, London

Pfeilschifter J, Seyedin SM, Mundy GR 1988. Transforming growth factor beta inhibits bone resorption in fetal rat long bone cultures. J Clin Invest 82:680-685.

Pfeilschifter J, D'Souza SM, Mundy GR 1987. Effects of transforming growth factor-ß on osteoblastic osteosarcoma cells. Endocrinol 121:212-218.

Pharoah MJ, Heersche JNM 1985. 1,25 dihydroxyvitamin D_3 causes an increase in the number of osteoclast-like cells in cat bone marrow cultures. Calcif Tiss Int 37:276-281.

Raisz LG. 1963. Stimulation of bone resorption by parathyroid hormone in tissue culture. Nature 197:1015.

Raisz LG 1965. Bone resorption in tissue culture. Factors influencing the response to parathyroid hormone. J Clin Invest 44:103-106.

Rao LG, Murray TM 1985. Binding of intact parathyroid hormone to rat osteosarcoma cells: major contribution of binding sites for the carboxy-terminal region of the hormone. Endocrinology 117:1632-1638.

Reynolds JJ, Dingle JT 1970. A sensitive in vitro method for studying the induction and inhibtion of bone resorption. Calcif Tiss Res 4:339-349.

Rico AG, Bernard P, Braun JP, Burgat-Sacaze V 1980. Whole body autoradiography in metabolic studies of drugs and toxicants. Adv Vet Sci Comp Med 24:291-311.

Robertson WR, Lambert A, Loveridge N (1987). The role of modern in clinical endocrinolgy. Clin Endocrinol 27:259-278.

Rodan GA, Martin TJ 1981. Role of osteoblasts in hormonal control of bone resorption: a hypothesis. Calcif Tiss Int 33:349-351.

Rodan GA, Rodan SB 1984. Expression of the osteoblastic phenotype. In; Bone and Mineral Research Annual vol 2 (Peck WA ed), Elsevier, Amsterdam, pp 244-285.

Rosen DM, Stempien SA, Thompson AY, Seyedin SM 1988. Transforming growth factor-beta modulates the expression of osteoblast and chondroblast phenotypes in vitro. J Cell Physiol 134:337-346.

Rosenblatt M, Callahan EN, Mahaffey JE, Pont A, Potts JT Jr 1977. Parathyroid hormone inhibitors. Design, synthesis and biological evaluation of hormone analogues. J Biol Chem 252:5847-5851.

Rouleau MF, Warshawsky H, Goltzman D 1986. Parathyroid hormone binding in vivo to renal, hepatic and skeletal tissues of the rat using a radioautographic approach. Endocrinol 118:919-931.

Rouleau MF, Mitchell J, Goltzman D 1988. in vivo distribution of parathyroid hormone receptors in bone: evidence that a predominant osseous target cell is not the mature osteoblast. Endocrinol 123:187-191.

Salmon DM, Azria M, Zanelli JM 1983. Quantitative cytochemical responses to exogenously administered calcitonins in rat kidney and bone cells. Mol Cell Endocrinol 33:293-304.

Saphier PW, Stamp TCB, Kelsey, CR, Loveridge N 1987. PTH bioactivity in osteoporosis. Bone and Mineral 3:75-83.

Scheven BAA, Kawilarang-de Hass EWM, Wassenaar A-M, Nijweide PJ 1986a. Differentiation kinetics of osteoclasts in the periosteum of embryonic bones in vivo and in vitro. Anat Rec 214:418-423.

Scheven BAA, Visser JWM, Nijweide PJ 1986b. in vitro osteoclast generation from different bone marrow fractions, including a highly enriched haematopoietic stem cell population. Nature 321:79-81.

Scheven BAA, Hamilton NJ 1990. Retinoic acid and 1,25-dihydroxyvitamin D_3 stimulate osteoclast formation by different mechanisms. Bone in press

Seshadri MS, Chan YL, Wilkinson MR, Mason RS Posen S 1985a. An adenylate cyclase bioassay for parathyroid hormone: some clinical experiences. Clin Sci 68:321-326.

Seshadri MS, Chan YL, Wilkinson MR, Mason RS Posen S 1985b. Some problems associated with adenylate cyclase bioassays for parathyroid hormone. Clin Sci 68:311-319.

Skerry TM, Bitensky L, Chayen J, Lanyon LE 1988. Loading related reorientation of bone proteoglycan in vivo. Strain memory in bone tissue? J Orthop Res 6:547-551.

Sporn MB, Roberts AB, Wakefield LM, deCrombrugghe B 1987. Some recent advances in the chemistry and biology of transforming growth factor-beta. J Cell Biol 33:105:1039-1045.

Stamp TCB, Jenkins MV, Loveridge N, Saphier PW, Katakity M, MacArthur S 1988. Fluoride therapy in osteoporosis: acut effects on parathyroid and mineral homeostasis. Clin Sci 75:143-146.

Stewart AF, Insogna KL, Goltzman D, Broadus AE 1983. Identification of adenylate cyclase and cytochemical glucose 6-phophate dehydrogenase stimulating activity in extracts of tumours from patients with humoral hypercalcaemia of malignancy. Proc Natl Acad Sci USA 80:1451-1458.

Strewler GJ, Stern PH, Jacobs JW, Eveloff J, Klein RF, Leung SC, Rosenblatt M, Nissenson R 1987. Parathyroid hormone-like protein from human renal carcinoma: structural and functional homology with parathyroid hormone. J Clin Invest 80:1803-1805.

Sudo H, Kodama H, Amagai Y, Yamamoto S Kasai S 1983. in vitro differentiation and calcification in a new clonal osteogenic cell line derived from newborn mouse calvaria. J Cell Biol 96:191-198.

Tashjian AH, Levine L 1978. Epidermal growth factor stimulates prostaglandin production and bone resorption in cultured mouse calvaria. Biochem Biophys Res Commun 85:966-975.

Tashjian AH, Hohman EL, Antoniades HN, Levine L 1982. Platelet-derived growth factor stimulates bone resorption via a prostaglandin-mediated mechanism. Endocrinol 111:118-124.

Tashjian AH, Voekel EF, Lazzaro M, Goad D, Bosma T, Levine L 1987. Tumour necrosis factor α (cachechtin) stimulates bone resorption in mouse calvaria via a prostaglandin-mediated mechanism. Endocrinol 120:2029-2036.

Tashjian AH, Voekel EF, Lazzaro M, Singer FR, Roberts AB, Derynck R, Winkler ME, Levine L 1985. α and ß human transforming growth factors stimulate prostaglandin production and bone resorption in cultured mouse calvaria. Proc Natl Acad Sci USA 82:4535-4538.

Testa NG, Allen TD Lajtha LG, Onions D, Jarret O 1981. Generation of osteoclasts in vitro. J Cell Sci 47:127-137.

Teitelbaum AP, Strewler GJ 1984. Parathyroid hormone receptors coupled to cyclic adenosine monophosphate formation in an established renal cell line. Endocrinol 114:980-986.

Thiede MA, Rodan GA 1988. Expression of a calcium-mobilizing parathyroid hormone-like peptide in lactating mammary tissue. Science 242:278-280.

Ullberg S 1977. The technique of whole body autoradiography. Cryosectioning of large specimens. Science Tools, LKB Instrument Journal 2-29.

Vaes G 1968. On the mechanisms of bone resorption. The action of parathyroid hormone on the excretion and synthesis of lysosomal enzymes and on the extracellular release of acid by bone cells. J Cell Biol 39:676-697.

Van de Velde JP, Loveridge N, Vermeiden JPW 1984. Parathyroid hormone responses to calcium stress during egg-shel calcification. Endocrinol 150:1901-1904

Van de Wijngaert FP, Tas MC, Burger EH 1987. Characteristics of osteoclast precursor-like cells grown from mouse bone marrow. Bone and Mineral 3:111-123.

Warshowsky H, Goltzman D, Rouleau MF, Bergeron JJM 1980. Direct in vivo demonstration by radioautography of specific binding sites for calcitonin in skeletal and renal tissues of the rat. J Cell Biol 85:682-694.

Webber D, Braidman IP, Robertson WR, Anderson DC 1989. The effect of tartrate on bone cell acid phosphatase; a quantitative cytochemical study. J Bone Min Res in press.

Wong GL 1984. Paracrine interactions in bone-secreted products of osteoblasts permit osteoclasts to respond to parathyroid hormone. J Biol Chem 259:4019-4022.

Wong GL, Cohn DV 1974. Separation of parathyroid hormone and calcitonin sensitive cells from non-responsive bone cells. Nature 252:713-715.

Wong GL, Cohn DV 1975. Target cells in bone for parathormone and calcitonin are different: enrichment for each cell type by sequential digestion of mouse calvaria and selective adhesion to polymeric surfaces. Proc Natl Acad Sci USA 72:3167-3170.

Wergedal JE, Baylink DJ 1969. Distribution of acid and alkaline phosphatase activity in undemineralised sections of the rat tibial diaphysis. J Histochem Cytochem 17:799-806.

Zanelli JM, Lane E, Kimura T, Sakakibara S 1985a. Biological activities of synthetic human parathyroid hormone (PTH) 1-84 relative to natural bovine 1-84 PTH in two different in vivo bioassay systems. Endocrinol 117:1962-1967.

Zanelli JM, Salmon DM, Azria M, Salmon GD 1985b. A rat model for resistance to chronic treatment with salmon calcitonin; application of quantitative cytochemistry. In: Calcitonin 1984. Chemistry, Physiology, Pharmacology, and Clinical Aspects, (ed Pecile A), Excerpta Medica, Amsterdam, pp 223-230.

Zanelli JM, Lea DJ, Nisbet JA 1969. A bioassay method in vitro for parathyroid hormone. J Endocrinol 43:33-46.

Zanelli JM, Parsons JA 1980. Bioassay of Parathyroid Hormone. In: Handbuch der inneren Medizin vol 1A (eds Kuhlencordt F, Bartelheimer H), Springer-Verlag, Berlin Heidelberg, New York, pp 599-621.

Zapf J, Schoenle E, Jagers E, Sand I, Froesch ER 1979. Inhibition of the action of non-suppressible insulin-like activity on isolated rat fat cells by binding to its carrier protein. J Clin Invest 63:1077-1084.

CALCIUM REGULATING HORMONES AND HORMONE-LIKE PEPTIDES PARTICIPATE IN BRAIN CONTROL OF BEHAVIOUR

A. Pecile, C. Netti, F. Guidobono, V. Sibilia,
P. Bettica, F. Pagani, and I. Villa

Dept.of Pharmacology, Chemotherapy and Medical Toxicology
University of Milan - Milan, Via Vanvitelli n. 32, Italy

In recent years a number of experimental data have suggested that calcium regulating hormones and hormone-like peptides participate in brain control of behaviour. The peptides directed by the calcitonin gene have been particularly thoroughly studied but immunoreactive PTH material has also been discovered in the brain and has also been suggested to be a neuromodulator within the nervous system. We will consider first the peptides directed by the calcitonin gene and then the brief story of IR PTH in the CNS.

Immunochemical studies have demonstrated the presence of a calcitonin-like substance in the nervous systems of several species including man (Deftos et al., 1978; Cooper et al., 1980; Girgis et al., 1980; Galan Galan et al., 1981; Fischer et al., 1983). The presence of calcitonin-like material demonstrated by immunochemical evidence was not corroborated by the identification in neural tissue of CT mRNA, as shown by recent studies with hybridization with specific calcitonin cDNA probes (Rosenfeld et al., 1982). The gene of calcitonin also appears to encode for calcitonin gene-related peptide (CGRP) in the brain and production of CGRP messenger RNA and CGRP in multiple locations within the nervous system has been demonstrated (Breimer et al., 1988).

Despite the evidence for the existence only of CGRP mRNA in the brain, distinct binding sites for calcitonin and CGRP have been found in the nervous system (Goltzman and Mitchell, 1985). Despite the absence of immunochemical cross-reactivity, each peptide inhibited binding to the high affinity receptor site for the other. Such cross-reactivity was not seen with unrelated peptides and may have reflected in part conformational similarities of CT and CGRP. In the nervous system there appears to be a family of receptors for calcitonin and CGRP. These have been extensively mapped throughout the nervous system by both biochemical and autoradiographic methods (Fischer et al., 1981a; Rizzo and Goltzman, 1981; Olgiati et al., 1983a; Skofitsch and Jacobowitz, 1985; Tschopp et al., 1985; Guidobono et al., 1986b; Guidobono et al., 1987). The demonstrated binding sites for CTs in the central nervous system in physiological terms are for an as yet unknown endogenous ligand. In fact, only binding sites in circumventricular organs of the nervous system may be accessible to circulating levels of CT, but binding sites in other neural regions would predictably not be able to interact with circulating CT of peripheral origin.

The hypothesis that CGRP might have central nervous system actions previously ascribed to CT, in addition to altering neural function at its own receptors, seems unlikely in physiological terms. In fact, CGRP interacts with CT receptors only in very high concentrations. In addition althrough effects of CT on adenylate cyclase were found in neural tissues containing high affinity binding sites for CT, no evidence of CGRP effects has been found in tissues containing high affinity binding sites for CGRP but without high affinity binding sites for CT. Consequently, CT and CGRP may function via separate second messenger systems. Nevertheless, CGRP was able to influence the adenylate cyclase system, apparently through the CT receptors in tissue containing predominantly high affinity CT binding sites (Goltzman and Mitchell, 1985). Therefore, CT and CGRP appear to have discrete target-tissue receptors, with a potential for heterologous interactions, and to have different second messenger systems. With CT binding sites and their endogenous ligand and with CGRP binding sites specific for this peptide biosynthesized in brain, the localization in a variety of discrete brain areas suggests possible neuromodulatory functions.

To discover functions for these neuropeptides in the brain is a formidable task, but they can give clues to still unknown mechanisms of control of central nervous system. Peptides from the calcitonin genes in several species including man have been shown to produce profound effects on physiological behaviour and metabolism mediated by the central nervous system (Breimer et al., 1988). The basic mechanism for these effects appears to be modulation of neuronal excitability (Gerber et al., 1985; Twery and Moss, 1985). Both peptides (CT and CGRP) have been found to depress firing, predominantly when applied iontophoretically to individual neurons of the hypothalamus, thalamus, cortex and other forebrain areas. However, few neurons have been shown to be stimulated. The CTs have been found to inhibit phosphorylation of a number of proteins present in the crude synaptic membrane of brain tissue. These proteins appear to be phosphorylated by calmodulin-dependent protein kinase, since the addition of exogenous calmodulin enhances their phosphorylation and calmodulin antagonists (such as trifluoroperazine, W-7 calmidazolium (R2 4571)) inhibit it. The effects of CT may be the result of a specific interaction of the peptide with calmodulin. Since calmodulin and protein phosphorylation have been implicated in the regulation of calcium mobilization, it is conceivable that CT may inhibit calcium uptake by interfering with calmodulin-dependent protein phosphorylation.

In conclusion, the finding that calcitonin is a potent inhibitor of phosphorylation of selective synaptic membrane proteins suggests a possible basic mechanism for some of the neural actions of this peptide (Patel et al., 1985). The potency of CT noted in Patel's paper was about 100 times less than those noted for sCT binding and behavioural effects of the hormone, but is well within the concentration range at which CT inhibits calcium uptake by neuronal tissue.

CALCITONINS AND CONTROL OF PAIN PERCEPTION

That calcitonin may elicit antinociception through an action in the CNS was shown in our earlier study demonstrating that injection of CT into rabbit brain ventricles enhanced the threshold to the licking reaction elicited by electrical stimulation of the pulp of the upper incisors (Pecile et al., 1975). Autoradiographic studies have shown a wide distribution of CT receptors in structures of the CNS subserving nociceptive transmission or modulation, such as mesencephalic PAG, raphe nuclei and dorsal horns of the spinal cord (Fischer et al., 1981a; Olgiati et al., 1983a; Guidobono et al., 1987). Therefore, CT may act upon specific neurons in these regions.

It was reported recently that microinjection of sCT into the periaqueductal grey matter (PAG) and medial pontine reticular formation induced a dose-dependent increase in hot-plate latencies in the rat (Fabbri et al., 1985). A modulatory function of CT on the electrophysiology of neural pathways involved in the transmission of signals elicited by noxious stimuli has been observed in various animal species. In the rabbit, i.c.v. administration of pCT inhibited the development of the long latency cortical potential evoked by electrical stimulation of both the tooth pulp and sciatic nerve (Yamamoto et al., 1981). In the rat, intracerebroventricular administration of sCT attenuates the nociceptive responses of thalamic neurons to mechanical and thermal peripheral stimuli (Braga et al., 1985). In the cat too, the microinjection of sCT into the mesencephalic periaqueductal grey or the medullary raphe regions reduced noxious heat-evoked responses of lumbar dorsal horn neurons (Morton et al., 1986). Dorsal horn nociceptive responses were unaffected by high doses of systemic sCT, demonstrating that only CT available at specific brainstem sites influences the spinal transmission of nociceptive information. The effectiveness of sCT administered into specific brainstem regions to produce descending inhibition of spinal dorsal horn neurons indicated activation by CT of the descending inhibitory control of spinal nociceptive pathways.

Since CT antinociception shares some CNS sites of action with the endogenous opioid system known to be important inhibitors of the perception of pain, it was hypothesized that CT might elicit analgesia through enhancement of opioid peptide activity. This hypothesis is now completely negated by several lines of evidence. First of all, the opiate antagonist, naloxone, does not reverse either the inhibitory activity of sCT on neuronal firing evoked by noxious stimuli (Yamamoto et al., 1981; Braga et al., 1985) or the analgesic effect of sCT after intraventricular injection into the rabbit (Braga et al., 1978) or intrathecal injection into rats (Spampinato et al., 1984) or microinjection into the PAG of rats (Fabbri et al., 1985). Moreover, another opioid antagonist, levallorphan, did not modify the increase in the pain threshold to pressure stimuli on the tail of mice consequent to intraventricular pCT (Yamamoto et al, 1979). Selective K and opioid receptor antagonists (MR 1452 and ICI 154, 129) also did not antagonize the increase in the hot-plate latencies elicited in the rat by intrathecal sCT (Candeletti et al., 1985). Besides the "in vivo" studies showing opioid-independent mechanisms for CT analgesia, there is evidence "in vitro" that CT does not interact with opiate receptors. In fact, our previous studies demonstrated that CT does not alter electrically-induced contractions longitudinal muscle of guinea-pig after stimulation of the myenteric plexus and that CT does not displace the binding of 3H-dihydromorphine to brain opiate receptors (Braga et al., 1978).

Unlike the opioids, CT antinociception does not develop tolerance since repeated injections of sCT into the cerebral ventricle of rabbits (Braga et al., 1978) or long-term treatment of rats (Spampinato et al., 1984; Guidobono et al., 1985b) are still active in enhancing pain thresholds. Furthermore, sCT induces analgesia in morphine-tolerant rats (Spampinato et al., 1984), thus indicating that the type of CT antinociception is quite different from that produced by opiates. In addition, comparisons between the antinociceptive effects of CT and opiates assessed by various algesic tests show that the antinociceptive behavior of CT is different from that of morphine. In fact, unlike morphine, CT is not able to enhance the nociceptive threshold in the tail-flick spinal reflex in the rats (Spampinato et al., 1984; Fabbri et al., 1985; Pecile et al., 1987), suggesting that CT evokes analgesia predominantly by its action at supraspinal sites.

All these data support the hypothesis that CT antinociception is primarily mediated by the activation of descending inhibitory pathways originating in the brain stem. Since the descending inhibitory systems have been reported to be in part noradrenergic and serotonergic (Yaksh, 1978) and since CT binding sites are located in brain areas rich in catecholamine cell bodies (such as the locus coeruleus) and serotonergic neurons (such as the raphe nuclei), we considered the possibility that CT might exert its antinociceptive activity through modulation of the serotonergic (5-HT)or the catecholaminergic (CA) system. This suggestion was supported by the observation that 5,7-DHT, the neurotoxin of both 5-HT and CA neurons, when administered directly into the raphe dorsalis (Clementi et al., 1985) or i.c.v. or intrathecally in the rats (Guidobono et al., 1986a) completely blunted the antinociceptive effects of sCT. Possible links between CT and the central serotonergic system were demonstrated in our earlier study showing that i.c.v. injection of CT causes an increase in 5-hydroxyindoleacetic acid (5-HIAA) in several brain areas of the rat (Guidobono et al., 1984) and by Bourgoin et al. (1988) of a stimulatory effect of pCT and sCT on K^+ evoked $|^3H|$5-HT overflow from slices of the rat spinal cord. Therefore, we investigated whether or not the action of CT on the serotonergic system might be related to its antinociceptive effect. Selective neurotoxin damage of the central serotonergic neurons (assessed by measurements of 5-HT and NA in brain and spinal cord) was obtained after protecting NA neurons with desipramine administered i.p. 4 h and 1 h prior to i.c.v. or intrathecal

196

injection of 5,7-DHT neurotoxin. Under these conditions, sCT administered i.c.v. or intrathecally was still able to elicit analgesia. Thus the participation of the serotonergic system in CT antinociception seems to be of minor importance. Additional evidence that confirmed these conclusions was obtained with the specific neurotoxin for 5-HT neurons (5,6-DHT), or with an inhibitor of 5-HT biosynthesis, para-chloro-phenylalanine (pCPA) or with 5-HT receptor blockers (metergoline, methysergide, ketanserine). The reduction of serotonergic tone obtained with these pharmacological manipulations failed to modify the increase in hot-plate latencies consequent to i.c.v. or intrathecal administration of sCT in rats (Pecile et al., 1984; Candeletti et al., 1985; Guidobono et al., 1986a).

On the basis of these results and since noradrenergic system has also been shown to modulate the spinal processing of nociceptive transmission we examined the possible involvement of the CA system in sCT induced analgesia. The i.c.v. administration of 6-hydroxydopamine (6-OHDA), a selective neurotoxin to CA neurons, caused a significant reduction in the NA content in various brain areas and complete inhibition of sCT antinociception assessed by the hot-plate test in the rat (Pecile et al., 1984). When 6-OHDA was administered intrathecally to rats, the antinociceptive effect of intrathecal sCT was also significantly reduced (Candeletti et al., 1985), although to a lesser extent than previously. Since 6-OHDA depletes both noradrenergic and dopaminergic neurons, the reduced effectiveness of sCT by 6-OHDA could indicate that both NA and DA systems are involved in CT antinociception. The participation of the NA system is supported by the evidence that propranolol (β_{1-2} antagonist) and atenolol (β_1 antagonist) inhibited the analgesic effect of i.c.v. sCT in the hot-plate test in rats (Guidobono et al., 1985a). The finding that the blocker phentolamine does not change sCT analgesia suggests that β adrenergic receptors are important to CT analgesia. When sCT is administered intrathecally, the α-blocker phentolamine also does not attenuate the analgesic response of the peptide, whereas the dopaminergic antagonist, haloperidol causes a slight but significant decrease in CT analgesia(Candeletti et al., 1985). These results toghether with the observation that 6-OHDA is more effective than ß receptor antagonists in removing sCT analgesia suggest noradrenergic and dopaminergic mediation of CT induced antinociception. However, considering that the neural basis of pain-signalling differs with the type and the duration of the noxious stimuli used, it is possible that there is an involvement of the serotonergic system in the antinociceptive activity of sCT in the abdominal constriction test in mice. In fact, in that case, the inhibitor of serotonin synthesis, pCPA, antagonized the analgesic effect of intracerebral sCT and the blocking effect of pCPA was overcomed by the simultaneous administration of sCT and 5-HT (Bates et al., 1983).

The modulatory effects of sCT on the neurotransmitters participating in pain processing might be attributed to alterations in Ca^{++} flux in the CNS. In this regard, Morley and Levine (1981) reported that i.c.v. sCT decreases $^{45}Ca^{++}$ levels in the rat hypothalamus. The importance of Ca^{++} in CT analgesia was first shown by Satoh et al.(1979), who reported that the analgesic effects of pCT administered intracisternally to mice was inhibited by the simultaneous injection of Ca^{++}. Besides Ca^{++}, drugs that facilitate calcium movement across the membrane, such as the ionophore A 23187, are also able to antagonize the analgesic effects of sCT assessed by the acetic acid abdominal constriction test in mice (Bates et al., 1981). Furthermore in a comparative study by the hot-plate test, we observed that the analgesic potencies of different calcitonins (sCT, hCT, pCT) administered i.c.v. to rats parallel their hypocalcemic activities (Olgiati et al., 1983b), suggesting that modulation of brain Ca^{++} by CTs may account for the inhibitory activity of the peptides on pain perception, at least in part.

CGRP AND CONTROL OF PERCEPTION

The distribution of CGRP in the spinal cord, particularly in laminae containing neurons responsive to both noxious and innocuous stimuli and in ganglia giving rise to C and A (S) afferent fibres (Gibson et al., 1984), its co-localization with the tachykinins and its depletion by capsaicin (Zaidi et al., 1985; Diez Guerra et al., 1988) suggest that CGRP may modulate or transmit sensory impulses. The experimental data are conflicting. Our most recent results (Pecile et al., 1987) show that CGRP administered centrally has an antinociceptive activity that has a different profile from that of sCT. CGRP prolongs tail-flick latencies which are not influenced by sCT and in the hot-plate test CGRP is active but at a higher dose than sCT. In the electrophysiological study, too, the two peptides behaved differently. CGRP completely inhibited the thalamic firing evoked by peripheral noxious mechanical stimuli while inhibition by sCT was only partial. Furthermore, the effect of CGRP was longer-lasting than that of sCT. Bates et al., (1984) also found CGRP to be effective in inhibiting the nociceptive response in mice, but with a different profile from that of sCT, in the acetic acid-induced abdominal constriction test. Antinociceptive activity of CGRP was also found by Welch et al., (1988) but the profile of this action was not clear.

It has been reported that CGRP applied by iontophoresis causes a rather slow and prolonged activation of a subpopulation of dorsal horn neurons. It is possible that the peptide activates dorsal horn neurons by facilitating the excitatory action of substance P (Miletic and Tan, 1988). Recently Kuraishi et al., (1988) reported that an intrathecal injection of an anti-CGRP antiserum increased the nociceptive threshold, thus indicating that endogenous CGRP probably has a facilitating function in nociceptive transmission in the spinal dorsal horn. It is too early to draw conclusions about the action of CGRP on sensory processes. Probably the action of the peptide is complex and depends on the neural structure involved, namely the spinal or the supraspinal areas. Although the exact functions of CGRP are still uncertain, this peptide also encoded by the calcitonin gene, seems to be a candidate for a modulator in the response to nociceptive stimuli.

CALCITONIN AND CGRP IN CONTROL OF NEUROENDOCRINE FUNCTION

The presence of CT-like immunoreactivity in the anterior pituitary of the rat (Deftos et al., 1978) and in the central nervous systems of humans (Fischer et al.,1981b) and the existence of a selective distribution of binding sites for calcitonin (CT) in the hypothalamus, particularly in the medio-basal region, (Olgiati et al., 1983a; Guidobono et al., 1986b) suggest that the peptide is involved in the neuroendocrine control of pituitary hormone secretion. The effects of exogenous CT on anterior pituitary hormone release have been studied: there are only a few studies on the role of CT in the control of TSH and LH secretion (Leicht et al., 1974; Isaac et al., 1980; Mitsuma et al., 1984), whereas the influence of CT on prolactin (PRL) and on growth hormone (GH) secretion has been evaluated, in both humans and animals.

CALCITONINS AND CGRP IN NEUROENDOCRINE CONTROL OF PROLACTIN

The administration of salmon (s) CT, eel (e) CT and $|ASU^{1-7}|$ eCT, into the lateral cerebral ventricle (i.c.v.) of unanaesthetized male rats decreased baseline PRL levels and blocked the PRL release induced by morphine and stress (Olgiati et al., 1980; Olgiati et al. 1981). Furthermore, the inhibitory effect of sCT on PRL release is particularly striking in lactating rats (Olgiati et al., 1982). This enhanced inhibitory effect is probably due to differences in the neuroendocrine mechanisms involved in PRL secretion or to enhanced sensitivity to CT of the pathways mediating the PRL surge in lactation. Since, participation of PRL has been proposed. In the regulation of calcium methabolism, during lactation, it is possible that the potent inhibitory effect of CT on PRL in this condition could serve as a part of the complex mechanism that prevents bone loss and protects the maternal skeleton. An analogue of eCT, ASU^{1-7} eCT, when administered intravenously (i.v.) at high doses in rats, was also able to suppress suckling-induced PRL release, whereas porcine CT did not (Chihara et al., 1981).

The inhibitory effect of CT on PRL seems to be due to a direct action on the central nervous system. In fact, this effect disappeared when CT was administered to median eminence-lesioned rats, in which the central nervous system control of anterior pituitary is disrupted (Olgiati et al., 1981). Further support for this view was obtained by an in vitro approach, incubating sCT with anterior pituitary halves. The spontaneous release of PRL from hemisected pituitaries was reduced only by doses of CT greater than the circulating levels of the hormone reached after i.c.v. administration (Pecile et al., 1980).

Since the hypothalamus is the locus of origin of the tubero-infundibular neurons involved in the regulation of PRL release from the anterior pituitary, it has been suggested that CT-induced reduction of PRL secretion might involve modulation of this dopaminergic pathway. This suggestion is supported by the data showing the complete abolishment of the inhibitory action of CT on PRL by pretreatment with a dopamine receptor blocker (Haloperidol) or with a blocker of cathecolamine biosynthesis (α-MpT) (Olgiati et al., 1980). Furthermore CT is able to counteract the stimulatory effects of morphine and stress on PRL, both conditions which increase PRL release through inhibition of dopamine release from tuberoinfundibular neurons (Gudelsky and Porter, 1979).

Another mechanism that could explain the inhibitory effect of CT on PRL secretion could be alteration of extra and/or intracellular calcium levels. It is well known that calcium is important in neurosecretory processes and that hormone release depends on acute alterations of extracellular calcium concentration (Moriarty, 1978; Isaac et al., 1984). However, the lack of hypocalcemic effects in clinical and animal studies of a dose of CT able to markedly reduce basal PRL levels suggests that CT-induced impairment of PRL secretion is not related to changes in extracellular calcium concentration (Pecile et al., 1980; Pun et al., 1987). Furthermore the reduction of extracellular calcium concentration resulting from larger doses of CT (Pecile et al., 1980; Goltzman and Tannenbaum, 1987) became evident only one hour after treatment, when the inhibitory effect of CT on stimulated PRL secretion was already well established, thus indicating, once more, a dissociation between the two actions.

The influence of sCT on PRL secretion has also been well documented also in man. While neither human or porcine CT altered basal PRL secretion (Stevenson et al.,1977; Barreca et al.,1980), the injection or infusion of sCT always reduced PRL secretion (Carman and Wyatt 1977; Pun et al., 1987). In addition to modifying the baseline plasma PRL levels, sCT reduced the plasma PRL concentrations in hyperprolactinemic patients and caused a rapid fall of the peak TRH-induced PRL release (Isaac et al., 1980). These results do not seem to be related to the different hypocalcemic activities of the CTs used, since ASU^{1-7} eCT which has hypocalcemic activity and stability similar to sCT, did not modify basal or TRH-stimulated PRL in normal subjects and did not suppress hyperprolactinemia in patients with prolactinoma (Kaji et al., 1985). The different activities of mammalian and fish CTs in the control of PRL (mammalian being ineffective) might be explained by the different affinities of these peptides for CT binding sites in the CNS. Autoradiographic studies have shown that human CT has very low affinity for CNS binding sites (Guidobono et al., 1986b), and it is less active in eliciting central activities than fish CTs (Yamamoto et al., 1982; Pecile et al., 1983). There is only one study showing that the central administration of ASU^{1-7} eCT to the rat stimulated PRL release (Iwasaki et al., 1979; Chihara et al. 1982).

These conflicting indications of the role of central CT in the control of PRL secretion might be due to differences in the experimental conditions. In this regard, it has been reported that sCT inhibited PRL secretion in low doses and from 30 min after injection, whereas the stimulatory action on PRL is evident at high doses and within 10 min of injection (Chihara et al., 1982). It is important to recall that CT is able to stimulate PRL release only in urethane-anesthetized rats, and it has been reported that urethane administration modifies the central control of PRL release (Findell et al., 1981), thus indicating that urethane anesthesia is not a useful tool in the identification of the effects of CT on PRL. This assumption is confirmed by the data obtained in conscious rats. In fact, when ASU^{1-7} eCT was administered to freely mooving rats, it reduced basal and morphine- or stress-induced PRL secretion in a dose-dependent manner (unpublished data).

All these observations are in favour of an inhibitory action of CT on PRL secretion. The effect of the peptide involves a specific interaction with its own receptors and not a cross-interaction with the CGRP receptors identified in the CNS (Rosenfeld et al., 1983). In fact, administration of CGRP into the brain cerebral ventricle of rats did not modify baseline PRL levels but significantly enhanced PRL secretion induced by stress or β-endorphin. Since during stress PRL secretion is under the control of PRL releasing factors (PRF), it is possible that CGRP might act through PRF to enhance PRL secretion (Sibilia et al., 1989). Consistent with such an hypothesis is the evidence that CGRP coexists and has a functional synergism with substance P (Gibbins et al., 1985) and VIP (Shin, 1979), considered to be a number of the PRF family.

CALCITONINS AND CGRP IN THE NEUROENDOCRINE CONTROL OF GROWTH HORMONE

CT has been reported to modulate the control of GH secretion also. Studies in humans demonstrated that sCT was able to reduce the GH response to arginine (Cantalamessa, 1978) or to insulin hypoglycemia (Petralito et al., 1979) or to growth hormone-releasing hormone (Lengyel et al., 1989), without influencing baseline GH levels . When sCT was injected i.c.v. into rats, inhibition of morphine-induced GH secretion was observed (Olgiati et al., 1981). The evidence that low doses of sCT or ASU$^{1-7}$ eCT i.c.v. completely suppress the pulsatile GH secretion in rats (Minamitani et al., 1985; Tannembaum and Goltzman, 1985) suggests a possible physiological role of CT in the control of GH secretion. Since CT had no effect on GH release from rat anterior pituitary tissues perfused in vitro (Minamitani et al., 1985), a central site of action has been proposed for the inhibitory activity of the peptide on GH response observed in vivo.

The mechanisms through which CT reduces spontaneous GH secretion as well as GH stimulated by GHRH are still not clear. It is possible that the inhibitory effect of CT on GH might occur through an increase in hypothalamic somatostatin (SRIF) release and/or a decrease in GHRH secretion from the hypothalamus. Since passive immunization with specific antiserum to SRIF failed to restore the amplitude of GH pulses to normal values in CT-treated rats and sCT did not increase hypothalamic SRIF release from hypothalamic fragments in vitro, it is possible that CT blocks spontaneous GH secretion by a mechanism independent of hypothalamic SRIF and this could be the consequence of an alteration of the response to growth hormone releasing factor (Lengyel and Tannenbaum, 1987).

Recently it has been reported that CGRP given to rats i.c.v. also inhibits spontaneous GH secretory episodes and GH release induced by various stimuli, such morphine, clonidine, β-endorphin and GHRH (Netti et al., 1989). CGRP appears to act within the brain to regulate GH secretion, since no effects were seen when the peptide was administered peripherally. The mechanism by which CGRP acts in the brain to reduce the GH secretion elicited by various stimuli differs from that of CT. It seems to be mediated through an increase in SRIF release because in cysteamine-treated rats, when SRIF is depleted, CGRP did not modify GHRH-induced GH secretion (Netti et al., 1989).

Another unique central action of calcitonins is in the control of blood calcium by the nervous system. (Goltzman and Tannenbaum, 1987). A dose-dependent reduction in plasma calcium levels was observed after injection of calcitonin into the brain. They feel that leakage of even a moderate quantity of sCT could not account for the marked hypocalcemic effects of the 250 ng and 2500 ng doses of the peptide administered centrally, inasmuch as central administration of these doses of sCT produced greater effects than the same doses of peripherally administered peptide. Consequently, the hypocalcemia appeared to be a result of a direct action of centrally administered sCT on brain tissue. The physiologic significance of this central effect of sCT is uncertain. To date, we still have no evidence for the biosynthesis of CT within the rat nervous system, despite the presence of CT receptors that are fairly widely distributed in neural tissue, especially within the hypothalamus. CGRP, a peptide known to be synthesized in neuronal tissue may cross-react at CT receptors. Consequently, CGRP may mimic the central hypocalcemic effect as well as other central effects of sCT, but the concentration of CGRP for effective interaction at the CT receptors was found to be very high. To what extent the variety of CNS actions of centrally administered CT may be dependent on the central hypocalcemic action of CT remains to be determined.

CALCITONINS AND BRAIN CONTROL OF FOOD INTAKE AND GASTROINTESTINAL FUNCTIONS

Both the major products of the calcitonin (CT) gene, calcitonin and calcitonin gene-related peptide (CGRP), contribute to the nervous system control of food intake and gastrointestinal functions (such as gastric secretion and gastrointestinal motility). CT inhibits food intake by the rat (Fargeas et al., 1984). Food intake was reduced by 34% in rats treated intracerebroventricularly (i.c.v.) with 4 ng of sCT. This action seems to be elicited by sCT acting directly on the hypothalamus (De Beaurepaire and Freed, 1987), since microinjection of sCT into areas of the hypothalamus such as the supraoptic nucleus, the paraventricular nucleus and the perifornical area significantly reduced food intake, while there was no reduction microinjection into areas not involved in the control of food intake, such as the olfactory tract. Fargeas et al., (1984) showed that the action of sCT is prevented by pretreatment with indomethacin i.c.v., which suggested that this central effect is mediated by prostaglandins.

Binding sites specific for CT can be detected in many areas of the central nervous system (CNS); (Guidobono et al., 1986b) and their distribution in the rat CNS shows high density in the hypothalamus (except the N.Ventromedialis) and the amygdala, which are both very important areas in the regulation of gastric functions. sCT is able to inhibit gastric acid secretion when centrally or peripherally injected. The peptide inhibits gastric acid secretion after i.c.v. administration (Morley and Levine, 1981) or injection into the cisterna magna (Taché et al., 1988), or when microinjected into the lateral and periventricular hypothalamus (Ishikawa and Taché, 1988). After an i.c.v. administration to the rat, 250 ng of sCT a dose that evoked a marked hypocalcemia, Goltzman and Tannembaum (1987) could not detect sCT in the peripheral blood, using a RIA technique without previous extraction. On the contrary, Morimoto et al., (1985) detected a rapid increase of radioactivity in plasma after an i.c.v. injection of ^{125}I-sCT (200 ng/rat). However they did not control by chromatographic analysis whether the radioactivity corresponded to the peptide. Finally, Sabatini et al., (1985) demonstrated a leakage of the peptide into the peripheral plasma after an i.c.v. injection of ^{125}I-sCT (224 ng/kg); in tissues there was a significant concentration of the peptide only in the kidneys and none in the stomach. The same was true also after i.v. injection of the peptide. The plasma levels were 11.1±0.42 fmol/g after i.c.v. and 7.85±1 fmol/g after i.v. administration of CT.

CT inhibits both basal and stimulated gastric secretion. Morley and Levine (1981), using the pylorus-ligation technique, showed that a dose as low as 41 pg/rat of sCT given i.c.v. was active and that the central administration was 1000 times more potent than the peripheral one. On the contrary, our data, while the same for the peripherally active dose, disagree about the centrally active dose of the peptide. In our experiments, in fact, central administration was only 5-6 times more potent than peripheral. However, there are some differences in the methodology used by Morley and Levine and by us, i.e. the duration of experiment, 2 h by Morley and Levine and 3 h by us, urethane-anesthetized rats by Morley and Levine and freely moving rats by us. In our experience, urethane by itself inhibits gastric acid secretion, therefore the discrepancy in the results might be due to the anesthetic used during the Shay test.

sCT administered i.c.v. inhibits gastric acid secretion induced by many vagus-dependent stimuli, such as insulin in fistula-implanted rats (Bueno et al, 1983), TRH (Morley and Levine, 1981) and muscimol (Levine et al., 1981), in the Shay test. The peptide is also very effective in inhibiting gastric acid secretion stimulated by pentagastrin in fistula-implanted rats (Bueno et al., 1983). On the other hand, sCT is not active when the gastric secretion is stimulated by either histamine or bethanecol but it is active on baclofen stimulation of acid gastric secretion measured every 10 min after saline lavage of the stomach (Goto et al., 1986).

It is very interesting that CT prevents gastric ulcer formation Taché et al., (1988) demonstrated that sCT (5 μg/rat) injected into the cisterna magna prevents the formation of gastric ulcers induced by cold-restraint stress, aspirin or TRH. This action of CT might be linked to the inhibition of gastric acid secretion ; CT, in fact, should not be cytoprotective, since it increases, rather than prevents, ulcer induction by HCl and ethanol, probably because it inhibits gastric emptying. Since centrally administered CT inhibits gastric acid secretion but no binding sites for the peptide can be detected in the gastric mucosa, many efforts have been made to explain the mechanisms by which centrally administered CT affects gastric activity.

Despite its marked inhibition of gastric activity induced by vagus-dependent stimuli, CT does not require the integrity of the vagus to exert its control on gastric secretion. The inhibition caused by sCT (416 ng/rat) administered centrally to the rat, in fact, is not prevented by acute vagotomy (Hughes et al., 1985). The action of CT does not even require peripheral catecholamines; pretreatment with bretilium (25 mg/kg), in fact, does not prevent the inhibition of gastric secretion in rats by sCT (416 ng/rat) (Hughes et al., 1985). On the other hand ganglionic blockade prevents CT activity; Lenz et al.,(1986b) demonstrated in the dog that pretreatment with chlorisondamine, (0.5 mg/kg, i.v.) prevents the inhibition by either human calcitonin (hCT) or rat calcitonin (rCT) (3.2 µg/kg, i.c.v.) of pentagastrin (4 µg/kg/h for 180')-stimulated gastric secretion.

The action of CT does not depend on its control of calcemia; Goltzman and Tannenbaum (1987) demonstrated that a dose of 25 ng/rat, of sCT i.c.v. is the lowest dose that induces significant hypocalcemia, while 1 ng/rat is, in our hands, able to significantly inhibit gastric acid secretion in the Shay test. CT does not alter plasma concentrations of gastrin; Lenz et al., (1986b) could detect no change in the post-prandial peak of gastrin in dogs treated with hCT or rCT (3.2 µg/kg, i.c.v.) and even a double dose of hCT (6.4 µg/kg, i.c.v.) does not change basal gastrin plasma concentrations (16). Local changes in Ca^{++} or gastrin concentrations cannot be totally excluded, since it was demonstrated that Asu-eCT inhibits gastrin release in the isolated stomach (Chiba et al., 1980). However the experimental conditions used were questionable (perfusion flow 2 ml/min in gastric artery).

It remains to be clarified whether CT regulate prostaglandin production in the stomach. While Taché et al., (1988) could find no change after an i.c.v. administration of sCT (5 µg/rat) in the gastric mucosal levels of PGE_2 and 6-keto-PGF_1 the major catabolite of prostacyclin, in the duodenal mucosa, they (Taché et al., 1987) found enhanced levels of Keto PGF_1 after sCT (5 µg/rat, intracisternally).

Finally, CT inhibits intestinal motility. Bueno et al., (1983) reported that sCT (4 ng/rat, i.c.v.) given to rats either fed or infused with pentagastrin (6 µg/kg/h) restored the fasted pattern of intestinal motility measured by intestinal electromyograms. CT is not active when the intestinal motility is stimulated by insulin. This action is probably induced via a change in the Ca^{++} fluxes in the CNS. The inhibition of intestinal motility caused by sCT (4 µg/rat, i.c.v.), in fact, is not prevented by i.c.v. injection of piroxicam (30 µg/rat), while it is completely abolished by pretreatment with indomethacin (0.5 mg/rat) (Fargeas et al., 1985a). However it has been demonstrated that indomethacin inhibits fatty acid cyclooxygenase but also inhibits Ca^{++} accumulation by mitochondria and microsomes (Burch et al., 1983). Furthermore Fargeas et al., (1985a) demonstrated that a pretreatment with a calcium channel antagonist TMB-8 (150 µg/rat, i.c.v.), completely prevented the sCT (4 ng/rat, i.c.v.) action on intestinal motility.

CGRP AND NERVOUS CONTROL OF FOOD INTAKE AND GASTROINTESTINAL FUNCTIONS

Calcitonin gene-related peptide (CGRP), the major product of the calcitonin gene in the CNS, is like CT, able to regulate food intake and gastrointestinal activities. CGRP (10 µg/rat, i.c.v.) inhibits food intake in 24 h-fasted rats for as long as 24 h, while a higher dose (20 µg/rat, i.c.v.) is necessary in another experimental model to inhibit spontaneous nocturnal food intake for 3 h (Krahn et al., 1984); this activity is probably elicited through an action on the CNS, since the peripheral administration of CGRP (20 µg/rat, s.c.) is not able to inhibit food intake, even in the first hour after treatment. In a later study (Krahn et al., 1986), it was shown that CGRP may inhibit food intake through an aversive mechanism. The peptide, in fact, in the "Differential Starvation Method" and in the "One-Bottle Conditioned Aversion Method", two tests commonly used to differentiate aversive from satiating effects, clearly behaved like an aversive factor. It is interesting to note that CT, on the contrary, does not cause a conditioned taste aversion (Freed et al., 1979).

While there are still controversial data on the presence of CT in the CNS, many investigators have demonstrated the presence of CGRP in the CNS by immunohistochemical and RIA techniques. Many CGRP immunoreactive fibers have been localized in the lateral hypothalamus and in the amygdala (Skofitsch and Jacobowitz, 1985). Moreover Seifert et al., (1985) demonstrated specific binding sites, in the rat brain, in areas involved in the control of the gastrointestinal activity, such as the dorsomedial hypothalamus and the amygdala. CGRP induces gastrointestinal effects when centrally or peripherally injected. The peptide, in fact, inhibits gastric acid secretion when it is injected into the cerebral ventricles (Hughes et al., 1984) or into the cisterna magna (Taché et al., 1984a) as well as when administered peripherally (Taché et al., 1984b). Moreover, it inhibits intestinal motility when injected into the cerebral ventricles or intrathecally (Fargeas et al., 1985b).

It seems likely, however, that the central and peripheral actions of CGRP are separate. I.c.v. administration of CGRP to the dog, in fact, is not followed by any increase in plasma CGRP immunoreactivity (Lenz et al., 1986a). Lenz et al., (1984) showed that i.v. administration of CGRP antiserum completely prevents the inhibition of gastric acid output induced by i.v. administration of 8.1 µg/rat of CGRP, but could not affect the inhibition caused by the same dose of the peptide injected i.c.v.

CGRP is active on both basal and stimulated gastric acid secretion. Using the pylorus ligation technique, many investigators have demonstrated that the peptide inhibits gastric acid output. 3.7 ng/rat, i.c.v. of rat CGRP (rCGRP) is the lowest effective dose when the gastric acid output is measured by a 2 h Shay test (Lenz et al., 1985). However, there is disagreement in the literature about the lowest effective dose; Taché et al., (1984a) showed that the lowest dose is 973 ng/rat intracisternally (i.c.), while Hughes et al., (1984) assess that a dose lower than 5 µg/rat i.c.v. is ineffective. One possible explanation for these discrepancies, is that the last two papers did not specify which

CGRP was used (rat or human) and, moreover, Hughes et al., used a 1 h Shay test instead of a two hrs test.

CGRP inhibits gastric acid output stimulated by many secretagogues, rCGRP (8.1 μg/rat, i.c.v.) inhibits gastric acid secretion stimulated by TRH (3 nmoles/rat, i.c.v.), pentagastrin (16 μg/kg/h, i.v., for 2 hrs), histamine (4 mg/kg/h, i.v., for 2 hrs) and bethanecol (4 mg/kg/h, i.v., for 2 hrs) (Lenz et al., 1985). In dogs, the lowest effective dose of rCGRP on pentagastrin (8 μg/kg, s.c.)-stimulated gastric acid secretion was 37 ng/kg, i.c.v. and rCGRP (3.7 μg/kg, i.c.v.) inhibited gastric acid output induced by 2-deoxy-D-glucose (100 mg/kg/3 mins, i.v.), but did not reduce the gastric acid secretion induced by a submaximal dose of histamine (80 μg/kg/h, i.v.) (Lenz et al., 1985).

The entire peptide seems to be necessary to inhibit gastric acid secretion. CGRP (1-14), the N-terminal fragment, (Tyr^{23})CGRP(23-37), the C-terminal residue, and (acetoamidomethyl-Cys^{2,7})CGRP, the linear peptide molecule devoid of the disulfide bridge, each at doses of 1 nmole/kg, were not able to reduce the gastric acid output induced by pentagastrin (4 μg/kg/h, i.v. for 3 hrs) (Lenz et al., 1985).

The action of the peptide does not seem to depend on the sympathetic system. Even through CGRP stimulated noradrenergic sympathetic outflow in rat (Fisher et al., 1983), both adrenalectomy and a pretreatment with either bretylium tosylate (25 mg/kg) or guanethidine (40 mg/kg, i.p., 5 days a week for 5 weeks) did not prevent the inhibition of gastric acid secretion caused by CGRP (9.7 μg/rat, i.c.v.) in a 2 hrs Shay test in rats (Lenz et al., 1985; Taché et al., 1984a).

It is still not clear whether the inhibition by CGRP of gastric acid output depends on the vagus. While CGRP (20 μg/rat, i.c.v.) is still able to inhibit gastric acid secretion in pylorus-ligated rats after acute vagotomy (Hughes et al., 1984), the inhibition caused by rCGRP (370 ng/rat) (Lenz et al., 1985) or CGRP (not stated whether rat or human) (973 ng/rat) (Taché et al. 1984a) of pentagastrin (16 μg/kg/h, i.v.)-stimulated gastric acid secretion was completely prevented by acute vagotomy. The differences in the data reported in the literature might be due to the fact that CGRP from different species and different experimental models have been used. While it is not clear whether vagotomy prevents CGRP's action on gastric acid secretion in rats, it seems likely that CGRP does not act through the vagus in dogs. After acute vagotomy, rCGRP (3.7 μg/kg, i.c.v.) is still able to inhibit gastric acid output stimulated by pentagastrin (4 μg/kg/h, i.v.) (Lenz et al., 1986a) and the action of both human CGRP (hCGRP) and rCGRP (3.7 μg/kg, i.c.v.) on an 8% peptone meal-stimulated gastric acid secretion was not prevented by truncal vagotomy (Lenz and Brown, 1987).

The action of CGRP is not altered by ganglionic blockade, since the inhibition by rCGRP (3.7 μg/kg, i.c.v., in dog) of 8% peptone stimulated gastric acid secretion is still present after pretreatment with chlorisondamine (0.5 mg/kg, i.v.) (Lenz et al., 1985) In dogs, it does not depend on opiates or vasopressin, since pretreatment with either naloxone (1 mg/kg, i.v.) or (1-deaminopenicillamine,0-Me-Tyr^2,Arg^8)

vasopressin (200 nmoles/kg, i.v.), a vasopressin antagonist, does not prevent the reduction in pentagastrin (4 µg/kg/h, i.v.)-stimulated gastric acid output elicited by rCGRP (3.7 µg/kg, i.c.v.) (Lenz et al., 1986a). Finally CGRP does not affect the secretion of gastrin, since after hCGRP (3.7 µg/kg, i.c.v.) there are no changes in the plasma levels of gastrin stimulated by an 8% peptone meal in dogs (Lenz and Brown, 1987).

CGRP, like CT, affects intestinal motility. The peptide dose-dependently inhibits the intestinal motility induced by a meal in rat, 0.5 µg/rat, i.c.v. being the lowest effective dose. CGRP is also active after intrathecal injection, but it is not active when injected peripherally (5 µg/rat, i.v.) (Fargeas et al., 1985b).

CALCITONIN AND LOCOMOTOR ACTIVITY

The hypermotility induced by amphetamine has been found to be inhibited by intracerebroventricular injection of sCT (Twery et al., 1983 and 1986). The decreases in amphetamine-induced locomotor activity can be obtained by localized intracerebral infusions of salmon calcitonin into the prefornical area, the paraventricular nucleus, the floor of the hypothalamus, the zona incerta and the nucleus accumbens (De Beaurepaire and Freed, 1987).

The activity of sCT in attenuating the response to amphetamine suggests an interaction of sCT with the dopaminergic system, inasmuch as this system is important for amphetamine-induced motor activity.

CALCITONIN AND TEMPERATURE REGULATION

The intracerebroventricular administraton of sCT or hCT (0.125, 0.250, ng and 1, 2.5 µg) induces an increase of body temperature (up to 1.5 degree with sCT and 1.2 degree with hCT). The effect of sCT is 4 times greater than that produced by hCT (Sibilia et al., unpublished observation). A maximum increase of $2.3 \pm 0.6°C$ was noticed 15-20 min after the i.c.v. administration of 0.02 U of calcitonin to the rat (Fargeas et al., 1985a). Such hyperthermia is prevented by piroxicam, an inhibitor of the cyclooxygenase, suggesting an involvement of prostaglandins.

PARATHYROID HORMONE-LIKE IMMUNOREACTIVE MATERIAL IN BRAIN, WITH A PUTATIVE ROLE AS NEUROTRANSMITTER OR NEUROMODULATOR

Peptides closely resembling mammalian PTH appear to be present ubiquitously in vertebrate pituitary glands and the results of the most recent studies suggest that it may also be present in brain (Pang et al., 1988). The widespread presence of IR-PTH in brain and pituitary tissue suggests that it serves an important although still mysterious physiological function in the vertebrates. The terminal loci of the IR-PTH neurons in the different vertebrate species would appear to be similar to those that secrete hypophysiotropic hormones. PTH-like peptides may be secreted into the hypophysial circulation. These results would therefore suggest that PTH-like peptides may participate in the regulation of adenohypophysial function.

Since PTH has been shown to stimulate prolactin release (Isaac et al., 1978), the PTH-like peptide neurosecretory system may participate in prolactin regulation. The IR-PTH material in the brain may play a role as neurohormone in calcium regulation, but it is also possible that it may act as a neurotransmitter or neuromodulator within the neuronal system. PTH has been found to reduce the pain threshold in male rats (Clementi et al., 1984). The hyperalgesic activity of PTH seems to be located in the fragment 44-68 of the molecule, which possesses hyperalgesic properties similar to those of the whole molecule.

CONCLUSION

From the reported observations, we may conclude that calcium regulating hormone-like peptides participate in brain control. These experimental advances have shed new light on brain functions that may be under the inflence of peptides such as calcitonins and CGRPs. These functions are sensory perception, neuroendocrine regulation, ingestive behaviour, gastric acid secretion, gastrointestinal motility, locomotor activity, temperature regulation, blood calcium control. IR-PTH seems, at present, to be mainly involved in the neuroendocrine regulation of prolactin.

The peptides encoded by the calcitonin gene serve as experimental tools for basic science studies of neuropeptide involvement in brain control. New research projects are under way and new interesting results are expected. In this context, it seems of particular interest that one analogue separates the biological effects of salmon calcitonin on brain and on renal cortical membranes (Twery et al., 1988). This analogue (Gly^8 D-Arg^{24} des Leu^{16} sCT) has selective effects on adenylate cyclase-linked binding sites in brain but not in kidney. This and similar analogues will be useful pharmacological probes for studies designed to characterize the actions of salmon calcitonin-like peptides - the endogenous misterious ligands - in the brain control systems.

In view of the clinical aspects and the therapeutic prospectives, it is clear that the central action of CT may contribute to the interpretation of the overall analgesic activity of the compound and it is the basis for the use of subaracnoid or epidural sCT injection in patients with chronic intractable pain (Fraioli et al., 1982; Hindley et al., 1982; Fiore et al., 1983; Gennari et al., 1985; Serdengecti et al., 1986; Szanto et al., 1986; Kessel and Wörz, 1987)

It is reasonable to believe that the studies on calcium-regulating hormone-like peptides will offer wider insight into the brain control systems and provide unpredictable possibilities for developing new drugs.

REFERENCES

Barreca, T., Milesi, G.M., Magnani, G., Sannia, A. and Rolandi, E., 1980,

Failure of calcitonin to modify prolactin and TSH secretion, Horm.Metab.Res., 12: 174-175.

Bates, R.F.L., Buckley, G.A., Eglen, R.M. and Srettle, R.J., 1981, Antagonism of calcitonin induced analgesia by ionophore A23187, Br.J.Pharmacol., 74: 857.

Bates, R.F.L., Buckley, G.A., Eglen, R.M. and McArdle, C.A., 1983, Calcitonin antinociception and serotonergic transmission, Br.J. Pharmacol., 80 (suppl): 518.

Bates, R.F.L., Buckley, G.A. and McArdle, C.A., 1984, Comparison of the antinociceptive effects of centrally administered calcitonins and calcitonin gene-related peptide, Br.J.Pharmacol., 82: 295.

Bourgoin, S., Pohl, M., Hursch, M., Mauborgne, A., Cesselin, F. and Hamon, H., 1988, Direct stimulatory effect of calcitonin on $|^3H|$5-hydroxytryptamine release from the rat spinal cord, Eur.J.Pharmacol., 156: 13-23.

Braga, P.C., Ferri, S., Santagostino, A., Olgiati, V.R. and Pecile, A., 1978, Lack of opiate receptor involvement in centrally induced calcitonin analgesia, Life Sci., 22: 971-978.

Braga, P.C., Biella, G., Tiengo, M., Guidobono, F., Pecile, A. and Fraschini, F., 1985, Comparative study on the electrophysiological responses at thalamic level to different analgesic peptides, Int.J.Tiss.Reac., VII: 85-91.

Breimer, L.H., MacIntyre, I. and Zaidi, M., 1988, Peptides from the calcitonin genes: molecular genetics, structure and function, Biochem.J., 255: 377-390.

Bueno, L., Fioramonti, J. and Ferre, J.P., 1983, Calcitonin CNS action to control the intestinal motility in rats, Peptides, 4: 63-66.

Burch, R.M., Wise, W.C. and Halushka, P.V., 1983, Prostaglandin-independent inhibition of calcium transport by nonsteroidal anti-inflammatory drugs: differential effects of carboxylic acids and piroxicam J.Pharmacol.Exp.Ther., 227: 84-91.

Candeletti, S., Romualdi, P., Spadaro, C., Spampinato, S. and Ferri, S., 1985, Studies on the antinociceptive effect of intrathecal salmon calcitonin, Peptides, 6 Suppl.3: 273-276.

Cantalamessa, L., Catania, A., Reschini, E. and Peracchi, M., 1978, Inhibitory effect of calcitonin on growth hormone and insulin secretion in man, Metabolism, 27: 987-992.

Carman, J.S. and Wyatt, R.J., 1977, Reduction of serum prolactin after subcutaneous salmon calcitonin, The Lancet, 1: 1267-1268.

Chihara, K., Iwasaki, J., Minamitani, N., Kobayashi, Y. and Fujita, T., 1981, Suppression by intravenous injection of $|ASU^{1-7}|$eel calcitonin of suckling-induced prolactin release on rats, Horm.Metab.Res., 13: 535-536.

Chihara, K., Iwasaki, J., Iwasaki, Y., Minamitani, N., Kaji, H. and Fujita, T., 1982, Central nervous system effect of calcitonin: stimulation of prolactin release in rats, Brain Res., 248: 331-339.

Chiba, T., Taminato, T., Kadowaki, S. Goto, Y., Mori, K., Seino, Y., Abe, K., Chihara, K., Matsukura, S., Fujita, T. and Kondo, T., 1980, Effects of $|ASU^{1-7}|$eel calcitonin on gastric somatostatin and gastrin release, Gut, 21: 94-97.

Clementi, G., Amico-Roxas, M., Nicoletti, F., Fiore, C.E., Prato, A. and

Scapagnini, U., 1984, Hyperalgesic activity of parathyroid hormone and its fragments in male rats, Brain.Res., 295: 376-377.

Clementi, F., Amico-Roxas, M., Rapisarda, E., Caruso, A., Prato, A., Trombadore, S., Priolo, G. and Scapagnini, U., 1985, The analgesic activity of calcitonin and the central serotonergic system, Eur.J.Pharmacol., 108: 71-75.

Cooper, C.W., Peng, T.C., Obie, J.F. and Garner, S.C., 1980, Calcitonin-like immunoreactivity in rat and human pituitary glands: histochemical, in vitro and in vivo studies, Endocrinology, 107: 98-107.

De Beaurepaire, R. and Freed, W.J., 1987, Anatomical mapping of the rat hypothalamus for calcitonin-induced anorexia, Pharm.Bioch.Behav., 27: 177-182.

Deftos, L.J., Burton, D., Bone, H.G., Catherwood, B.D., Parthermore, J.G., Moore, R.Y., Minick, S. and Guillemin, R., 1978, Immunoreactive calcitonin in the intermediate lobe of the pituitary gland, Life Sci., 23:743-748.

Diez Guerra, F.J., Zaidi, M., Bevis, P., McIntyre, I. and Emson, P.C., 1988, Evidence for release of calcitonin gene-related peptide and neurokinine A from sensory nerve endings in vivo, Neuroscience, 25: 839-846.

Fabbri, A., Fraioli, F., Pert, C.B. and Pert, A., 1985, Calcitonin receptors in the rat mesencephalon mediate its analgesic actions: autoradiographic and behavioural analyses, Brain Res., 343: 205-215.

Fargeas, M.J., Fioramonti, J. and Bueno, L., 1984, Prostaglandin E2: a neuromodulator in the central control of gastrointestinal motility and feeding behavior by calcitonin, Science, 225: 1050-1052.

Fargeas, M.J., Fioramonti, J. and Bueno, L., 1985a, Central actions of calcitonin on body temperature and intestinal motility in rats: evidence for different mediations, Reg.Pept., 11: 95-103.

Fargeas, M.J., Fioramonti, J. and Bueno, L., 1985b, Calcitonin gene-related peptide: brain and spinal actions on intestinal motility, Peptides, 6: 1167-1171.

Findell, P.R., Larsen, B.R., Benson, B. and Blask, D.E., 1981, Mechanism of the effect of urethane on the secretion of prolactin in the male rat, Life Sci., 29: 1515-1522.

Fiore, C.E. Castorina, F., Malatino, L.S. and Tamburino, C., 1983, Antalgic activity of calcitonin: effectiveness of the epidural and subarachnoid routes in man, Int.J.Clin.Pharm.Res., 3: 257-260.

Fischer, J.A., Sagar, S.M. and Martin, J.B., 1981a, Characterization and regional distribution of calcitonin binding sites in the rat brain, Life Sci., 29: 663-671.

Fischer, J.A., Tobler, P.H., Kaufmann, M., Born, W., Henke, H., Cooper, P.E, Sagar, S.M. and Martin, J.B., 1981b, Calcitonin: regional distribution of the hormone and its binding sites in the human brain and pituitary, Proc.Nat.Acad.Sci., 78: 7801-7805.

Fischer, J.A., Tobler, P.H., Henke, H. and Tschopp, F.A., 1983, Salmon and human calcitonin-like peptides coexist in the human thyroid and brain, J.Clin.Endocrinol.Metab., 57: 1314-1316.

Fisher, L.A., Kikkawa, D.D., Rivier, J.E., Amara, S.G., Evans, R.M.,

Rosenfeld, M.G., Vale, W.W. and Brown, M.R., 1983, Stimulation of noradrenergic sympathetic outflow by calcitonin gene-related peptide, Nature, 305: 534-536.

Fraioli, F., Fabbri, A., Gnessi, L., Moretti, C., Santoro, C. and Felici, M., 1982, Subarachnoid injection of salmon calcitonin induces analgesia in man, Eur.J.Pharmacol., 78: 381-382.

Freed, W.J., Perlow, M.J. and Wyatt, R.J., 1979, Calcitonin: Inhibitory effect on eating in rats, Science, 206: 850-852.

Galan Galan, F., Rogers, R.M., Girgis, S.M. and MacIntyre, I., 1981, Immunoreactive calcitonin in the central nervous system of the pigeon, Brain.Res., 212: 59-66.

Gennari, C., Chierichetti, S.M., Piolini, M., Vibelli, C., Agnusdei, D., Civitelli, R. and Gonnelli, S., 1985, Analgesic activity of salmon and human calcitonin against cancer pain: a double blind placebo controlled clinical study, Current Ther.Res., 38: 298-308.

Gerber, U., Felix, D., Felder, M. and Schaffner, W., 1985, The effects of calcitonin on central neurons in the rat, Neurosci.Lett., 60: 343-348.

Gibbins, B.L., Furnes, J.B., Costa, M., MacIntyre, I., Hillyard, C.J. and Girgis, S., 1985, Co-localization of calcitonin gene-related peptide-like immunoreactivity with substance P in cutaneous vascular and visceral sensory neurons of guinea pigs, Neurosci.Lett., 57: 125-130.

Gibson, S.J., Polak, J.M., Bloom, S.R., Sabate, I.M., Mulderry, P.M., Ghatei, M.A., McGregor, G.P., Morrison, J.F.M., Kelley, J.S., Evans, R.M. and Rosenfeld, M.G., 1984, Calcitonin gene-related peptide immunoreactivity in the spinal cord of man and of eight other species, J.Neurosci., 4: 3101-3111.

Girgis, S.I., Galan Galan, F., Arnet, T.R., Rogers, R.M., Bone, Q., Ravazzola, M. and MacIntyre, I., 1980, Immunoreactive human calcitonin-like molecule in the nervous systems of protochordates and a cyclostome, Myxine, J.Endocrinol., 87: 375-382.

Goltzman, D. and Mitchell, J., 1985, Interaction of calcitonin and calcitonin gene-related peptide at receptor sites in target tissues, Science, 227: 1343-1345.

Goltzman, G. and Tannenbaum, G.S., 1987, Induction of hypocalcemia by intracerebroventricular injection of calcitonin: evidence for control of blood calcium by the nervous system, Brain Res., 416: 1-6.

Goto, H., Hagiwara, H. and Taché, Y., 1986, Calcitonin as a selective inhibitor of vagal-mediated gastric acid secretion in rats, Gastroenterology, 90: 1434.

Gudelsky, G.A. and Porter, J.C., 1979, Morphine and opioid peptide-induced inhibition of the release of dopamine from tubero-infundibular neurons, Life Sci., 25: 1697-1702.

Guidobono, F., Sibilia, V., Pecile, A., Tirone, F., Parenti, M. and Groppetti, A., 1984, Calcitonin modulation of serotonergic system, In: "Neuromodulation of brain function", G. Biggio, P.F. Spano, G. Toffano and G.L. Gessa, eds., Advances in Biosci. 48: Pergamon Press, Oxford, pp 231-236.

Guidobono, F., Netti, C., Sibilia, V., Olgiati, V.R. and Pecile, A.,

1985a, Role of catecholamines in calcitonin-induced analgesia, Pharmacology, 31: 342-348.

Guidobono, F., Netti, C., Sibilia, V., Zamboni, A. and Pecile, A., 1985b, Behavioral changes and selective decreases in binding capacity to the rat CNS after long-term treatment with calcitonin, in: "Calcitonin 1984", A. Pecile Ed., Excerpta Medica, Amsterdam, pp. 253-260.

Guidobono, Netti, C., Pagani, F., Sibilia, V., Pecile, A., Candeletti, S. and Ferri, S., 1986a, Relationship of analgesia induced by centrally injected calcitonin to the CNS serotonergic system, Neuropeptides, 8: 259-271.

Guidobono, F., Netti, C., Sibilia, V., Villa, I., Zamboni, A, Pecile, A., 1986b, Eel calcitonin binding sites distribution and antinociceptive activity in rats, Peptides, 7: 315-322.

Guidobono, F., Netti, C., Pecile, A., Gritti, I. and Mancia, M., 1987, Calcitonin binding site distribution in the cat central nervous system: a wider insight of the peptide involvement in brain functions, Neuropeptides, 10: 265-273.

Hindley, A.C., Hill, E.B., Leyland, M.J. and Wiles, A.E., 1982, A double-blind controlled trial of salmon calcitonin in pain due to malignancy, Cancer Chemother.Pharmacol., 9: 71-74.

Hughes, J.J., Levine, A.S., Merley, J.E., Gosnell, B.A. and Silvis, S.E., 1984, Intraventricular calcitonin gene-related peptide inhibits gastric acid secretion, Peptides, 5: 665-667.

Hughes, J.J., Gosnell, B.A., Morley, J.E., Levine, A.S., Krahn, D.D. and Silvis, S.E., 1985, The localization and mechanism of the effect of calcitonin on gastric acid secretion in rats, Gastroenterology, 88(5): 1424.

Isaac, R., Merceron, R.E., Caillens, G.P., Raymond, J.P. and Ardaillou, R., 1978, Effect of parathyroid hormone on plasma prolactin in man, J.Clin.Endocrinol.Metab., 47: 18-23.

Isaac, R., Merceron, R., Caillens, G., Raymond, J.P. and Ardaillou, R., 1980, Effects of calcitonin on basal and thytotropin-releasing hormone-stimulated prolactin secretion in man, J.Clin.Endocr.Metab., 50: 1011-1015.

Isaac, R., Raymond, J., Ramfrey, H. and Ardaillou, R., 1984, Effects of an acute calcium load on plasma ACTH, cortisol aldosterone and renin activity in man, Acta Endocrinol., 105: 251-257.

Ishikawa, T. and Taché, Y., 1988, Intrahypothalamic microinjection of calcitonin prevents stress-induced gastric lesions in rats, Br.Res.Bull., 20: 415-419.

Iwasaki, I., Chihara, K., Iwasaki, J., Abe, H. and Fujita, T., 1979, Effect of calcitonin on prolactin release in rats, Life Sci., 25: 1243-1248.

Kaji, H., Chihara, K., Minamitani, N., Kodama, H., Kita, T. and Fujita, T., 1985, Effect of |ASU$^{1-7}$|eel calcitonin on prolactin release in normal subjets and patients with prolactinoma, Acta Endocr., 108: 297-304.

Kessel, C. and Wörz, R., 1987, Immediate response of phantom limb pain to calcitonin, Pain, 30: 79-87.

Krahn, D.D., Gosnell, B.A., Levine, A.S. and Morley, J.E., 1984, Effects of calcitonin gene-related peptide on food intake, Peptides, 5: 861-864.

Krahn, D.D., Gosnell, D.A., Levine, S.E. and Morley, J.E., 1986, The effect of calcitonin gene-related peptide on food intake involves aversive mechanisms, Pharm.Bioch.Behav., 24: 5-7.

Kuraiski, Y., Nanayama, T., Ohno, H., Minami, M and Satoh, M., 1988, Antinociception induced in rats by intrathecal administration of antiserum agonist calcitonin gene-related peptide, Neurosci.Lett., 92: 325-329.

Leicht, E., Birö, G. and Weings, K.F., 1974, Inhibition of releasing hormone-induced secretion of TSH and LH by calcitonin, Horm.Metab.Res., 6: 410-414.

Lengyel, A.M. and Tannenbaum, G.S., 1987, Mechanisms of calcitonin-induced growth hormone (GH) suppression: roles of somatostatin and GH-releasing factor, Endocrinology, 120: 1377-1383.

Lengyel, A.M.J., Toledo, A.L.G., Czepielewki, M.A., Vieira, J.G.H. and Chacra, A.R., 1989, Calcitonin suppresses growth hormone (GH) response to growth hormone-releasing hormone (GHRH) in man, J.Endocrinol.Invest., 12: 25-29.

Lenz, H.J., Mortrud, M.T., Vale, W.W., Rivier, J.E. and Brown, M.R., 1984, Calcitonin gene-related peptide acts within the central nervous system to inhibit gastric acid secretion, Reg.Pept., 9: 271-277.

Lenz, H.J., Mortrud, M.T., Rivier, J.E. and Brown, M.R., 1985, Central nervous system actions of calcitonin gene-related peptide on gastric acid secretion in rat, Gastroenterology, 88: 539-544.

Lenz, H.J., Hester, S.E., Saik, R.P. and Brown, M.R., 1986a, CNS actions of calcitonin gene-related peptide on gastric acid secretion in consciuos dogs, Am.J.Physiol., 250: G742-G748.

Lenz, H.J., Klapdor, R., Hester, S.E., Webb, V.J., Galyean, R.F., Rivier, J.E. and Brown, M.R., 1986b, Inhibition of gastric acid secretion by brain peptides in dog, Gastroenterology, 91: 905-912.

Lenz, H.J. and Brown, M.R., 1987, Intracerebroventricular administration of human calcitonin and human calcitonin gene-related peptide inhibits meal-stimulated gastric acid secretion in dogs, Dig.Dis.Sci., 32(4): 409-416.

Levine, A.S., Morley, J.E., Kneip, J., Grace, M. and Silvis, E.S., 1981, Muscimol induces gastric acid secretion after central administration, Brain Res., 229: 270-274.

Miletic, V. and Tan, H., 1988, Iontophoretic application of calcitonin gene-related peptide produces a slow and prolonged excitation of neurons in the cat lumbar dorsal horn, Brain Res., 446: 169-172.

Minamitani, N., Chihara, K., Kaji, H., Kodama, H. and Fujita, T., 1985, Inhibitory effect of |ASU$_{1-7}$|eel calcitonin on growth hormone secretion in conscious, freely mooving male rats, Endocrinology, 117: 347-353.

Mitsuma, T., Nogimori, T. and Chaya, M., 1984, Peripheral administration of eel calcitonin inhibits thyrotropin secretion in rats, Eur.J.Pharmacol., 102: 123-128.

Moriarty, C.M., 1978, Role of calcium in the regulation of adenohypophyseal hormone release, Life Sci., 23: 185-194.

Morimoto, T., Ikamoto, M., Koida, M., Nakamuta, H., Stahl, G.L. and Orlowski, R.C., 1985, Intracerebroventricular injection of ^{125}I-salmon calcitonin in rats: fate, anorexia and hypocalcemia, Jpn.J.Pharmacol., 37: 21-29.

Morley, J.E. and Levine, A.S., 1981, Intraventricular calcitonin inhibits gastric acid secretion, Science, 214: 671-673.

Morton, C.R., Maisch, B. and Zimmermann, M., 1986, Calcitonin: brainstem microinjection but not systemic administration inhibits spinal nociceptive transmission in the cat, Brain Res., 372: 149-154.

Netti, C., Guidobono, F., Sibilia, V., Pagani, F., Braga, P.C. and Pecile, A., 1989, Evidence of a central inhibition of growth hormone secretion by calcitonin gene-related peptide, Neuroendocrinology, 49: 242-247.

Olgiati, V.R., Guidobono, F., Netti, C., Pagani, F., Bianchi, C. and Pecile, A., 1980, Calcitonin inhibition of prolactin secretion: mechanism of action and possible significance in calcium metabolism, In: "Mineral Metabolism Research in Italy", Wichting Ed., pp 25-29.

Olgiati, V.R., Guidobono, F., Netti, C., Sibilia, V. and Pecile, A., 1981, Calcitonin and pituitary secretion, in: "Monoclonal antibodies and developments in immunoassay", A. Albertini and R. Ekins, Eds., pp. 343-357.

Olgiati, V.R., Guidobono, F., Netti, C. and Pecile, A., 1982, High sensitivity to calcitonin of prolactin-secreting control in lactating rats, Endocrinology, 111: 641-644.

Olgiati, V.R., Guidobono, F., Netti, C. and Pecile, A., 1983a, Localization of calcitonin binding sites in rat central nervous system: evidence of its neuroactivity, Brain Res., 265: 209-215.

Olgiati, V.R., Pecile, A. and Sibilia, V., 1983b, Attività analgesica di calcitonine di diversa origine, in: "Gli effetti delle calcitonine nell'uomo" C. Gennari and G. Segre, Eds., Masson Italia, pp. 205-211.

Pang, P.K.T., Kaneko, T. and Harvey, S., 1988, Immunocytochemical distribution of PTH immunoreactivity in vertebrate brains, Am.J.Physiol., 255: R 643-R 647.

Patel, J., Fabbri, A., Pert, C., Gnessi, L. Fraioli, F. and McDevitt, R., 1985, Calcitonin inhibits the phosphorylation of various proteins in rat brain synaptic membranes, Bioch.Biophys.Res.Comm., 130: 669-676.

Pecile, A., Ferri, S., Braga, P.C. and Olgiati, V.R., 1975, Effects of intracerebroventricular calcitonin in the conscious rabbit, Experientia, 31: 332-333.

Pecile, A., Olgiati, V.R., Luisetto, G., Guidobono, F., Netti, C. and Ziliotto D., 1980, Calcitonin and control of prolactin secretion, in: "Calcitonin 1980", A. Pecile Ed., Excerpta Medica, Amsterdam, pp. 183-198.

Pecile, A., Olgiati, V.R. and Sibilia, V., 1983, Calcitonin and pain perception, in: "The pharmacological basis of anaesthesiology", M. Tiengo and M.J. Cousins, Eds., Raven Press, New York, pp. 157-165.

Pecile, A., Guidobono, F., Sibilia, V. and Netti, C., 1984, Calcitonin induced analgesia: role of monoaminergic systems, in: "Endocrine control of bone and calcium metabolism", D.V. Cohn, T. Fujita, J.T. Pots and R.V. Talmage, Eds., Excerpta Med., Amsterdam, pp. 176-179.

Pecile, A., Guidobono, F., Netti, C., Sibilia, V., Biella, G. and Braga P.C., 1987, Calcitonin gene-related peptide: antinociceptive activity in rats, comparison with calcitonin, Regul.Pept., 18: 189-199.

214

Petralito, A., Lunetta, M., Liuzzo, A., Mangiafico, R.A. and Fiore, C.E., 1979, Effects of salmon calcitonin on insulin-induced growth hormone secretion in man, Horm.Metab.Res., 11: 641-642.

Pun, K.K., Varghese, Z. and Moorhead, J.F., 1987, Reduction of serum prolactin after salmon calcitonin infusion in patients with impaired renal function, Acta Endocr., 115: 243-246.

Rizzo, A.J. and Goltzman, D., 1981, Calcitonin receptors in the central nervous system of the rat, Endocrinology, 108: 1672-1677.

Rosenfeld, M. G., Chijen, R. L., Amara, S.G., Stolarsky, L., Roos, B.A., Ong, E.S. and Evans, R.M., 1982, Calcitonin mRNA polymorphism: peptide switching associated with alternative RNA spicing events, Proc.Natl.Acad.Sci., 79: 1717-1721.

Rosenfeld, M.G., Mermod, J. and Amara S.G., 1983, Production of a novel neuropeptide encoded by the calcitonin gene via tissue-specific RNA processing, Nature, 304: 129-135.

Sabatini, F., Fimmel, C.J., Pace, F., Tobler, P.H., Hinder, R.A., Blum, A.L. and Fischer, J.A., 1985, Distribution of intraventricular salmon calcitonin and suppression of gastric secretion, Digestion, 32: 273-281.

Satoh, M., Amano, H., Nakazawa, T. and Takagi, H., 1979, Inhibition by calcium of analgesia induced by intracisternal injection of porcine calcitonin in mice, Res.Commun.Chem.Pathol.Pharmacol., 26: 213-216.

Seifert, H., Chesnut, J., De Souza, E., Rivier, J. and Vale, W., 1985, Binding sites for calcitonin gene-related peptide in distint areas of rat brain, Brain Res., 346: 195-198.

Serdengecti, S., Serdengecti, K., Derman, U. and Berkarda, B., 1986, Salmon calcitonin in the treatment of bone metastases, Int.J.Clin.Pharm.Res., 6: 151-155.

Shin, S.H., 1979, Prolactin secretion in acute stress is controlled by prolactin releasing factors, Life Sci., 25: 1829-1836.

Sibilia, V., Netti, C., Guidobono, F., Cazzamalli, E. and Pecile, A., 1989, Effect of calcitonin gene-related peptide on prolactin secretion, Pharmacol.Res., 21: 97-98.

Skofitsch, G. and Jacobowitz, D.M., 1985, Calcitonin gene-related peptide: detailed immunohistochemical distribution in the central nervous system, Peptides, 6: 721-745.

Spampinato, S., Candeletti, S., Cavicchini, E., Romualdi, P., Speroni, E. and Ferri, S., 1984, Antinociceptive activity of salmon calcitonin injected intrathecally in the rat, Neurosci.Lett., 45: 135-139.

Stevenson, J.C., Evans, I.M.A., Colston, K.W., Gwee, H.M. and Mashiter, K., 1977, Serum prolactin after subcutaneous human calcitonin, Lancet, 2: 711-712.

Szanto, J., Jozsef, S., Radõ, J., Juhos, E., Hindy, I. and Eckardt, S., 1986, Pain killing with calcitonin in patients with malignant tumours, Oncology, 43: 69-72.

Taché, Y., Gunion, M., Lauffenberger, M. and Goto, Y., 1984a, Inhibition of gastric acid secretion by intracerebral injection of calcitonin gene-related peptide in rats, Life Sci., 35: 871-878.

Taché, Y., Pappas, T., Lauffenberger, M., Goto, Y., Walsh, J.H. and Debas, H, 1984b, Calcitonin gene-related peptide: potent peripheral inhibitor of gastric acid secretion in rat and dogs, Gastroenterology, 87: 344-349.

Taché, Y., Kolve, E. and Kauffman, G., 1987, Potent CNS action of calcitonin to inhibit cysteamine-induced duodenal ulcers in rat, Life Sci., 41: 651-655.

Taché, Y., Kolve, E., Maeda-Hagiwara, M. and Kauffman, G. Jr., 1988, Central nervous system action of calcitonin to alter experimental gastric ulcer in rats, Gastroenterology, 94: 145-150.

Tannenbaum, G.S., Goltzman, D., 1985, Calcitonin gene-related peptide mimics calcitonin action in brain on growth hormone release and feeding, Endocrinology, 116: 2685-2687.

Tschopp, F.A., Henke, H., Petermann, J.B., Tobler, P.H., Jangzer, R., Hokfelt, T., Lundberg, J.M., Cuello, C. and Fischer, J., 1985, Calcitonin gene-related peptide and its binding sites in human central nervous system and pituitary, Proc.Natl.Acad.Sci., USA, 82: 248-252.

Twery, M.J., Cooper, C.W. and Mailman, R.B., 1983, Calcitonin depresses amphetamine-induced locomotor activity, Pharmacol.Biochem.Behav., 18: 857-862.

Twery, M.J. and Moss R.L., 1985, Calcitonin and calcitonin gene-related peptide alter the excitability of neurons in rat forebrain, Peptides, 6: 373-378.

Twery, M.J., Kirkpatrick, B., Lewis, M.H., Mailman, R.B. and Cooper, C.W., 1986, Antagonistic behavioural effects of calcitonin and amphetamine in the rat, Pharmacol.Biochem.Behav., 24: 1203-1207.

Twery, M.J., Seitz, P.K. Allen Nickols, G., Cooper, C.W., Gallagher, J.P. and Orlowski, R.C., 1988, Analogue separates biological effects of salmon calcitonin on brain and renal cortical membranes, Eur.J.Pharmacol. 155: 285-292.

Yaksh, T.C., 1978, Direct evidence that spinal serotonin and noradrenaline terminalis mediate the spinal antinociceptive effects of morphine in the periacqueductal gray, Brain Res., 160: 180-185.

Yamamoto, M., Kumagai, F., Tachikawa, S. and Maeno, H., 1979, Lack of effect of levallorphan on analgesia induced by intraventricular application of porcine calcitonin in mice, Eur.J.Pharmacol., 55: 211-213.

Yamamoto, M., Tachikawa, S. and Maeno, H., 1981, Evoked potential studies of porcine calcitonin in rabbits, Neuropharmacology, 20: 83-86.

Yamamoto, Y, Nakamuta, H., Koida, M., Seyeler, J.K. and Orlowski, R.C., 1982, Calcitonin induced anorexia in rats: a structure-activity study by intraventricular injections, Japan.J.Pharmacol., 32: 1013-1017.

Welch, S.P., Cooper, C.W. and Dewey, W.L., 1988, An investigation of the antinociceptive activity of calcitonin gene-related peptide alone and in combination with morphine: correlation to $^{45}Ca^{++}$ uptake by synaptosomes, J.Pharmacol.Exp.Ther., 244: 28-33.

Zaidi, M., Bevis, P.J.R., Girgis, S.I., Lynch, C., Stevenson, J.C. and McIntyre, I., 1985, Circulating CGRP comes from the perivascular nerves, Eur.J.Pharmacol., 117: 283-284.

DIET AND LIFESTYLE FACTORS IN OSTEOPOROSIS

F. Loré

Institute of Clinical Medicine
University of Siena
53100 Siena, Italy

INTRODUCTION

Osteoporosis represents a prominent public health problem, responsible for very high direct and indirect social costs in western countries.

Osteoporosis can be secondary to diseases or to the use of drugs that cause bone loss, but it occurs more commonly in primary form, particularly in postmenopausal women. The incidence of osteoporosis has increased along with the longer duration of life, that allows most women to spend a significant part of their existence after menopause.

It is generally acknowledged that the main causative factor of postmenopausal osteoporosis is the estrogen deficiency occurring after menopause. However, although all postmenopausal women are estrogen deficient only a proportion of them will experience osteoporosis. Thus, a number of factors must cooperate with estrogen deficiency to determine individual susceptibility.

It is not completely clear what differentiates the women who will develop osteoporosis from the majority who will not. There is no doubt that genetic and constitutional factors play an important role in this perspective: it is well known that black women rarely develop osteoporosis, that osteoporotic patients manifest a familial tendency to the disease and that obesity is a protective factor.

Some of these influences can probably be explained by their effects on initial bone density: blacks have a greater bone density at maturity (1) and genetically determined variations in bone mass can explain the familial pattern of certain cases of osteoporosis (2), although the influence of factors related to the environment and lifestyle of families cannot be ruled out. On the other hand obesity is considered to be protective for two main reasons: more endogenous estrogen is metabolized by the peripheral conversion of androstenedione in fat cells and excessive weight provides a greater stress on the skeleton, thereby stimulating new bone formation.

Therefore, white women with fair complexions or who are short and thin are at greater risk (3) of osteoporosis; these characteristics cannot be modified.

There is a number of other factors, mainly related to diet and lifestyle, that can influence the accretion or loss of bone mineral. Their role in the development of osteoporosis is probably relevant, but their influence in patients with established osteoporosis is likely to be of secondary importance.

Actually, the effectiveness of the pharmacological treatments so far available for established osteoporosis is also often questioned. In fact, an ideal treatment should lead to the complete restoration of the conditions existing before the onset of the disease. This is not possible at present: the best therapies available are effective in blocking the progression of the disease and in increasing bone mineral significantly but the original bone structure cannot be restored.

In postmenopausal osteoporosis, and, to a lower extent, in the process of ageing) spongy bone loss results in a progressive thinning and reduction in number of trabeculae. If we look at the structural changes occurring with advancing age we will notice that a regular trabecular pattern is replaced by a certain degree of thinning of horizontal trabeculations. Later, there is a clear loss of horizontal trabeculae, possibly accompanied by a thickening of vertical trabeculae. Progression of bone loss leads to further disruption of trabecular structure. In advanced osteoporosis the only visible remnant of the original structure may be represented by bone spicules.

Pharmacological agents influencing bone remodelling may thicken remnant structures and increase bone mass but, due to the fact that new bone can only be deposited on preexisting surfaces, the transected structures will never be repared. Thus, despite the encouraging results claimed in terms of increases in bone mineral content, the resistance of bone to compressive forces will not necessarily improve, so that the risk of facture will not automatically decrease.

This is particularly true when the bone mineral content is severely reduced, so that even remarkable increases in bone mass may offer little advantage with respect to the risk of fracture, if the final bone mass remains far below the so called 'fracture threshold'.

Moreover, treatment with inhibitors of bone turnover, such as calcitonin or bisphosphonates, might interfere with the repair processes of the microfractures occurring in trabecular structure, which are believed to represent important determinants of clinically relevant fractures. If this is true such agents, by decreasing the rate of bone turnover, would paradoxically increase at the same time both bone mass and liability to fractures due to delayed repair of 'fatigue' damage.

On the other hand, it should be borne in mind that increasing the trabecular thickness does not necessarily mean improving the mechanical resistance of bone. There are treatments, e. g. fluoride, capable of altering the quality of bone, so that the increase in bone mass achieved is not always accompanied by a parallel improvement of the ability of bone to withstand compressive forces.

For all the aforementioned considerations treatment of osteoporotic patients should begin as early as possible since the lesions of established osteoporosis can hardly be reversed.

However, an early pharmacological treatment of all the subjects at risk for osteoporosis is not feasible. The real problem is the identification of those subjects who will actually develop the disease.

In a simplified view of the problem one could assume that the amount of bone existing in a given women in a given moment of her postmenoausal life is the result of two main factors:
- the bone mass present at skeletal maturity (around age 40);
- the subsequent rate and duration of bone loss.

It appears that two characteristic groups may be distinguished: a proportion of postmenopausal women would lose significant amounts of bone ('fast losers'), whereas the majority of them would lose only about one per cent per year ('normal losers').

Several screening procedures have been suggested for the identification of fast losers. Most of them are based on bone mass measurements and determination of biochemical estimates of bone formation and resorption. In our opinion, however, none of them has revealed to be both easily feasible and effective.

What we can safely do is to identify the risk factors for osteoporosis related to diet and lifestyle. These can be easily avoided and these preventive measures can be applied to all the potential osteoporotic individuals safely and with no adverse effects.

Several of these factors have been identified: many commonly ingested substances, apart from drugs, have been found to influence the calcium economy of the organism in varying ways and to varying degrees.

A high caffeine intake increases the urinary calcium excretion by an unidentified mechanism (5), but the effect is small, so that at moderate coffee intake levels is probably of little importance.

Smoking is associated with reduced bone mass (6-8), but it is not known whether this is due to the lower weight of smokers, to the common occurrence of chronic pulmonary disease with consequent system acidosis or to the earlier menopause usually experienced by these women (6,9).

Alcohol excess also leads to bone loss (8,10). The mechanism of alcohol effect has only been partly worked out, but its importance can hardly be doubted. A combination of factors have been implicated: poor nutrition, including an inadequate intake of calcium and vitamin D; gastro-intestinal and pancreatic malfunction, inhibition of intestinal calcium absorption (11). A depression of bone formation by a direct effect on osteoblasts has also been suggested (12,13).

Other nutritional factors seem to be less important: among them a high protein intake, responsible for increases in urinary calcium excretion through the inhibition of renal tubular resorption exerted by acid radicals (5), or the excess of dietary phosphorus resulting from a large consumption of soft drinks (14).

The actual relevance of the above nutritional and behavioural elements as risk factors in the development of osteoporosis, however, is still controversial.

Apart from them, three main factors related to diet and lifestyle appear of major importance: calcium intake, vitamin D and exercise.

DIETARY CALCIUM

A person wanting to find out in the literature information about the role of dietary calcium in the development or treatment of osteoporosis would be bewildered and confused by the variety of experimental approaches used and results obtained.

Actually, many investigators have looked at this issue over the past 30 years and a great variety of studies have been carried out in order to assess the relationship between calcium intake and bone health: current bone mass has been related to current calcium intake in cross-sectional epidemiological studies; changes in bone mass have been related to current calcium intake in longitudinal studies; rate of change in bone mass has been related to direct calcium supplementation in prospective, controlled studies; calcium requirement has been assessed by metabolic balance studies; etc.

Of the cross-sectional studies the majority showed a positive correlation between current bone mass and current calcium intake, but some did not. Among longitudinal studies a proportion showed a positive correlation between changes in current bone mass and calcium intake, but others failed to find such a relationship. Prospective trials demostrated a decrease in the rate of bone loss with high dose oral calcium supplementation, but other studies showed no effect. Finally, metabolic balance studies showed a positive correlation between calcium intake and calcium balance (15).

Let us put some order in this controversy.

Calcium is absorbed primarily in the small intestine with a maximum in the duodenum and proximal jejunum. Calcium absorption depends on the combination of three processes: passive diffusion, binding to a protein carrier, active transport. In normal individuals there is a 'adaptation' of this process to the level of calcium intake: in the presence of low dietary calcium intake the absorption of calcium becomes more efficient and higher percentages of this mineral are absorbed from the gut.

The mechanism of this adaptation is based on the regulation by parathyroid hormone of the synthesis of 1,25-dihydroxyvitamin D (1,25(OH)2D), the active vitamin D metabolite, which is the main or sole determinant of the active calcium transfer.

Intestinal calcium absorption decreases in elderly women and the adaptation mechanism does not operate in women with osteoporosis.

There is no doubt that postmenopausal osteoporosis is associated with decreased calcium absorption (16). It has also been demonstrated that the dietary calcium intake of osteoporotic women is lower than that of non osteoporotic controls (17) and the calcium deficiency model is still considered the most credible one, but this view does not imply that osteoporosis can be cured by increasing the dietary intake of calcium.

In fact, a very recent trial has examined the influence of dietary intake of calcium on bone in a large group of women early in the menopause and the possible additive effect of calcium intake in treatments that could prevent bone loss (18). No correlation was found between current intake of calcium and either total calcium in the body or the density of trabecular or cortical bone in the forearm or vertebral trabecular lone. The dietary intake of calcium did not influence the rate of postmenopausal bone loss in the women who completed 12 months of active or placebo treatment.

A possible explanation of this finding is that in postmenopusal osteoporotic women there is a defect of calcium absorption that cannot be overcome only by increasing the dietary calcium intake.

It seems that the role of dietary calcium in postmenopausal osteoporotic women has been overemphasized.

In 1984 the Consensus Development Conference on Osteoporosis concluded that the daily requirement for maintenance of skeletal mass was 1,000 mg per day in postmenopausal and 1,500 mg in untreated postmenopausal women.

This recommendation was mainly based on a study (19) of calcium balance in which the authors hypothesized that if calcium balance were a linear function of calcium intake, zero calcium balance would occur at a daily calcium intake of 989 mg in premenopausal and 1,504 mg in postmenopausal women.

This model has not been confirmed experimentally and a subsequent report (20) revealed no correlation between dietary calcium intake and calcium balance for intakes higher than 1000 mg per day: in this new model optimal calcium intake is asymptotically approached at 1,000 mg per day; estrogen (and 1,25-dihydroxyvitamin D) deficiency in postmenopausal women results in negative balance, which is not fully corrected even by extraordinarily high dietary calcium intake (21).

The conclusion can be drawn that, even if, obviously, a minimum requirement of dietary calcium must be met, a high calcium intake alone is not an effective treatment of postmenopausal osteoporosis, probably because its intestinal absorption is impaired.

A different problem is that of the role of calcium in the prevention of osteoporosis. Several studies have supported the view that the dietary intake of calcium may modify the peak bone mass. A study carried out in Yugoslavia a few years ago (22) has obtained a certain popularity among calcium metabolism researchers. In this study individuals from a "high calcium" and a neighboring "low calcium" area were compared. It was found that women from the region where dietary calcium intake was high (940 mg per day) had half the femoral fracture rate of women in the areas with a lower calcium intake (470 mg per day).

In other words epidemiologic data support the concept that higher calcium consumption during growth and early adulthood is associated with a higher peak bone density.

VITAMIN D

The role of vitamin D and its metabolites in postmenopausal osteoporosis is considered in another part of this volume. I would like to report here the results of a study, recently carried out in this Institute, about the occurrence and characteristics of vitamin D deficiency in the elderly and its possible consequences on bone.

It is generally agreed that the serum levels of 25-hydroxyvitamin D (25OHD) represent a good index of the so called 'vitamin D status' of the organism, resulting from both the physiological sources of the vitamin: endogenous synthesis in skin, as a result of ultraviolet sunlight irradiation, and dietary intake through the intestinal absorption. Indeed, it has been shown that more than 80% of the vitamin D entering the circulation is rapidly taken up by the liver, where it undergoes C-25 hydroxylation, and is released in the blood stream as 25OHD (23).

Vitamin D status is known to vary according to a number of factors such as the duration, intensity and wavelenght of sunlight exposure, the characteristics of the skin, and also diet, intestinal absorption, etc.

We have studied 318 healthy subjects (161 males, 157 females), of both sexes and all ages, from 6 months to 96 years; there were 69 children, 189 adults and 60 elderly subjects (24).

The method used for 25OHD determination can be summarized as follows: protein precipitation and lipid extraction of samples, column chromatography on Sep-pak silica cartridges (Millipore, Stillwater, Minn., USA), competitive protein binding assay using rat serum as the source of binding protein (25).

Children and young adults up to the age of forty showed similar mean values, but the range was remarkably wide. It is likely that this was mainly a consequence of differences amongst individual subjects in open air activities, and, therefore, in sunlight exposure. After the age of forty there was a progressive decrease up to the extreme age of life.

A similar pattern is shown by females. However, the decrease in serum 25OHD appears to begin earlier than in men. The levels observed in elderly women are sometimes very low.

Our results confirm that age is an important determinant of vitamin D status in man.

Concerning sex-related differences a comparison of the correlations between serum 25OHD and age indicate that females generally exhibit slightly lower levels than males.

The examination of the results obtained in the oldest subjects of both sexes reveals a pattern that can only be described as a subclinical condition of vitamin deficiency.

The distribution of 25OHD values in our 60 subjects aged 81 or more reveals some interesting aspects. It is known that 25OHD values usually show a distribution which is quite different from the 'normal' distribution. However, a significant logarithmic pattern can rarely be demonstrated. This aspect is more evident in groups of subjects with low 25OHD levels. Our elderly subjects showed an asymmetrical distribution of 25OHD values, in which the majority of values fell below the mean. After logarithmic transformation the values showed a pattern very similar to a normal distribution. The statistical significance of the similarity of this distribution to a Gaussian curve has been demonstrated by the Shapiro and Wilk test (26).

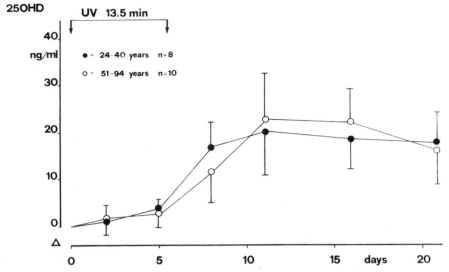

Fig. 1. 25OHD response to artificial ultraviolet irradiation (UV) in normal subjects aged 24-40 or 51-94 years.

As to the causes of the decrease in 25OHD levels with increasing age, it has been suggested that the main steps of vitamin D synthesis and metabolism might be impaired in the elderly and in particular, cutaneous synthesis, intestinal absorption, and liver hydroxylation. A clear demonstration of such an impairment, however, is still lacking.

We have considered this aspect and have designed a few studies aimed at ascertaining the ability of elderly subjects to synthesize vitamin D, absorb it from food and hydroxylate it in the liver. In these studies we have failed to demonstrate any significant difference between young and elderly normal subjects, concerning 25OHD response to whole-body irradiation with artificial ultraviolet light (27). This indicates that neither cutaneous synthesis nor liver hydroxylation of vitamin D are grossly impaired in healthy elderly subjects (Fig. 1).

Similarly, the intestinal absorption of vitamin D, after administration of a known oral dose, was not found to be significantly less efficient in young as compared with elderly subjects, in a study aimed to evaluate the effect of age on vitamin D absorption (28) (Fig.2).

Therefore, although it cannot be excluded that reduced intestinal absorption or impaired liver hydroxylation might play a role in some individual case, it seems likely that reduced sunlight exposure and low dietary intake of vitamin D are the main determinants of the impairment of vitamin D status in the elderly.

In fact, geriatric subjects are often confined indoors;

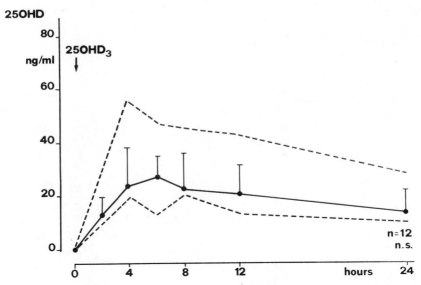

Fig. 2. 25OHD response to the oral administration of 25OHD3 (4 µg/Kg body weight) in a group of elderly subjects. Dotted lines indicate the range in young adults.

particularly in winter, when the low external temperature prevents outdoor activities. Moreover, the diet of elderly subjects is often poor and unbalanced.

Reduced sunlight exposure is certainly the predominant factor, since it is generally agreed that ultraviolet irradiation contributes more to serum 25OHD than does oral vitamin D.

Another aspect of vitamin D physiology is represented by the circannual variation of 25OHD levels as a consequence of seasonal changes in sunlight irradiation. Experimental evidence indicates that there is no such rhythm in the serum levels of 1,25(OH)2D (29, 30). This fact is considered to result from the tight regulation of the synthesis of the hormonal form of vitamin D, according to the calcium demand of the organism (31).

In a cross-sectional study we have considered 227 individuals divided into two groups. The first group included 107 subjects aged 20 to 55. The second group consisted of 120 elderly subjects aged 66 to 95. None of them suffered from endocrine diseases or from diseases known to affect vitamin D or calcium metabolism. Renal function, as assessed by blood urea nitrogen and serum creatinine, was normal according to age. They were not taking any medication known to interfere with calcium metabolism and did not take calcium or vitamin D supplements. In these subjects we measured serum 25OHD, 1,25(OH)2D, calcium, phosphate and alkaline phosphatase throughout one year.

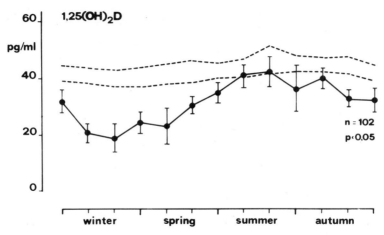

Fig. 3. 1,25(OH)2D levels throughout one year in 102 subjects aged
66-95 years. The mean $\pm$ 1 standard error (M $\pm$ SE) is indicated
for each month. Dotted lines indicate the M $\pm$ SE interval in
subjects aged 20-55.

The headlines of the methods used for 25OHD and 1,25(OH)2D were
the following: protein precipitation and lipid extraction of samples,
column chromatography on Sep-pak C-18 cartridges, high pressure liquid
chromatography on silica columns, competitive protein binding assay
using rat serum (25OHD) or radioreceptor assay using the thymus
receptor from calves (1,25(OH)2D) (32). Serum calcium, phosphate and
alkaline phosphatase were measured by standard methods.

In the younger group the serum levels of 25OHD showed a clear
seasonal variation with a maximum in late summer and a minimum in
winter.

Elderly subjects showed lower mean levels, and the seasonal
variation was less pronounced. The difference can be quantitated by
examining the equations of the respective best fitting sinusoidal
functions. In these equations the values of the variables M and W,
which denote the mean annual level and the width of variation
respectively, were the following: in the younger group M = 17,9 ng/ml,
W = 5,9 ng/ml. In the elderly M = 9,2 ng/ml; W = 2,9 ng/ml.

The serum values of 1,25(OH)2D were grouped according to month
and the statistical significance of the seasonal variation was tested
by one-way analysis of variance using the months as factors.

No significant seasonal variation was observed in the group of
controls, but, surprisingly, 1,25(OH)2D concentrations showed a marked
seasonal fluctuation in older subjects: the serum levels reached their
maximum in September and their minimum in February and March (Fig. 3).

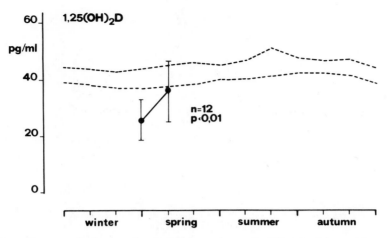

Fig. 4. Effects of the oral administration of 25OHD3 (10 µg/day for 1 month) on 1,25(OH)2D serum levels in a group of elderly subjects (age range 66-79).

There is no other study in the literature for comparison of our data except that carried out by Bouillon in Belgium (33): the results reported in that study are very similar to our own data; this indicates that the influence of our relatively low latitude on vitamin D rhythms is probably lower than expected.

The question arises as to the causes of the 1,25(OH)2D seasonal variation. It is not likely that the low 1,25(OH)2D levels we found in winter in elderly subjects might result from a decrease in renal func-tion (this was excluded in the selection of subjects), by a deficiency in renal 1alpha-hydroxylase activity, or by a lack of stimulators of this enzyme, since these factors do not seem to vary cyclically, so that they are not a good explanation of a cyclic phenomenon.

We hypothesized that the winter deficiency in substrate concentrations we found in the same subjects was the most likely explanation of the simultaneous decrease in the serum levels of the active vitamin D metabolite; in fact, in summer, when 25OHD levels increase, there is a rapid restoration of normal 1,25(OH)2D concentra-tions. Moreover, the oral administration of 25OHD3 in winter causes a significant increase in 1,25(OH)2D levels (Fig. 4). In other words the senile kidney is not able to adapt 1,25(OH)2D synthesis any more in the presence of low substrate levels.

The presence of normal serum concentrations of vitamin D metabolites only for one period of the year is probably not sufficient for a normal bone and mineral homeostasis. Therefore, we believe that this temporary vitamin D deficiency may cause alterations in the process of bone formation and may be responsible for the high frequency of subclinical conditions of osteomalacia or, more often, of mixed patterns of osteoporosis and osteomalacia in the elderly. The observation of the effectiveness of 25OHD3 in restoring normal levels of 1,25(OH)2D in these subjects could be of some practical value.

In conclusion:
- age is an important determinant of vitamin D status;
- vitamin D deficiency is a rather common condition in geriatric subjects, even in the absence of clinically manifest osteomalacia;
- the seasonal variation of 25OHD is less pronunced in elederly subjects than in controls, but this does not seem to result from reduced ability to synthesize vitamin D in skin or to absorb it from the intestine;
- geriatric subjects show a winter decrease in serum 1,25(OH)2D, which is, most likely, a consequence of the relative deficiency of the precursor compound 25OHD, occurring at this time of the year;
- low doses of 25OHD3 rapidly restore normal levels of serum 1,25(OH)2D in elderly subjects.

EXERCISE

Mechanical forces are essential for the development and maintenance of bone mass and strenght. It is well known that simple bed rest can result in loss of bone mineral. Several observations have confirmed this concept, that was well described by Whedon et al. in their famous experiment: in a group of volunteers immobilized in plaster casts nitrogen and calcium balances rapidly turned to negative and the effect persisted for several weeks after the end of immobilization (34).

It has been hypothesized that a dose response relationship exists between exercise and bone status, so that immobilization leads to severe bone loss, whereas loading and adequate strain magnitudes can result in bone hypertrophy. The latter effect, however, appears to occur to a significant extent in growing rather than in mature bone (35).

Therefore, exercise performed at an appropriate age can be included among the factors influencing peak bone mass at maturity. There is a direct relationship between muscle mass and bone mass (1), not only systemically, but also locally since it has been found that the cortical thickness of female professional tennis players was greater in the playing arm than in the non-dominant one (36).

However, excessive and prolonged activity can lead to bone fatigue with microfracture and finally stress fractures, as has been observed in long-distance runners. On the other hand women excercising intensely, who develop exercise-induced amenorrhea, were found to have a reduced amount of trabecular bone in their lumbar vertebrae (37). This finding has been related to estrogen deficiency resulting from reduced peripheral conversion of steroids, as a consequence of decreased body fat.

The mechanism whereby exercise stimulates new bone formation has not yet been clearly established. Intermediaries, through which mechanical load results in a stimulus for bone cell growth and differentiation, include the generation of piezo-electricity.

This has been hypothesized to act by stimulating cyclic nucleotide activity, prostaglandin synthesis and other bone growth factors. The result of these processes is the laying down of new matrix in the remodelling bone surfaces.

The effects of exercise on bone mass in postmenopausal women are not well established. Some investigators have reported that exercise does not lead to any significant increase in bone mass in these subjects (38,39), while others report positive results (40,41).

A very recent study (42) indicates that a moderate brisk walking program of one year duration does not prevent the loss of spinal lone density in early-postmenopausal women (43).

An interesting model of the skeletal changes occurring in the absence of mechanical forces is offered by space flights.

After the first human space missions American scientists hypothesized that the lack of gravity could cause a significant decrease in bone mass during long-term flights.

In space bone and muscles, particularly those of the lower limbs, which usually bear body weight, are not adequately utilized. In fact, astronauts in space never assume an erect posture, but, in defiance of gravity, float in the space in the most comfortable position or tie themselves to the apparatus with which they have to work. This lack of 'stress and strain' may result in bone loss and muscle atrophy, if the duration of flights is long enough.

Actually, the most impressive medical observations made during space missions are represented by progressive calcium loss and muscular and skeletal involution.

Metabolic studies carried out in the 'Skylab' space laboratory have shown an often dramatic increase in urinary calcium excretion in all the crew members, with a mean net calcium loss of about 140 mg per day. A remarkable variability was noticed among different subjects concerning the degree of hypercalciuria. The loss of bone mineral was highest in the lower extremities, particularly in tarsal bones, but it was also relevant in the spine.

In addition to calcium, a significant loss of nitrogen and

phosphorus has been observed and related to the acceleration of muscular catabolism.

An intense program of physical activity using appropriate devices has been suggested for prevention of this 'space osteoporosis'.

The greatest experience on bone loss during space flights has been accumulated by Russian scientists, since the longest missions, more than one year, have been carried out by soviet astronauts.

The consequent scientific information, however, has not become widely available yet, due to several factors: most of the data obtained are still being processed, preliminary data have been published in soviet journals that have a limited diffusion abroad, the use of the Russian language does not allow a direct approach by most part of the scientific world.

I have obtained some interesting information on this subject from A. Le Blanc, a NASA researcher who recently met a group of Russian astronauts and scientists, who paid a visit to their American collegues.

The most interesting finding reported by soviet scientists was, apart from the confirmation of the severity of osteoporosis after long-term flights, that Russian astronauts never recovered completely after their return to earth, with the only possible exception of the lesions occurred at skeletal sites subjected to the highest mechanical stress.

It seems that the astronauts in these conditions simply reduced the rate of bone loss to a level similar to that of their age-matched peers, without recuperating the bone mass previously lost, so that their skeleton appears to be older than their chronological age (44).

Thus, in this model we are in the presence of a loss of bone mineral provoked in healthy, relatively young subjects by a unique and well identified cause, the absence of gravity. Well, when this cause ceases to operate a completely recovery is not possible.

This finding further emphasizes the importance of prevention in whatever kind of osteoporosis.

CONCLUSIONS

Dietary and lifestyle factors can play an important role in the preventive management of osteoporosis. Three essential factors emerge from the above discussion: physical activity to stimulate new bone formation; good nutrition, in terms of both calcium and vitamin D intake, to mineralize the newly formed osteoid; reduction of the minor risk factors, such as caffeine, alcohol, smoking, etc.

The observance of these simple recommendations, during growth and development and later on, will help maximize peak bone mass at maturity and maintain it in subsequent years.

REFERENCES

1. S.H. Cohn, C. Abesamis, S. Yasumura, J.F. Aloia, I. Zanzi and K.J. Ellis, 1977, Comparative skeletal mass and radial bone mineral content in black and white women. Metabolism, 26: 171.
2. D.M. Smith, W.E. Nance, K.W. Kang, J.C. Christian and C.C. Jr. Johnston, 1973, Genetic factors in determining bone mass. J. Clin. Invest., 52: 2800.
3. J.M. Lane and V.J. Vigorita, 1983, Current concepts review: osteoporosis, J. Bone Joint Surg. Am., 65: A:274.
4. C. Christiansen, B.J. Riis and P. Rodbro, 1987, Prediction of rapid bone loss in postmenopausal women, Lancet, 1: 1105.
5. R.P. Heaney and R.R. Recker, 1982, Effects of nitrogen, phosphorus and caffeine on calcium balance in women. J. Lab. Clin. Med., 99: 46.
6. J.F. Aloia, S.H. Cohn and A. Vaswani, 1985, Risk factors for postmenopausal osteoporosis, Am. J. Med., 78: 95.
7. H.W. Daniel, 1976, Osteoporosis of the slender smoker, Arch. Inter. Med., 136: 298.
8. E. Seaman, L.J. III Melton and W.M. O'Fallon, 1983, Risk factors for spinal osteoporosis in men, Am. J. Med., 75: 977.
9. A.R. Williams, N.S. Weiss, C.L. Ure, J. Ballard and J.R. Daling, 1982, Effect of weight, smoking and estrogen use on the risk of hip and forearm fractures in postmenopausal women. Obstet. Gynecol., 60: 695.
10. B.C. Labor, M.W. France and D. Powell, 1985, Bone and mineral metabolism and chronic alcohol abuse, Q.J. Med., 59: 497.
11. B. Lalar and T.B. Counihan, 1982, Metabolic bone disease in heavy drinkers, Clin. Sci, 63: 43.
12. D.T. Baran, S.L. Teitelbaum, M.A. Bergfeld, G. Parker, E.M. Cruvant and L.V. Avioli, 1980, Effect of alcohol ingestion on bone and mineral metabolism in rats, Am. J. Physiol., 238: E507.
13. J.R. Farley, R. Fitzsimmons, A.K. Taylor, U.M. Jorch and K.-H.W. Lau, 1985, Direct effects of ethanol on bone resorption and formation in vitro. Arch. Biochem. Biophys, 238: 305.
14. L.K. Massey and M.M. Strang, 1982, Soft drink consumption, phosphorus intake and osteoporosis, Perspectives in Practice, 80: 581.
15. R.P. Heaney, 1987, The role of nutrition in prevention and management of osteoporosis, Clin. Obst. Gynecol., 50: 833.
16. A. Caniggia, C. Gennari, V. Bianchi and R. Guideri, 1963, Intestinal absorption of 45Ca in senile osteoporosis, Acta Med. Scand., 173: 5.
17. F. Lenzi and A. Caniggia, 1962, Fisiopatologia delle Osteoporosi Diffuse, Edizioni L. Pozzi, Roma.

18. J.C. Stevenson, M.I. Whitehead, M. Padwick, J;A. Endacott, C. Sutton, L.M. Banks, C. Freemantle, T.J. Spinks and R. Hesp, 1988, Dietary intake of calcium and postmenopausal bone loss, Brit. Med. J. 297: 15.

19. R.P. Heaney, R.R. Recker and P.D. Saville, 1978, Menopausal changes in calcium balance performance, J. Lab. Clin. Med., 92: 953.

20. R.P. Heaney and R.R. Recker, 1985, The effect of milk supplementations on calcium metabolism, bone metabolism, and calcium balance, Am. J. Clin. Nutr., 41: 254.

21. A.C. Santora, 1987, Role of nutrition and exercise in osteoporosis, Am. J. Med., 82: 73.

22. V. Matkovic, K. Kostial, I. Simonovic, R. Buzina, A. Brodarec and B.E.C. Nordin, 1979, Bone status and fracture rates in two regions of Yugoslavia, Am. J. Clin. Nutr., 32: 540.

23. F. Ponchon, and H.F. DeLuca, 1969, The role of the liver in the metabolism of vitamin D., J. Clin. Invest. 48: 1273.

24. F. Loré, I. Caniggia and G. Di Cairano, 1986, Vitamin D status and age. In: Bernardi M, Facchini A, Labò G, eds. Nutritional and metabolic aspects of aging, Rijswijk: Eurage, 107: 112.

25. F. Loré, G. Di Cairano and G. Manasse, 1983, Metodo rapido per il dosaggio della 25-idrossivitamina D nel siero, Boll. Soc. It. Biol. Sper., 59: 119.

26. S.S. Shapiro and M.B. Wilk, 1965, An analysis of variance test for normality (complete samples), Biometrika, 52: 591.

27. F. Loré and G. Di Cairano, 1986, Vitamin D status in the extreme age of life, Ann. Med. Int. 137: 206.

28. F. Loré, G. Di Cairano and F. Di Perri, 1984, Intestinal absorption of 25-hydroxyvitamin D according to age and sex. Calcif. Tissue. Int., 36: 143.

29. R.W. Chesney, J.F. Rosen and A.J. Hamstra, 1981, Absence of seasonal variation in serum concentrations of 1,25-dihydroxyvitamin D despite a rise in 25-hydroxyvitamin D in summer. J. Clin. Endocrinol. Metab., 53: 139.

30. R. Bouillon, F.A. Van Assche and H. Van Baelen, 1981, Influence of the vitamin D-binding protein on the serum concentration of 1,25-dihydroxyvitamin D3. J. Clin. Invest., 67: 589.

31. A.W. Norman, 1979, Interrelation between vitamin D and other hormones. In: Vitamin D: the Calcium Homeostatic Steroid Hormone. New York: Academic Press, 274.

32. F. Loré, G. Di Cairano and M. Nobili, 1986, A new binding protein for the radioreceptor assay of 1,25-dihydroxyvitamin D. Nuclear Med., 25: 103.

33. R.A. Bouillon, J.H. Auwerx and W.D. Lissens, 1987, Vitamin D status in the elderly: seasonal substrate deficiency causes 1,25-dihydroxycholecalciferol deficiency. Am. J. Clin. Nutr., 45: 755.

34. G.D. Whedon, J.E. Deitrick and E. Shorr, 1949, Modification of the effects of immobilization upon metabolic and physiologic function of normal men by the use of an oscillating bed. Am. J. Med., 6: 684.

35. D.R. Carter, 1983, Mechanical loading histories and bone remodelling. Calcif. Tissue Int., 36: 519.

36. H.H. Jones, J.D. Priest, W.C. Hayes, C.C. Tichenor and D.A. Nagel, 1977, Humeral hypertrophy in response to exercise, J. Bone Joint Surg., 59A: 204.

37. B.L. Drinkwater, K. Nilson, C.H. Chestnut, W.J. Bremner, S. Chainholz and M.B. Southworth, 1984, Bone mineral content of amenorrhoeic and eumenorrheic athletes.

38. B. Krolner, B. Toft, S.P. Nielsen and E. Tondevold, 1983, Physical exercise as prophylaxis against involutional vertebral bone loss: a controlled trial. Clin. Sci., 64: 541.

39. M.K. White, R.B. Martin, R.A. Yater, R.L. Butcher and E.L. Radin: The effects of exercise on the bones of postmenopausal women, Int. Ortho., 7: 209.

40. E.L. Smith, P.E. Smith, C.J. Ensign and M.M. Shea, 1984, Bone involution decrease in exercising middle-aged women. Calcif. Tiss. Int., 36: S129.

41. G.P. Dalsky, A.A. Ehsani, K.S.Kleinheider and S.J. Birge, 1986, Effect of exercise on lumbar bone density, Gerontologist, Supp. 26: 16A.

42. D.J. Cavanaugh and C.E. Cann, 1988, Brisk walking does not stop bone loss in postmenopausal women, Bone, 9: 201.

43. M. Notelovitz, 1986, Post-menopausal osteoporosis, a practical approach to its prevention, Acta Obstet. Gynecol. Scand. Suppl., 134: 67.

44. A. Le Blanc, Personal Communication.

PATHOPHYSIOLOGY OF BONE FORMATION AND RESORPTION

Angelo Caniggia

Institute of Clinical Medicine
University of Siena
53100 Siena, Italy

BONE REMODELING

Bone remodeling exists at birth and continues until death: it does not cease at skeletal maturity.

The concept of continuous remodeling of bone in adults implies that living bone is constantly changing its matter.

The absorption of preexisting bone is a necessary accompaniement of bone remodeling:
- the multinucleated giant cells named osteoclasts are the agents by which bone destruction is brought about;
- the formation of new bone results from the activity of another kind of specialized cells, the osteoblasts.

The process of bone formation and bone resorption occurs at the mineralized interface between bone tissue and its ensheating. The structures involved include the surfaces of the trabeculae of cancellous bone, the resorption lacunae, the periosteal and endosteal surfaces.

Areas of bone destruction can be identified by the presence of osteoclasts located in eroded lacunae on the bone surface where osteoclasts may be arranged in clusters; the eroded bays are frequently more extensive than the accumulation of osteoclasts that evidently quickly disappear after eroding bone.

Areas of bone formation can be identified by the presence of active osteoblasts on the surface concerned and by the presence immediatly beneath these cells of a thin layer of osteoid tissue showing a microradiographic low density of calcification and a maximum uptake of the bone seeking radionuclides.

The sequential theory of bone remodeling (1) is becoming more and more popular:

- first step: activation of inactive bone surfaces covered by resting osteoblasts (the so called flat lining cells) which could release some proteolytic enzymes "uncovering" the mineralized bone surface so that it can be resorbed by osteoclasts;
- second step: bone resorption which involves differentiation and migration of osteoclasts, secretion of hydrogen-ions that dissolve bone mineral and lysosomal enzymes degrading bone matrix;
- third step: reversal phase characterized by the appearance of macrophages in the resorbing surface whom the exact role is not known.
- fourth step: formation phase in which osteoblasts replace resorbed bone; it depends on the release of local growth factors ("coupling factors"), on the ability of osteoblasts-precursors to differentiate and on the capacity of osteoblasts to lay down bone matrix.

Histological examinations of bone in primary hyperparathyroidism (HPT-1) as well as in Paget's disease support this theory.

This is a bone biopsy from the iliac crest in a patient with HPT-1 (Fig. 1): you can see an extension of osteoclasts and within a bay eroded by the osteoclastic activity a large part of the bone surface covered by active osteoblasts laying down newly formed bone matrix not yet mineralized.

In this patient both bone destruction and bone formation appeared to be occurring at an increased rate, probably in a sequential way.

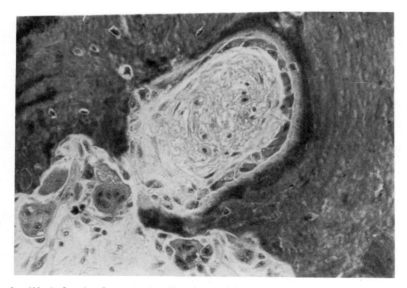

Fig. 1. Histological aspect of a bone biopsy from the iliac crest in a patient with HPT-1.

Everybody knows the bone findings in HPT-1: the osteoclastic stimulation by PTH is particularly strong so that osteoclasts frequently clusters in brown tumors as in patients of the present slides where osteoclastomata were evident clinically and at X ray.

The hyperactivity of osteoclasts leads to a generalized bone resorption because osteoblasts rarely keep the pace with the rate of osteoclastic activity: the bone mass rapidly decreases and patients experience severe bone pain and fractures by trivial trauma.

In other words the activity of osteoclasts prevails on the activity of osteoblasts.

A dramatic reversal of this situation follows parathyroid surgery:

the complete excision of the parathyroid adenoma is testified by the sudden fall of plasma calcium level and serum cyclic AMP;

the blocking effect on bone is indicated by the fall of urinary hydroxyproline, plasma alkaline phosphatase and osteocalcin.

A complete healing of bone occurs within years.

The bone findings in chronic hypoparathyroidism are opposite: the bone turnover becomes slower and slower, bone biopsies from iliac crest show an increase in bone mass with a diminution of resorption lacunae; no osteoclasts, no osteoblasts; increased bone mineral density at X ray and absorptiometry.

The confrontation between metacarpal bones in a patient with HPT-1 and another with chronic idiopatic hypoparathyroidism shows a very impressive difference in thickness of the compact bone; despite the low stimulation of osteoclasts in this patient osteoblasts did succeed in laying down large amounts of compact bone.

Provided the sequential theory of bone remodeling must be maintained, it is compulsatory considering some pathological conditions where the osteoblastic activity is florid despite a scarce presence of osteoclasts;

Other examples given: Albers/Schömberg's marble-bone disease, pachydermoperiostosis and other idiopathic hyperostoses with different uncommon localisations.

In further pathological conditions the activity of osteoblasts may prevail on the activity of osteoclasts:
- fluorosis is characterized by an enhanced activity of osteoblasts that leads to a significant bone formation; unfortunately the newly formed bone shows frequently an impairment in mineralisation; in this pathological condition the enhanced bone accretion has been

demonstrated to be the direct consequence of the stimulating effect
of fluoride on osteoblasts;

- in the osteoblastic metastases of prostatic cancer the
  hyperactivity of osteoblasts seems to be accounted for by the
  production of a "growth factor" which enhances the transformation
  of pre-osteoblasts in osteoblasts; this hypotesis has been
  suggested by the luxuriant proliferation of mesenchymal cells in
  the marrow spaces ensheating the newly formed bone (Fig. 2).

It must be kept in mind that fibrous bone marrow is
characteristic of several pathological conditions with osteoblastic
hyperactivity as primary and secondary hyperparathyroidism.

Paget's disease is another exemple of pathological sequential
formation of bone tissue.

The condition may affect any of the bones singly or in
combination; it may be discovered by the enlargement of the skull or
the bowing of a long bone.

These deformities are avidly uptaking the bone-seeker tracers
indicating a high local bone turnover; they are attributable to
remodeling of bone due to a previous endosteal resorption (V-shaped
advancing edge in long bones, "osteoporosis circumscripta" in the
skull) followed by a mainly periosteal compensatory apposition
enlarging the involved skeletal segment.

The enlargment of the pagetic bones is absolutely characteristic
and necessary for a positive X ray diagnosis.

The marked increase in bone matrix degradation associated with
an increase in osteoclastic activity, is reflected by a rise of the
urinary hydroxyproline content.

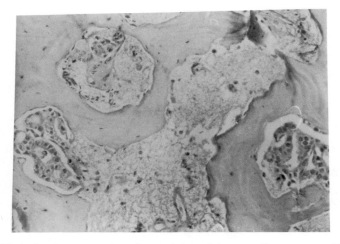

Fig. 2. Histologic aspect of a bone biopsy from a patient with
metastases of prostatic cancer.

The compensatory increase in osteoblastic bone repair is reflected both by elevated serum alkaline phosphatase and the serum levels of the bone GLA protein, that is osteocalcin.

Bone biopsies demonstrate that areas of active Paget's disease contain increased numbers of osteoclasts whereas the surrounding non pagetic bone is histologically normal.

Osteoclastic resorption is particularly evident at the advancing edge of the lesion, osteoblastic regeneration behind it.

Osteoclasts in Paget's disease frequently present an elevated number of nuclei containing characteristic virus-like inclusions.

This finding has been considered an index that Paget's disease might be possibly induced by a slow virus (perhaps the virus of measles) (2).

The resorptive phase is followed by marrow fibrosis similar to the osteitis fibrosa of primary hyperparathyroidism, with increased skeletal vascularity.

The compensatory increase in osteoblastic bone repair results in a distorsion of bone architecture leading to the so called "mosaic pattern" (Fig. 3).

Most of the pagetic bone tissue consists in small patches having scalloped contours, interlocked by policyclic lines.

Osteoblasts may lay down either lamellar or woven bone; polarized light inspection of histological preparations enables to ascertain the lamellar or woven quality of single patches of the pagetic bone tissue.

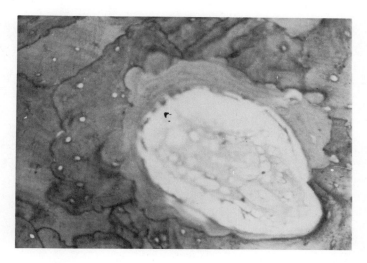

Fig. 3. Histologic aspect of a bone biopsy from a pagetic patient.

Then Paget's disease is a good model of chaotic remodeling of bone: in the osteolytic forms of the disease resorbing processes prevail whereas in the less aggressive hyperostotic forms a prevalence of osteoblastic activity may be observed.

The working hypothesis of bone remodeling states a parallel and proportional activity of osteoblasts and osteoclasts: but this is not the case in the majority of the aforementioned pathological conditions.

Moreover it must be stressed that in the adult normal bone areas of bone formation and bone destruction are quite infrequent, occupying only a small part of the bone surface.

OSTEOPOROSES

Osteoporoses show little evidence of bone remodeling except immobilisation osteoporosis that is associated with active osteoclastic bone resorption and the osteoporosis of hyperthyroidism where in some cases the increased osteoclastic activity parallels a significant activity of osteoblasts (3).

It is largely known that immobilisation leads to a rapid demineralisation of bone with increased hypercalciuria and elevated levels of urinary hydroxyproline.

As it concerns hyperthyroidism it is possible that thyroid hormones stimulate either osteoclasts and osteoblasts likeliwise parathyroid hormone excess, although finally the osteoclastic activity will prevail.

According to Nordin "Osteoporoses are characterized by a reduced volume of bone tissue relative to the volume of anatomical bone";

In osteoporosis the bone mass is decreased but the mineralization of the remaining bone is normal.

The bone loss may be due either to a defect in bone accretion as in "Fragilitas ossium hereditaria" (osteogenesis inperfecta), or to an excess in bone resorption as in post-menopausal osteoporosis and in that due to corticosteroid excess.

In both these varieties of osteoporosis the histological inspection of bone biopsies shows that osteoblasts and osteoclasts are exceedingly rare and I wonder to what extent in these pathological conditions it can be suggested a sequential treatment according to the bone remodeling hypothesis.

Osteogenesis imperfecta is characterized by fragility of bones associated with frequent fractures and blu sclera.

It may be accounted for to a mutation which can have a lethal result (Vrolik's disease) or not (Ekman-Lobstein's disease); it is transmitted generally as a dominant character not linked with sex, with a pleiotropic monogenic control (4).

The bones of such patients show thinned cortices, decreased trabeculation and little evidence of bone remodeling.

Nevertheless the healing of fractures is rapid and satisfactory, and bony callus is generally hypertrophic.

Despite the normal histological appearance of osteoblasts, biochemical studies of bone collagen in osteogenesis imperfecta led to the suggestion that the collagen has a deficiency in cross-linkage of the elementary fibrils; likeliwise the collagen synthesis by fibroblasts from patients with osteogenesis imperfecta is impaired, whence the blu sclera (5).

Scurvy osteoporosis seems to be correlated to a similar impairment of collagen synthesis due to the deficiency in vitamin C (6). And finally the heparin osteoporosis would be due to the formation of heparin complexes with collagen that break the collagen helicial structure by competing for the labile ester cross-links (7).

Knowledge of the pathophysiology and treatment of metabolic bone disease has been enhanced by accurate measurements of total bone mineral mass and precise estimations of bone mass change.

Since 98-99% of total body calcium is normally in the skeleton, bone mineral mass is consequently accurately assessed by measurement of total body calcium.

Total body calcium may be measured utilizing the technique of total body neutron activation analysis and at present by the computerized total body dual photon (or X ray) absorptiometry.

The computerized absorptiometric device gives us the exact mineral content of the entire skeleton, together with a significant visual display, and calculates the bone mineral density expressed in gr/cm2.

It must be kept in mind that "Bone Mineral Density" (expressed in gr/cm2) is not equivalent to "Bone Mass" but to the mineral content of the bone mass.

Low values of bone mineral density can be found in osteoporoses as well in osteomalacias, that is in two pathological conditions absolutely different from a pathophysiological and histological point of view.

Post-menopausal osteoporosis is a very common pathological

condition characterized by a reduction in bone mass that is mainly the result of bone resorption.

A spongy appearance of cortical bone is observed as a consequence of large resorption lacunae; a thinning of the trabeculae of cancellous bone is also apparent; no osteoid seams are present which are characteristic of osteomalacia.

Thus bone mass is reduced but the mineralisation of the remaining bone is normal, as it clearly appears at the microscopic inspection of undecalcified bone biopsies from the iliac crest (Fig. 4).

The skeletal changes are mostly evident in spine and lead to a progressive brittleness of bone with increased liability to fractures.

The painful crush fractures and cod-fishing of vertebrae lead to kyphotic deformity of the spine and reduction in stature.

Albright suggested an impairment in the activity of osteoblasts as pathogenetic factor in post-menopausal osteoporosis; nevertheless he showed that negative calcium balance in this pathological condition was mainly due to increased fecal losses of calcium: evidently calcium was not absorbed enough as we have been able to demonstrate later by the radiocalcium oral test.

The long-term negative calcium balance in these women was consistent with a resorptive pathogenetic mechanism: the disappearance of large amounts of bone tissue and particularly the spongy transformation of compact bone led to consider the possibility of an increased bone resorption for homeostatic purposes to preserving a normal level of calcium in plasma and interstitial fluids necessary for life.

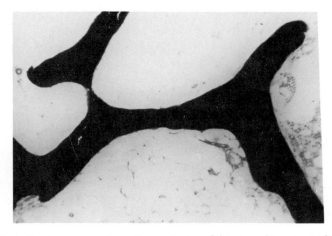

Fig. 4. Histologic aspect of a bone biopsy in a patient with post-menopausal osteoporosis.

The assessment of the total body retention of bone seeker tracers (as 99mTc-MDP) enabled to demonstrate the initial high turnover phase of post-menopausal osteoporosis (8,9) and recently Vattimo (10) pointed to the greater uptake of compact bone in appendicular skeleton at menopause despite the decreased bone mineral content measured by absorptiometric devices.

Fast bone losers present a rapid increase in bone resorption with hypercalciuria and increased urinary excretion of hydroxyproline; whereas in the slow bone loser women the velocity of the resorptive process is lower.

Nevertheless in both instances osteoclasts are scarce in comparison to other high turnover bone diseases.

If we consider that a post-menopausal woman with osteoporosis can loose within few years by 30 to 40% of the skeletal mass we must conclude that this is a very intriguing problem.

The starting loss near the time of menopause supports the view that oestrogens lack is particularly involved in post-menopausal osteoporosis, but the precise mechanism which is important in promoting bone resorption is still unknown.

Corticosteroid osteoporosis is another metabolic bone disease frequent in practice. Partly it shares the pathogenesis of post-me-nopausal osteoporosis, at least as it concerns the impairment in intestinal calcium transport.

Short-term courses of corticosteroid therapy in patients never treated before lead to the following biochemical consequences (11):
- impairment of the intestinal calcium transport;
- excessive urinary losses of calcium and phosphate;
- direct catabolic effect on bone that can be demostrated on patients pre-labelled with 45Calcium where the cyclic administration of steroids was accompanied by a significant release of radiocalcium from bone and an increase in urinary hydroxyproline (Fig.5, Fig.6).

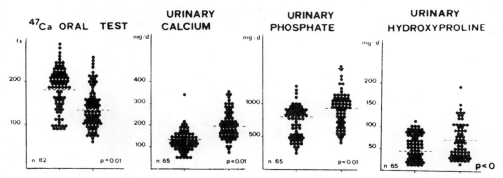

Fig. 5. 47Ca absorption and urinary calcium, phosphate and hydroxy-proline before and after (respectively left and right side of each panel) a short-term (30 days) treatment with steroids.

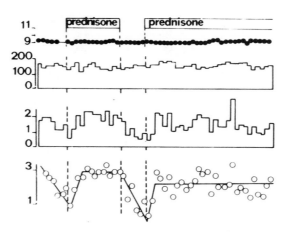

Fig. 6. Effects of two prednisone courses on: (from the top) plasma calcium (mg%), urinary calcium (mg/d) and 45Ca (cpm x 10^{-5}) excretion and urinary 45Ca specific activity (cpm/mg x 10^{-3}).

Because of the aforementioned pathogenetic effects in long-term corticosteroid treatments the onset of an overt osteoporosis is rapid.

It is surprising that such a rapidly resorptive bone disease does not show a proportional evidence of osteoclastic resorption (12).

It may be considered the possibility that in osteoporoses sustained losses of bone tissue may happen independently on parallel increases of osteoclasts.

OSTEOMALACIAS

Bone is first a tissue and secondly a mineralized tissue.

Osteoblasts lay down collagen, a macromolecular structure which becomes organized into precise arrays within the extracellular phase of the bone matrix.

Collagen elementary fibrils demonstrate an axial periodicity of 640 Angstrom; they have a characteristic aminoacid composition containing considerable proportion of glycine, proline and hydroxyproline, hydroxylysine being 1%. Collagen fibrils are surrounded by a mucopolysaccharide moiety.

In normal skeleton the newly formed, not yet mineralized bone tissue has been estimated 0 to 4%; it can be seen as a very thin layer involving few elementary lamellae, covering limited areas of the trabecular surface.

It is not always appreciated that osteoid is present in normal bone; for this it is important to measure the amount of osteoid tissue: its width on undecalcified bone biopsies and the extent of it on the bone surfaces.

Osteoporosis indicates a defect in the mechanism of bone formation and resorption without impairment in the mineralisation of the newly formed bone.

Osteomalacia indicates a defect in the mineralisation of bone with normal bone formation.

Frequently a mixed pattern of osteoporosis and osteomalacia can be observed namely in elderly people.

My personal opinion is that the cohexistence of osteoid seams with an histological pattern of osteoporosis cannot be considered as "high turnover osteoporosis" but rather as a particular variety of osteomalacia developing in patients with a parallel defect in the bone formation/resorption mechanism.

The mineralisation of newly formed bone needs adequate concentrations of calcium and phosphate. The Ca x P product has been regarded as a useful, empirical diagnostic test of osteomalacia despite some overlap with control subjects.

Bone mineralisation requires certain minimum values of calcium and phosphate in tissue fluid; in the majority of cases it is the depression of plasma phosphate which is proportionally the greatest and so mainly responsible of the presence of osteoid seams.

It may be interesting to remind that large osteoid seams are frequently found in bone biopsies of patients with HPT-1° who present high plasma calcium but a severe decrease in plasma phosphate. In these patients the Ca x P product does not reach the minimal threshold needed for normal mineralisation of bone that is largely laid down because of the luxuriant activity of osteoblasts (the so called "hyperosteoidosis") (Table I). Then, the characteristic feature of osteomalacia is a failure of new bone to calcify.

Today the total body calcium can be directly measured by total body absorptiometry.

In osteomalacia total body absorptiometry demostrates the lowest total mineral content of the skeleton; in these patients the total body calcium rises quickly on treatment:
recently in a woman, who had a completely disabling form of osteomalacia, the total body bone calcium rose by 12% within 3 months and at the some time this lady got up and did walk; within 1 year the bone mineral content rose up to the 50% of the basal values and the increase in total body bone mineral was easily seen in the visual display.

Table 1. Ca x P product in various conditions

	Ca mg%	P mg%	CaxP	Osteoid
Normals	10.2	4.1	41.8	No
Osteoporosis	9.8	4.2	41.1	No
Osteomalacia	8.5	1.5	12.7	Yes
HPT 1°a	11.5	2.8	32.2	No
HPT 1°b	11.5	1.5	17.2	Yes

Of course severe diminutions of the bone mineral density may be accounted for either to osteoporosis or osteomalacia and a differential diagnosis from this laboratory procedure only is impossible as we shall see this afternoon.

The histological pattern of osteomalacia is characterized by the presence of large osteoid seams covering extensive areas of bone trabeculae and the internal surface of Havers' channels (Fig. 7).

The clinical and radiological diagnosis of osteomalacia may be very easy in individual cases and very difficult in others.

Bone pain is generally more severe than in other demineralizing bone diseases; muscular weakness is paramount (disability in rising from a chair and in going up or down stairs), and can be accounted for to the myopathy of the pelvic girdle and thigh; the majority of patients show the "goose gait".

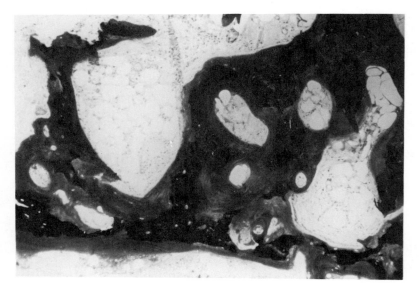

Fig. 7. Histologic aspect of a bone biopsy obtained from the iliac crest of a patient with osteomalacia.

The pseudofractures of Looser-Milkman are the radiological hallmark of osteomalacia: the commonest sites for these fractures are the ribs, the outher board of the scapulae, the metatarsal bones, the pubic rami, the upper end of the femur.

Unfortunately pseudofractures are not easily found, and a failure to find them does not rule out osteomalacia.

Fractures in the trabecular bone of the spine and their the cod-fish vertebrae are more commonly found, but appearance is not unique to osteomalacia being also frequently present in osteoporosis.

The main biochemical parameters in osteomalacia are the following:
- a defect in calcium absorption with negative calcium balance that can explain the usually low plasma calcium and the low urinary calcium excretion to be accounted for to a diminution in the calcium filtration load;
- a defect in phosphate metabolism: the intestinal radiophosphate absorption is usually decreased (13) and the phosphate balance is negative, but not only for the intestinal losses; an impaired renal tubular reabsorption of phosphate can be observed that results in elevated renal phosphate clearance;
- raised serum alkaline phosphatase and serum osteocalcin both indicating an increased activity of osteoblasts;

In other words a high bone turnover confirmed by the Whole body retention of 99mTc-MDP that is more elevated than in normals and in osteoporoses, and by the histological evidence of a secondary hyperparathyroidism (8).

Among the principal causes of osteomalacia there are nutritional vitamin D deficiency and errors in the metabolism of vitamin D.

The requirement of vitamin D in adult is less then 2.5 ug per day (100 I.U.) vitamin D being synthesized in the skin or absorbed by food in the duodenum and jejunum.

Its function is not activated unless it was given more than 10 hours prior: vitamin D must be converted first to 250H vit D in the liver and after 250H vit D to 1,25(OH)2 vit D in the kidney; daily production being 1 ug or so (14).

The serum levels of 250H vit. D give us a nice measure of the "vitamin D status" of the organism, being so particularly useful in the diagnosis of nutritional osteomalacias.

Here are the results of a large study on the vitamin D status in different sex and age; you can appreciate the progressive decrease of 250H vit. D levels in old people (15).

The serum 250H vit. D presents significant seasonal variations due to different U.V. exposure (16).

A nutritional deficiency of vitamin D can be accounted for to:
- a defect in sunlight exposure and vitamin D intake;
- a defect in the intestinal absorption of vitamin D.

The exposure of the skin to sunlight may be scorce because of
- the heavy clothing;
- the poor housing and the habit of spending much of the time inside dark room (usual among the elderly with or without personal handicaps;
- the air pollution and the obliquity of solar rays (latitude, season).

Patients with nutritional osteomalacia show very low serum levels of 250H vit. D indicating a poor vitamin D status; in extremely old subjects the levels of serum 250H vit. D can hardly be distinguishable from those of osteomalacia in elderly people that is often responsible for pathological fractures.

Vitamin D is mainly absorbed in the jejunum, and jejunal mucosa is the principal target for the vitamin D related absorption of phosphate.

Osteomalacia can be observed in any malabsorption syndrome, nevertheless it is uncommon in pancreatic disease despite the severity of steatorrhoea whereas it is particularly frequent in coeliac disease.

Despite a general opinion in gastrectomized patients osteomalacia can be demonstrated only in 2% of cases generally with a long interval between operation and the onset of the disease.

Osteoporosis is the most frequent bone complication in gastrectomized patients because the exclusion of duodenal loop leads to a substancial impairment in the intestinal calcium absorption whereas phosphate is still convenienty absorbed in jejunum.

Osteomalacia is particularly frequent in coeliac disease; its pathogenetic mechanism is twofold:
- malabsorption of vitamin D;
- damage of the intestinal receptors for calcitriol, the active metabolite of vitamin D.

Really osteomalacia is common after jejuno-ileal by pass for obesity: in these cases osteomalacia is insensitive to U.V. light exposure; hence factors other than simple vitamin D deficiency may contribute to its development, particularly the large resection of the phosphate absorptive intestinal tract.

In gluten-entheropathy the nutritional defect in vitamin D must not be considered the sole pathogenetic factor of osteomalacia; the severe involvement of the intestinal mucosa plays certainly an important role in the phosphate malabsorption independently of the vitamin D lack. The flattening of the intestinal villi and the inflammatory involvement of the intestinal mucosa eliminate the receptors for 1,25(OH)2 vit. D and can be considered the major responsibles for phosphate malabsorption (17). Vitamin D given orally or parenterally has no effect until gluten is excluded from the diet.

Osteomalacia may be due to defects in the renal tubular reabsorption of phosphate.

The hypophosphataemic rickets shows all the clinical, radiological, histological and biochemical features of deficiency osteomalacia, save that the plasma calcium tends to be normal whereas the plasma phosphate is particularly decreased. It is inherited as a sex linked dominant trait, being low plasma phosphate level better discriminant than the overt involvment of bone.

The cause of this disease is the poor responsiveness of the renal and intestinal targets for 1,25(OH)2 vit. D.

The consequent impairment of the renal reabsorption and intestinal absorption of phosphate (13) leads to hypophosphatemia with low CaxP product despite the normal plasma calcium levels.

Because of the receptors involvement the administration of calcitriol may result poorly effective in this disease. On the contrary the administration of high oral doses of phosphate can result in complete healing of this variety of osteomalacia.

Oncogenic osteomalacia is recognized as a vitamin D resistant hypophosphataemic osteomalacia that heals after resection of a coexisting mesenchymal tumor; generally "a strange tumor in a strange place" not easily detectable at the beginning of the disease.

Here is an example (Fig. 8): a sicilian volley ball player severely handicapped for osteomalacia with pseudo-fractures of Looser-Milkman and pelvic girdle myopathy: no familiar incidence, normal vitamin D status; calcitriol treatment led initially to an improvement while plasma calcium normalized and plasma phosphate rose to the lower limits of the normal range.

One year later he relapsed and a maxillary tumor became evident: despite the intensive calcitriol treatment and the persistently normal plasma calcium levels, the urinary phosphate clearance rose with a fall in the plasma phosphate.

Surgery and radiotherapy for this mesenchymal tumor: immediate fall of urinary phosphate clearance and rise in plasma phosphate with normalisation of Ca x P product and dramatic improvement of osteomalacia: at present, now two years later, he is perfectly recovered.

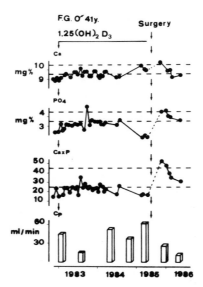

Fig. 8. Changes in the main biochemical parameters in a case of oncogenic osteomalacia

The discovery of the metabolites of vitamin D led to imagine:
- osteomalacias due to unvailability of vitamin D (the aforementioned nutritional osteomalacias;
- osteomalacias due to unavailability of 25OH vit. D;
- osteomalacias due to unavailability of 1,25(OH)2 vit. D.

It has been put forward the possibility of liver osteomalacias to be accounted for to a defect in 25OH vit.D synthesis. This is nothing than a theoretical hypothesis because osteomalacia is exceedingly uncommon in liver disease patients (except chronically jaundiced subjects for obstruction of biliary ducts: the pathogenesis in these cases being the intestinal malabsorption of vitamin D (18).

The osteomalacia associated with long-term anticonvulsant therapy can really be considered due to unvailability of 25OH vit D because a degradation of vitamin D to inactive product.

More important is the impaired renal conversion of 25OH vit. D to 1,25(OH)2 vit. D in patients with chronic renal insufficiency when the renal mass is below the 20% of that of the normal kidney.

This variety of osteomalacia is not relieved by dialysis though promptly corrected after renal transplantation (19). It is not easily understandable why in uraemic patients osteomalacia may be found despite the elevated plasma Ca x P product. It is largely known that chronic renal insufficiency is characterized by low plasma calcium and high plasma phosphate levels; probably other factors than 1,25(OH)2 vit. D participate in the pathogenesis of this variety of osteomalacia.

Nordin claimed the importance of metabolic acidosis (20); recently a possible relationship between aluminium accumulation and osteomalacic renal osteodystrophy was sought (21).

Bone aluminium was increased with a close correlation with the amount of unmineralized osteoid; it accumulates particularly on the calcification front interfering with bone mineralisation probably through the formation of insoluble phosphates; but this is a still debatatle point of view.

Apart from aluminium other local factors leading to defective bone crystal deposition have been considered:
- chronic fluoride intoxication: histologically fluorotic bone presents a luxuriant activity of osteoblasts but an increase in the width and number of osteoid seams;
- long-term treatment with diphosphonates which are quoted to operate through a stabilizing effect on the the normal content of pyrophosphate at surface of bony trabeculae.

To sum up:
Osteomalacias may be accounted for to the following main pathogenetic factors:
- unavailability of vit. D or impairment in vitamin D metabolism;
- defect in receptors for calcitriol either intestinal or renal;
- poisoning local factors leading to defective mineralisation of bone.

REFERENCES

1. H.M. Frost, (1963), Bone Remodelling Dynamics, Charles C. Thomas, Springfield.
2. F.R. Singer, B.G. Mills and D.L. Madden, 1983, Pathophysiological and etiological considerations on Paget's disease of bone, in: "Human Calcitonin", A. Caniggia ed., Ciba-Geigy S.p.A., Basel.
3. P.H. Adams, J. Jowsey, P.J. Kelly, B.L. Riggs, V.R. Kinney and J.D. Jones, 1967, Effects of hyperthyroidism on bone and mineral metabolism in Man, Quart. J. Med., 36: 1-15.
4. A. Caniggia, C. Stuart and R. Guideri, 1958, Fragilitas ossium hereditaria tarda, Acta Med. Scand., Suppl. 340.
5. M.J.O. Francis, R. Smith and D.C. MacMillan, 1973, Polymeric collagen of skin in normal subjects and in patients with inherited connective tissue disorders, Clin. Sci., 44: 429.
6. G.H. Bourne, 1956, Vitamini C and Bone in: "The Biochemistry and physiology of Bone", by G.H. Bourne, ed. Acad. Press. inc., New York.
7. A. Courts and B.G. Giles, 1965, Collagen polysaccarides interactions, in Fitton-Jackson et al., eds "Structure and function of connective and skeletal tissue". Butterwords, London.
8. A. Caniggia and A. Vattimo, 1980, Kinetics of 99mTc- -Methylene Diphosphonate in normal subjects and in pathological conditions: a simple index of bone metabolism, Calcif. Tissue, 30: 5.

9. A. Caniggia and A. Vattimo, 1979, Kinetics of 99mTc- -Methylene Diphosphonate in women with post-menopausal osteoporosis, in "Molecular Endocrinology" I. Mc Intyre et al., Elsevier, North Holland Biochemical Press.

10. A. Vattimo, 1989, Personal communication.

11. A. Caniggia and C. Gennari, 1973, Cortisone osteoporosis an approach to the metabolic problem, in: "Clinical aspects of metabolic bone disease", Boy Frame et al eds., Excepta Medica, Amsterdam.

12. H.A. Sisson, 1960, Osteoporosis of Cushing's syndrome in: "Bone as Tissue" Rodahl K. et al., eds. McGraw-Hill Book Co. inc., New York.

13. A. Caniggia, C. Gennari, M. Bencini and V. Palazzuoli, 1968, Intestinal absorption of radiophosphate in osteomalacia before and after vitamin D treatment, Calcif. Tissue Res., 2: 299.

14. H.F. DeLuca, (1984), The metabolism, physiology and function of vitamin D, in: "Vitamin D Basic and Clinical aspects", Kumar R ed., Martinus Nijhoff, Boston.

15. F. Loré, G. Di Cairano, A.M. Signorini and A. Caniggia, 1981, Serum levels of 25-hydroxyvitamin D in post-menopausal osteoporosis, Calcif. Tissue Int., 33: 467.

16. F. Loré, G. Di Cairano, G. Petrini, A. Caniggia, 1982, Effect of the administration of 1,25-dihydroxyvitamin D3 on serum levels of 25-hydroxyvitamin D in postmenopausal osteoporosis, Calcif. Tissue Int. 34: 539.

17. A. Caniggia, F. Loré, R. Nuti, G. Di Cairano, V. Turchetti, G. Righi, G. Martini, G. Manasse, 1988, Osteomalacias: a pathophysiological and clinical survey. In: "Calciotropic hormones and Calcium Metabolism", Bi & Gi, Verona, 37.

18. F. Loré, 1985, La vitamina D e i suoi metaboliti nelle malattie croniche del fegato, Fegato, 31: 85.

19. B. Lund, E. Clausen, M. Friedber, B. Lund, S.P. Nielsen and O.H. Soerensen, 1980, Serum 1,25(OH)2Vit.D in anephric, haemodialized and kidney-transplated patients, Nephron, 25: 30.

20. B.E.C. Nordin, 1973, Metabolic Bone and Stone Disease, Churchill Livingstone, Edimburg and London.

21. S.M. Ott, N.A. Maloney, J.W. Coburn, A.C. Alfrey, D.J. Sherrad, 1982, The prevalence of bone aluminium deposition in renal osteodystrophy and its relation to the response to calcitriol therapy, New. Engl. J. Med., 307: 709.

PATHOPHYSIOLOGICAL ASPECTS IN THE TREATMENT OF POST-MENOPAUSAL OSTEOPOROSIS

Angelo Caniggia, Ranuccio Nuti, and Fausto Loré

Institute of Clinical Medicine
University of Siena, Italy

DIAGNOSIS OF POST-MENOPAUSAL OSTEOPOROSIS

This is the most characteristic clinical finding in post-menopausal osteoporosis (p.m.o.p.): dorsal kyphosis with shortening of the trunk and diminution of the height accounted for by the anterior vertebral crushes.

Vertebral fractures are particularly significant because of pain: either anterior crushes responsible for dorsal kyphosis or the so-called "cod-fishing" due to weakness of the vertebral plates become no more resistant to the mechanical pressure of the intervertebral disks.

Vertebral plates are composed by compact bone and the cod-fishing of the vertebrae indicates a softening of the compact bone.

The compact bone of the appendicular skeleton is more and more involved as well by the resorptive process in p.m.o.p., as you can see in this slide that compares the section of a normal compact bone to that of an advanced case of p.m.o.p.: the spongy transformation of the compact bone is particularly evident.

This is the case in this biopsy from iliac crest in a woman with p.m.o.p.: below the periosteum you can see a characteristic spongy tranformation of compact cortical bone; only poor remnants of the former haversian systems persist that are transformed in thin bony trabeculae similar to those of cancellous bone; some new carved resorption lacunae are still present, but no osteoclasts!

Cancellous bone in p.m.o.p. shows very rare and thin bony trabeculae with a prevalence of bone marrow on bone tissue; likewise to the former case in this histological section neither osteoclasts nor osteoblasts were present.

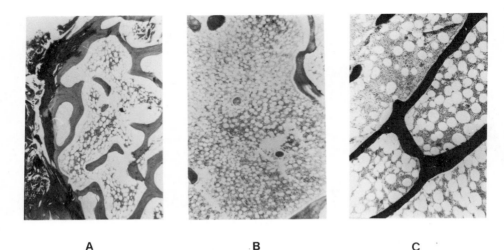

A   B   C

Figure 1. Biopsies from iliac crest in women with p.m.o.p.
A: spongy transformation of compact cortical bone;
B: scarse and thin trabeculae in cancellous bone;
C: thin trabeculae fully mineralized (preparations on undecalcified bone - Von Kossa stain).

Despite their thinning cancellous bone trabeculae in p.m.o.p. are fully mineralized as you can see in this histological preparation on undecalcified bone: black colour (von Kossa stain) indicates the complete mineralisation of the trabeculae (Figure 1).

Let me present the histological finding in a patient with osteomalacia and in another with a mixed pattern of osteoporosis and osteomalacia: red osteoid seams are evident in either cases being the trabecular thickness normally large in osteomalacia and thin in osteoporomalacia.

It is generally thought that the differencial diagnosis between osteoporosis and osteomalacia is easy.

Physicians generally believe that the most common biochemical parameters (as plasma calcium and phosphate, serum alkaline phosphatase, urinary hydroxyproline), are within the normal range in osteoporosis. But as matter of fact osteoporomalacia is frequently underestimated because of the lack of overt characteristic biochemistry of osteomalacia.

At X-ray a decrease in bone mineral content is appreciable both in osteoporosis and osteomalacia: but only when skeleton did loose more than 40% of its calcium content.

Vertebral fractures responsible of pain are evident in both pathological conditions either as crushes or as vertebral cod-fishing.

The Looser-Milkman pseudofractures characteristic of osteomalacia, are exceedingly rare and difficult to detect for their localisation that is some time strange.

This leads to overestimate the diagnosis of osteoporosis (particularly in post-menopausal women) and do not recognize osteomalacias.

Accounting vertebral pain to osteoporosis in post-menopausal women affected by spondyloarthritis is another very common mistake that leads to uncorrect conclusions on the effectiveness of some therapeutical procedures.

A correct clinical and radiological examination of these patients can easily avoid this mistake.

In the past years impressive advances have been made in non-invasive measurement of bone mass.

In the 1970's the advent of single photon absorptiometry (125I, 241Am) with its reasonable precision and accuracy allowed epidemiological studies in metabolic bone diseases.

The major problems for the clinical use of single-photon absorptiometry involve the precise localisation and relocation of the measurement site: this is a serious handicap for longitudinal studies to evaluating the effect of therapeutical procedures.

Of greater clinical relevance has been the measurement of bone mineral density using dual-photon 153Gd absorptiometry: this method enables measurements scans of lumbar spine and proximal femur.

But also in dual photon absorptiometry accurate location and relocation may represent a clinical problem particularly in patients with spinal deformities or fractures.

Total body calcium estimation by neutron activation analysis represents a reliable method to evaluate bone mass in vivo; but its clinical use is not practicable because of problems of elevated costs and radiation safety.

At present bone mineral content may be exactly measured by the dual-photon total body absorptiometry that can use either a 153Gd or an X-ray source (1).

This absorptiometric procedure enables to measure exactly total body bone mineral, total body calcium and total body bone-density that has been expressed in g/cm2. Moreover it is possible to obtain a hard copy of the skeletal image including cuts of regions of interest, as total spine for example.

In specialized papers frequently the expression "Bone Mineral Density" is considered equivalent to "Bone Mass"; this is absolutely uncorrect: low bone mineral density (BMD) is found in osteoporosis as well as in osteomalacia but the meaning of these results are

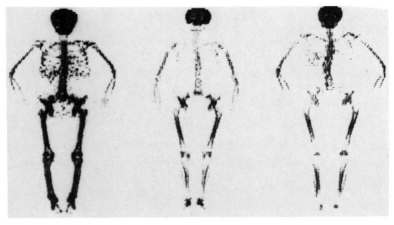

NORMAL   OSTEOPOROSIS   OSTEOMALACIA

Figure 2. Visual display of the total body bone mineral in a case with p.m.o.p. (in the middle) and in another with nutritional osteomalacia (on the right), compared to a normal subject (on the left).

completely different: low BMD in osteoporosis may really measure the degree of osteopenia that is the diminution of the fully mineralized bone mass, whereas low BMD in osteomalacia indicates the bone calcium content in a skeleton whom bone mass in normal.

Bone absorptiometry is an additional factor of diagnosis in osteoporoses and osteomalacias but in any case this cannot be founded only an the diminution of Bone Mineral Density which is decreased in either these pathological conditions (2).

PATHOGENESIS OF POST-MENOPAUSAL OSTEOPOROSIS

Post-menopausal osteoporosis is accounted for to the post-menopausal estrogen deficiency.

Such a decrease in bone mass can only result from a negative calcium balance.

Despite his theory of osteoblasts deficiency Albright demonstrated that negative calcium balance in p.m.o.p. was due to an increase in the faecal losses of calcium: evidently calcium was not sufficiently absorbed (3).

Since 1963 we demostrated that the intestinal transport of radioactive calcium was defective in women with p.m.o.p. (4); this finding has been largely confirmed afterwards (5-20).

The impairment in the intestinal calcium transport cannot be accounted for by the "vitamin D status" of these women in whom the administration of vitamin D is ineffective.

Serum levels of 25OHvit.D and 1,25(OH)2vit.D have been measured in a number of women with p.m.o.p., the basal concentrations of 25OHvit.D were found to be higher than in age matched controls or normal younger women so demostrating an excellent vitamin D status (21).

On the contrary the basal concentrations of 1,25(OH)2vit.D were lower, according to many authors (22-25).

1,25(OH)2 vit.D3 administered at physiological dose (1μg/day) was effective in restoring a normal radiocalcium absorption within 10 days in women with p.m.o.p. (26).

According to these data it could be suggested an impaired activity of 25OH-1-alpha-hydroxylase no longer stimulated by estrogens.

The findings we obtained many years ago in a double blind study carried out in women with p.m.o.p. given an oestrogen gestogen combination or placebo, are consistent with this hypothesis: the treatment was effective in restoring a normal radiocalcium absorption, whereas no change was observed in the placebo group (27).

Hence the following working hypothesis: estrogen lack ⟶ impaired calcium absorption ⟶ negative calcium balance ⟶ decrease in the bone mineral content considered as a necessary sequential reaction to preserve the calcium homeostasis in body fluids (28).

LONG-TERM CALCITRIOL TREATMENT OF POST-MENOPAUSAL OSTEO-POROSIS.

The present study was begun in 1980 and is still in progress (29).

240 women with p.m.o.p. entered the study: mean age 64 years.

The lenght of the treatment has been shown in the present slide.

Only women with symptomatic post-menopausal osteoporosis were admitted according to the following criteria:
- back pain and difficulty in walking;
- vertebral translucency with one or more edge crushes and/or cod-fishing;
- decreased bone mineral density;
- histological pattern of osteoporosis (osteomalacia and osteoporomalacia were ruled out);
- impaired intestinal radiocalcium transport as assessed by the measurement of the circulating fraction of the administered dose (fx);
- normal values of plasma calcium and phosphate, serum

alkaline phosphatase, 24hr. urinary calcium, phosphate
and hydroxyproline;
- normal renal function.
          Criteria of exclusion:
- other disease than osteoporosis;
- long-term treatments with glucoactive corticosteroids,
  anticonvulsant or heparin;
- spondyloarthritis.
          The patients were given calcitriol (1,25(OH)2
vitamin D3) at the oral dose of 1 microgram per day:
- patients were allowed to their usual diet without
  calcium supplementation;
- no interruption of the treatment since the beginnig of
  the trial;
- no other drug given, including analgesics;
          The probability density function has been
assessed by a sophisticated statistical method (30).
          In the patients of the present study the
probability density function for plasma calcium and
urinary hydroxyproline in basal conditions did coincide
with those of 103 age-matched non osteoporotic women (left
part of the panel). On the contrary the probability
density curves for fractional radiocalcium absorption and
the 24h. urinary calcium excretion in osteoporotic women
showed a significant shift toward lower values (right part
of the panel).
          On treatment: laboratory parameters have been
determined initially every other month.

Intestinal calcium absorption

          Intestinal calcium absorption was measured by
our radiocalcium oral test 10 μ Ci of Ca47 or Ca45 given
orally in 80 mg of calcium chloride as non radioactive
carrier, and expressed as circulating fraction of the
administered dose (fx) according to Marshall and Nordin
(31):
          The women of the present study showed basal fx
values lower than the normal range without significant
regression on age on the contrary of the normal
age-matched women (left part of the panel). This indicates
a severe impairment of the intestinal calcium transport
beginning soon after the menopause.
          The probability density function calculated 2-6
and 12 months after the beginning of calcitriol administration showed rapid and significant increases in the
fractional calcium absorption.
          This significant increase did persist 1 to 8
years after the beginning of treatment as long as
calcitriol was administered.
          The persistent normalisation of the intestinal
calcium absorption achieved on calcitriol treatment is
summarized in figure 3.

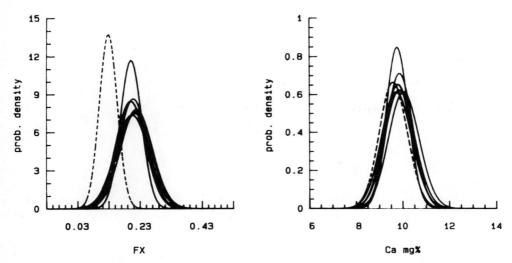

Figure 3. Left: Normalisation of the intestinal radiocalcium absorption on long-term calcitriol treatment (1 μg
per day).
Right: trivial increases in fasting plasma calcium.

        It must be stressed that calcitriol given at the
physiological dose of 1 microgram per day did succeed in
leading to normal values the intestinal calcium transport
in p.m.o.p. women; in other words it correct d
persistently the main pathophysiological defect in these
patients as a substitution therapy does.
        it must be stressed that this effect was
achieved provided calcitriol was administered at the dose
of 1 μg per day:
- no clearly cut results were obtained with 0.50 μg;
- 0.25 μg per day were an absolutely ineffective dose.
        In other words it was necessary to administering
calcitriol at its physiological dose.

Fasting plasma calcium

        Fasting plasma calcium showed a slight increase
in mean values on calcitriol treatment: this increase was
to be expect d due to the improved intestinal calcium
absorption.
        Here are the probability density functions since
1 to 8 years showing but trivial increases in fasting
plasma calcium.
        Actually transient plasma calcium levels above
11.5 mg% were only exceptionally observed: in any case the
treatment did not need to be discontinued.
        This result can be surely account d for to the
fact that we did avoid any calcium supplementation:

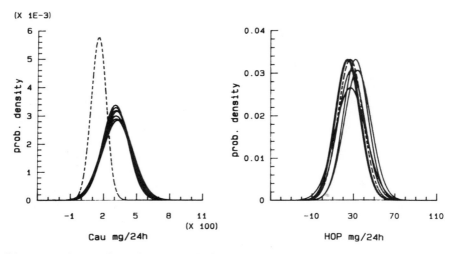

Figure 4. Left: hypercalciuria in p.m.o.p. on long-term calcitriol treatment.
Right: no parallel modifications in urinary excreation of hydroxyproline.

calcitriol "per se" enables a sufficient calcium absorption through a normalisation of the intestinal calcium transport.

Urinary calcium and hydroxyproline

        24 hour urinary excretion of calcium rose on calcitriol administration and hypercalciuria was observed throughout the treatment being a significant parameter of the patients compliance because urinary calcium excretion fell soon after calcitriol was discontinued.
        The increases in calcium excretion that were statistically significant are summarized in figure 4.
        It has been suggested that 1,25(OH)2vit.D3 administration results in an increase in bone resorption and that the hypercalciuria enhanced by calcitriol can be account d for to this mechanism.
        According to our experience this view is unt nable: in fact the 24 hr. urinary excretion of hydroxyproline did neither increase in the fir t year of calcitriol administration nor 1 ter.
        In basal conditions the regression of 24 hr. urinary calcium ver us fractional calcium absorption did not give significant results in the patients of the present study; whereas along with the calcitriol treatment, when individual levels of urinary calcium were plotted against the corresponding values of fractional calcium absorption, a highly significant positive correl tion was obtained.

260

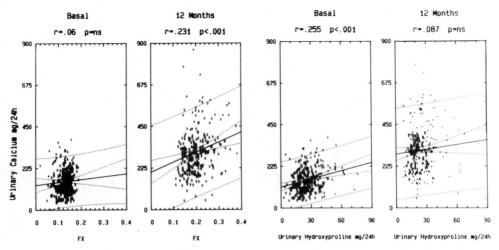

Figure 5. Left: regression of 24h. urinary calcium vs. fractional radiocalcium absorption; very significant on calcitriol treatment.
Right: no parallel regression of 24h. urinary calcium vs. 24h. urinary hydroxyproline.

The regression of 24 hr. urinary calcium ver us urinary hydroxyproline was statistically significant in basal conditions but it was no more on long-term calcitriol treatment (Figure 5).

No correl tion was observed between fasting plasma calcium and total urinary calcium.

It must be concluded that hypercalciuria was mainly due to the calcitriol effect on the intestinal calcium transport that is obviously more appreciable after the meals rather than after an overnight fast.

Renal function

Hypercalcemia and hypercalciuria are generally believed to be harmful to renal function and to increase the risk of renal stone formation.

Despite the hypercalciuria induced by long-term calcitriol administration:
- no patient showed changes in renal function as demonstrated by urinalysis,blood urea nitrogen, plasma creatinine levels and urinary creatinine clearance;
- no renal stone developed.

The conclusion can be drawn that in spite of a persistent hypercalciuria the long-term calcitriol administration at the dose of 1 µg/day did not result in any adver e effect on renal function.

Parathyroid function

The cAMP/creatinine ratio on 24 hr. urine collections is generally recognized as a good index of parathyroid function.

In the patients of the present study a slowly progressive but significant decrease in this parameter was observed; that is shown by the slight shifting of the probability density function curves toward left.

This could be account d for by parathyroid suppression and must be considered a favourable effect since it would reduce bone resorption.

Bone GLA Protein

Serum levels of osteocalcin in basal conditions and during long-term treatment with calcitriol have been evaluated in a small number of our patients.

Prior to the initiation of treatment osteocalcin levels averaged lower than in a group of age-matched non--osteoporotic women previously studied in our l boratory 3.8 ± 1.1 ng/ml and 6.8 ± 2.0 ng/ml respectively.

Treatment with calcitriol produced a significant increase in osteocalcin levels 4.5 ± 1.4 ng/ml, $p < 0.001$.

It is known that calcitriol is a physiological stimulator of bone GLA protein synthesis by osteoblasts (32).

Our results indicate that in p.m.o.p. osteoblasts had not lost their ability to respond to calcitriol.

Clinical results

We should like to emphasize that the treatment with calcitriol resulted in a significant and often dramatic relief from pain and improvement in motility: some of our women were practically bedridden or confined to wheel chair and after a few months of therapy they were able to walk again.

Patients compliance was testified by the fact that they came diligently from every part of Italy to our Institute for the periodical controls at their own expenses (travel nd housing). In simil r so long trials this can be considered a good measure of social compliance and is a confirmation of the beneficial effects of treatment as seen from the point of view of patients and their physicians.

The reduction in the occurrence of new non-traumatic fractures was significant as compared with the period preceding the initiation of therapy.

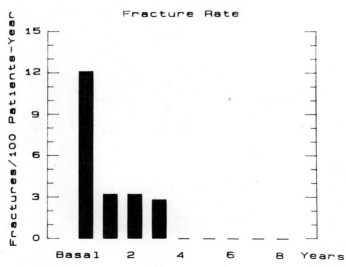

Figure 6. Occurrence of non traumatic fractures in the
patients of the present study before and on long-term
calcitriol treatment.

Bone absorptiometry

Longitudinal mineralometric studies on the
results achieved with the administration of anti-osteo-
porotic drugs are burden with repositioning difficulties
in single photon measures and with the exact
identification of single vertebrae in the lumbar spine
with dual photon procedures.

At the beginning of this trial we measured the
bone mineral density at the distal forearm.

In basal conditions a significant regression on
age was ascertained indicating the progressive worsening
of the disease.

On calcitriol treatment an improvement in bone
mineral density was checked: it was statistically
significant only after 10-12 months from the beginning of
treatment.

Bone mineral content and the Bone mineral
density may more exactly be measured by dual photon total
body absorptiometry that is in use in our Institute since
two years or so.

With this absolutely impartial device the
spectacular increases of BMC and BMD in successfully
treated patients with osteomalacia may be checked merely
looking at the visual display; for instance in this
patient the bone mineral content rose by 30% in 1 year and
you can see directly the progressive increase in bone
mineral density. In p.m.o.p. the improvement in BMD
achieved after long-term treatment with calcitriol has
never been of such an extent.

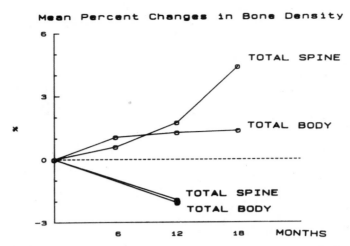

Figure 7. Bone Mineral Density measured by total body bone mineral absorptiometry in 44 women of the present study: after 1 year treatment with calcitriol an increase in BMD was ascertained in all cases (o), while in a control group (•) a decrease in BMD was appreciated.

Nevertheless after 1 year or more of calcitriol treatment an increase in total body bone density was ascertained almost in all patients.

In any case a reversal of the well known spontaneous decrease in bone mineral density was observed.

In postmenopausal osteoporotic women the decrease in BMD has been evaluated by 5% "per annum" or so; with total body dual photon absorptiometry we have been able to confirm such a decrease in a small placebo group in comparison to the patients of the present study.

The efficacy of the calcitriol treatment on Bone Mineral Density in total spine was greater than that in total skeleton, probably because of the prevalence of spongy bone.

The difference in the absorptiometric results achieved in osteoporosis and osteomalacia must be accounted for to the different mechanisms of the decreasing BMD in these pathological conditions:
- in osteomalacia bone is avid of calcium and thanks its normal mass it is able to uptaking larger calcium amounts;
- in osteoporosis the extensive disappearance of bone trabeculae led to substancial decreases of template for new bone accretion, so that a stop in the spontaneous progressive bone loss can be considered a real success whereas spectacular increases in bone mineral density cannot be expected.

Calcitriol treatment is a substitution therapy:

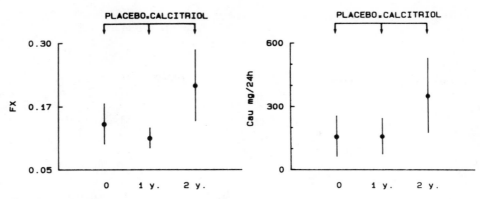

Figure 8. Double blind placebo control trial in 28 women
with p.m.o.p. Sequential study: placebo administration for
1 year, subsequent calcitriol treatment for the next year.

interrupting calcitriol administration leads rapidly to a
worsening of the intestinal calcium transport and -
within months - to the relapsing of pain and possibly of
fractures.

The patients of the present slide did interrupt
the calcitriol intake: they rapidly fell to very low
intestinal calcium transport with a parallel decrease in
urinary calcium.

But no problems, because calcitriol:
- is a physiological compound;
- given orally in physiological doses;
- devoid of untoward adverse effects;
 biochemically and clinically effective;
- unexpensive;
So that it can be administered safely for years.

Double blind placebo control study

The present study has been an open trial:
why we did not choose a double blind study?
For two reasons:
first: it was not ethical, considering the trial
lenght;
secondly: it would be only a partially blind
study, because of the overt biochemical responses in any
patient given calcitriol.
Recently we have been able to perform a
sequential study in a relatively small number of women
according to the following schedule:
- placebo adomistration for one year;
- subsequent calcitriol treatment for the next year.

You can see in figure 8 the striking differences between the first and the second part of this trial.

REFERENCES

1. Mazess R.B., Peppler R.W., Chesney R.W., Lange T.A., Lindgren U and Smith E. Jr., 1984, Total body and regional bone mineral by dual-photon absorptiometry in metabolic bone disease, Calcif. Tissue Int., 36: 8.
2. Nuti R., Righi G., Martini G., Turchetti V., Lepore C. and Caniggia A., 1987, Methods and clinical applications of Total Body Absorptiometry. J. Nucl.Med.All. Sciences, 31: 213.
3. Albright F. and Reifenstein B.C., 1948, "The parathyroid glands and metabolic bone disease", Williams & Wilkins Co. Baltimore.
4. Caniggia A., Gennari C., Bianchi V. and Guideri R., 1963, Intestinal absorption of 45Ca in senile osteoporosis, Acta Med. Scand., 173: 613.
5. Kinney V.R., Tauxe V.N. and W.H. Dearing, 1966, Isotopic tracer studies of intestinal calcium absorption, J. Lab. Clin. Med. 66: 187.
6. Parson V., Veall N. and Butterfield W.J.H., 1968, The clinical use of orally administered 47Ca for the investigation of intestinal calcium absorption, Calcif. Tissue Res., 2: 83.
7. Bullamore J.R., Wilkinson R., Gallagher J.C., Nordin B.E.C. and Marshall D.H., 1970, Effects of age on calcium absorption, Lancet, II: 535.
8. Szymedera J., Heaney R.P. and Saville P.D., 1979, Intestinal calcium absorption: concurrent use of oral and intravenous tracers and calculation by the inverse convolution method, J. Lab., Clin. Med. 79: 570.
9. Alevizaki C.C., Ikkos D.C. and Singhelakis P., 1973, Progressive decrease of true intestinal calcium absorption with age in normal man. J. Nucl. Med., 14: 760.
10. Gallagher J.C., Aaron J., Horsman A., Marshall D.H., Wilkinson R. and Nordin B.E.C., 1973, The crush fracture syndrome in postmenopausal women, Clinic Endocrinol. Metabol., 2: 293.
11. Ireland P. and Fordtran S., 1973, Effect of dietary calcium and age on jejunal calcium absorption in humans studied by intestinal perfusion, J. Clin., Invest., 52: 2672.
12. Nordin B.E.C., Williams R., Marshall D.H., Gallagher J.C., Williams A. and Peacock M., 1976, Calcium absorption in the elderly. IIth European Symposium on Calcified Tissues, Calcif. Tissue Res., 215: 422.
13. Lindholm T.S., Sevastikoglou J.A. and Lindgren U., 1977, Treatment of patients with senile

post-menopausal and corticosteroid-induced osteoporosis with 1-alpha-hydroxyvitamin D3 and calcium: short and long-term effects, Clin. Endocrinol., 7, Suppl. 183.

14. Sorensen O.H., Andersen R.B., Christiansen M.S., Friis T., Hjorth L., Jorgensen F.S., Lund B., Melsen F. and Mosekilde L., 1977, Treatment of senile osteoporosis with 1 alpha-hydroxyvitamin D3. Clin. Endocrinol. (Oxf), 7: 169.

15. Heaney R.P., Recker R.R. and Saville P.D., 1978, Menopausal changes in calcium balance performance, J. Lab. Clin. Med., 92: 953.

16. Gallagher J.C., Riggs B.L. and DeLuca H.F. 1980, Intestinal Calcium Absorption and Serum Vitamin D Metabolites in Normal Subjects and Osteoporotic Patients, J. Clin. Invest., 64: 729.

17. Gallagher J.C., Riggs B.L. and DeLuca H.F., 1980, Effect of estrogen on calcium absorption and serum vitamin D metabolites in postmenopausal osteoporosis, J. Clin. Endocrinol. Metab., 53: 833.

18. Riggs B.L., Hamstra A., DeLuca H.F., 1981, Assessment of 25-hydroxyvitamin D-1-hydroxylase reserve in postmenopausal osteoporosis, J. Clin. Endocrinol. Metab., 53: 833.

19. Nordin B.E.C. and Peacock M., 1982, The relation between bone calcium flow, plasma 1,25(OH)2D3 and calcium absorption in post-menopausal women. In: Fifth Workshop on Vitamin D, Historic Williamsburg, Virginia, p. 335, Abstracts.

20. Riggs B.L., 1982, Vitamin D metabolism in involutional osteoporosis: evidence for etiologic heterogeneity. In: Fifth Workshop on vitamin D, Historic Williamsburg, Virginia, p. 324, Abstracts.

21. Loré F., Di Cairano G. Signorini A.M. and Caniggia A., 1981, Serum levels of 25-hydroxyvitamin D in post-menopausal osteoporosis, Calcif.Tissue Int., 33: 467.

22. Gallagher J.C., Riggs B.L., Eisman J., Hamstra A., Arnaud S.B. and DeLuca H.F., 1979, Intestinal calcium absorption and serum vitamin D metabolites, J. Clin. Invest, 64: 729.

23. Lund B., Sorensen O.H. and Lund B., 1982, Serum 1,25-dihydroxyvitamin D in normal subjects and in patients with postmenopausal osteopenia, Horm. Metab. Res., 14: 271.

24. Loré F., Nuti R., Vattimo A., Caniggia A., 1984, Vitamin D metabolites in postmenopausal osteoporosis, Hormone and Metabolic Research, 16: 58.

25. Caniggia A., Loré F., Di Cairano G., Nuti R., 1987, Main endocrine modulators of vitamin D hydroxylases in human pathophysiology. The Journal of Steroid Biochemistry, 27: 815.

26. Caniggia A. and Vattimo A., 1979, Effects of 1,25-dihydroxycholecalciferol on 47Calcium absorption on post-menopausal osteoporosis, Clin. Endocrinology 11: 99.
27. Caniggia A. and Vattimo A., 1979, Effects of 1,25-dihydroxycholecalciferol on 47Calcium absorption in post-menopausal osteoporosis, Clin. Endocrinology, 11: 99.
28. Caniggia A., Gennari C., Borrello G., Bencini M., Cesari L., Poggi C. and Escobar S., 1970, Intestinal absorption of calcium 47 after treatment with oral oestrogen-gestogen in senile osteoporosis, Brit. Med. J., 4: 30.
29. Caniggia A., 1965, Medical problems in senile osteoporosis, Geriatrics, 20: 300.
30. Scala C., 1985, Funzioni di densità di probabilità: atlante descrittivo. Tipi Monotypia Franchi. Società Artigiana Tipografica, Lama (PG).
31. Marshall D.H. and Nordin B.E.C. 1969, Kinetic analysis of plasma radioactivity after oral ingestion of radiocalcium, Nature, 222: 797.
32. Price P.A., Williamson M.K. and Lothringer J.W., 1981, Origin of the vit. K-dependent bone protein found in plasma and its clearance by kidney and bone, J. Biol. Chem., 256: 12760.

RECENT TRENDS IN THE USE OF BONE REGULATORY

FACTORS AS THERAPEUTIC AGENTS

D. Harold Copp

Department of Physiology, University of British Columbia

Vancouver, B.C., Canada V6T 1W5

I.   INTRODUCTION

Bone is a highly dynamic tissue with a blood flow in the rat which has been estimated at 5-10% of the resting cardiac output (Copp and Shim, 1965). There is also continuing osteogenesis and osteolysis occurring in the modelling of new bone in the growing animal and in the remodelling of trabecular and cortical bone in the adult. This is clearly shown by Raisz (1988a) in Figure 1, which illustrates the sequence of activation of osteolysis, a transition period and subsequent osteogenesis. In this way, the bone continually renews

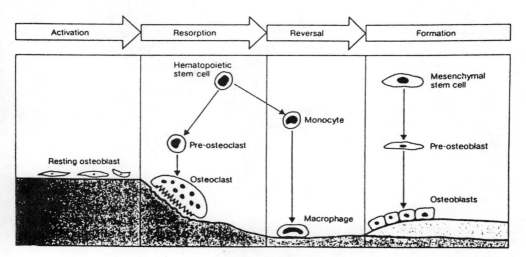

Figure 1.   Dynamic cycle of bone remodelling. From Raisz (1988a)
Reproduced courtesy of author and publisher.

269

itself. As discussed by Raisz in a recent review (1988b), the bone
regulatory factors act as modulators of these dynamic processes, and
include a) the systemic hormones involved in homeostasis of calcium in
body fluids; b) other systemic hormones which affect bone, c) local
factors, and d) inorganic ions (Ca, P, F). Their therapeutic
effectiveness depends on these effects.

A. HORMONES INVOLVED IN CALCIUM HOMEOSTASIS

The level of ionic calcium in the extracellular fluid is a
critical factor in many important biological systems, including
neuronal excitability, muscle contraction, cell division, cell
permeability, hormone release, blood clotting and the normal
mineralization of bones and teeth (Copp, 1969). Thus it is not
surprising that vertebrates have very efficient homeostatic mechanisms
for its regulation. The factors involved are shown in Figure 2, and
include the organ systems of the gut, kidney and bone and the actions
of the specific calcium-regulating hormones (parathyroid hormone,
calcitonin and calcitriol).

1. Parathyroid Hormone (PTH)

MacCallum and Voegtlin (1909) showed that removal of the
parathyroids in the dog resulted in hypocalcemia and symptoms which
could be corrected by injection of calcium salts. They correctly
concluded that the glands prevented hypocalcemia and were involved in
calcium homeostasis. Indeed, until 1961, it was assumed that they were
solely responsible for this critical role (McLean, 1957) in view of
their action on bone and kidney and the effective feedback control by
which the level of plasma calcium regulated the secretion of
parathyroid hormone (Copp and Davidson, 1961). An active extract of

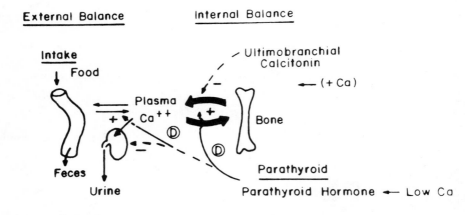

Fig. 2. Factors involved in the homeostatic regulation of ionic
calcium in extracellular fluid. Calcitriol is indicated by a circled
D. From Copp (1969). Reproduced coutesy of J.Endocrinology.

the glands was prepared by Collip (1925), and pure bovine PTH was
finally prepared and characterized by Niall et al. (1970). It is a
straight chain peptide with 84 amino acids, but the biological activity
resides in the first 34 amino acid sequence from the N terminal (Marcus
and Aurbach, 1969) and the human 1-34 sequence has been synthesized and
used in human therapy (Slovik et al., 1986). Recently, a PTH-like
peptide from tumor tissue has been isolated and characterized (Moseley
et al., 1987).

     Parathyroid hormone acts primarily on kidney and bone cells,
specifically osteoblasts. The latter release a local factor which
stimulates the activity and proliferation of osteoclasts, and the
resulting osteolysis mobilizes calcium and phosphate from the skeleton,
thus raising their level in plasma. In the kidney, PTH is phosphaturic
(thus disposing of the phosphate mobilized from bone) and stimulates
tubular reabsorption of calcium in the kidney. In appropriate doses,
PTH stimulates osteogenesis (Hock et al.,1989)- an action which has led
to its use in osteoporosis (Slovik et al., 1986). In addition, it
stimulates the activity of the l-alpha hydroxylase in the kidney cells
which converts 25-hydroxycholecalciferol into the active hormone,
calcitriol (Boyle et al., 1971).

2. Calcitonin (CT)

     In 1961, a second peptide hormone involved in calcium homeostasis
was discovered (Copp et al., 1961, 1962) and given the name CALCITONIN
because of its evident role in controlling the level or "tone" of
calcium in body fluids. There is a recent review by Wolfe (1982), and
a very comprehensive monograph by Azria (1989). In addition, in this
volume, Wimalawansa has given a very comprehensive survey of the
molecular biology, physiology and pathophysiology of this hormone along
with some important therapeutic applications.

     Shortly after the discovery of calcitonin, Hirsch et al. (1964)
found that simple acid extracts of rat and hog thyroid had a potent and
log-dose related hypocalcemic effect in young rats and proposed the
alternative name for the hormone, THYROCALCITONIN, to indicate its
gland of origin. Their simple rat assay is still the basis for the
determination of biological potency of calcitonin preparations used in
human therapy, which is expressed in terms of the International
Standard for Calcitonin (Parsons and Reynolds, 1968). Pearse (1966)
found that the calcitonin producing cells, which he labelled "C" cells,
were distinct from the regular follicular cells, and were, in fact,
derived from the ultimobranchial body of the embryo (Pearse and
Carvalheira, 1967) which merges with the thyroid in mammals, but
remains a distinct and separate gland in lower vertebrates. The
ultimobranchial origin of CT in chickens was demonstrated by Copp et
al. (1967) and Tauber (1967). In a brilliant series of experiments, Le
Douarin and Le Lievre (1970) showed that these cells were originally
derived from the neural crest of the embryo, clearly linking calcitonin
with the neuroendocrine system.

     Early studies clearly showed that the hypocalcemic effect of
calcitonin in young animals was the result of inhibition of osteolysis
(Friedman and Raisz, 1965; Reynolds, 1968). This stimulated interest
in a number of pharmaceutical companies (Armour, Ciba, Merck, Sandoz,
etc.) in its potential for treating diseases associated with bone
loss. However, the first report on the purification and determination

of the amino acid sequence of porcine calcitonin, published in 1967, was from Potts' laboratory at Harvard (Potts et al., 1968). It proved to be a straight chain peptide of 32 amino acids with a 7 membered disulfide ring at the N terminal and prolinamide at the C terminal. Unlike PTH, the entire molecule appears to be necessary for biological activity (Guttmann et al., 1981). Shortly after, the structure of human CT was determined (Neher et al., 1968), from hormone extracted from a medullary carcinoma of thyroid (a tumor of the C cells). Inspired by the discovery of calcitonin in the ultimobranchial glands of lower vertebrates, we collected 200kg. of these glands from over half a million pacific salmon. In an international collaborative effort, the glands were bulk processed by the Armour Pharmaceutical Company, pure salmon calcitonin was isolated in our laboratory (O'Dor et al., 1969), the amino acid sequence was determined by John Potts' group in Boston (Niall et al., 1969) and the hormone was synthesized by the Sandoz Company in Basel, Switzerland (Guttmann et al., 1969). Of particular interest was the very high potency of the salmon hormone (5,000 U/mg) compared to human and porcine CT (100-200 U/mg). Because of this high potency, and its greater analgesic effect, salmon calcitonin is now the form commonly used in human therapy, along with eel calcitonin, first isolated by Otani et al. (1975), which has similar potency. A year later, Morikawa et al. (1976) prepared a synthetic derivative (elkatonin) in which the disulfide bridge (-S-S-) was replaced by (-C-C-) which is almost as potent, and is thought to be more stable. Based on the amino acid sequences, the calcitonins whose structures have been determined fall into 3 classes: 1) artiodactyl (ox, sheep and hog); 2) human and rat; and 3) non-mammalian vertebrates (chicken, salmon and eel). MacIntyre and Craig (1981) traced the evolution of the calcitonins and demonstrated molecules immunoreactive with human CT in the brains of primitive chordates and even in unicellular organisms such as E. coli and C. albicans.

2B. Calcitonin Gene-Related Peptide (CGRP)

One of the most exciting developments of the past 6 years has been the isolation of the calcitonin gene from a transplantable medullary carcinoma of the thyroid of the rat. Alternative mRNA processing in the thyroid C cells, produced calcitonin as the major product, and in the hypothalamus produces a new biologically active product referred to as calcitonin gene-related peptide or CGRP (Amara et al., 1982). The latter consists of 37 amino acids, with a six membered disulfide ring at the N terminal and an amide at the C terminal, so that it bears some resemblance to calcitonin. The gene has also been identified in the human, where it is located on the short arm of chromosome 11 (Kittur et al., 1985). While the thyroid does produce some CGRP, particularly in older rats, the main source of circulating CGRP appears to be the perivascular nerves (Zaidi et al., 1986). Two forms of human CGRP have been characterized and appear to be equally potent biologically (Brain et al., 1986). In addition to the hypothalamus, CGRP has been demonstrated in the peripheral nervous system and, in particular, in the dorsal horn of the spinal cord where its distribution corresponds with that of substance P (Lee et al., 1985). Sectioning of the dorsal root on one side resulted in a 95% reduction in the CGRP in the dorsal horn, leading to the conclusion that it was probably derived from neurons in the dorsal root ganglion (Gibson et al., 1984). Gene processing in the thyroid C cells produces not only calcitonin, but equimolecular amounts of a second biologically active peptide which has been referred to as PDN 21 (MacIntyre et al., 1982) or katacalcin (MacIntyre, 1984). It consists of a straight chain peptide of 21 amino acids with no disulfide ring, and is hypocalcemic, although at a dose level a thousand times higher than for calcitonin.

The first observed action of calcitonin was inhibition of osteolysis (Friedman and Raisz, 1965; Reynolds, 1968) and this was associated with a fall in plasma calcium and an increase in urinary hydroxyproline (Klein and Talmage, 1968). Receptors for calcitonin are present in kidney and bone (Marx et al., 1972). Kallio et al. (1972) observed with electron microscopy a marked inhibitory response, including loss of the ruffled border, within 15 minutes of adding salmon calcitonin to a culture of 6 day old mouse calvaria.

The early studies clearly indicated a homeostatic role in controlling hypercalcemia. This requires an efficient negative feedback control, as was demonstrated by Care et al. (1975) in sheep. However, its most important function in mammals may be the protection of the calcium stores of the body during periods of stress, such as pregnancy and lactation (Lewis et al., 1970), particularly when the calcium intake is low. Gray and Munson (1969) also produced evidence for a role in controlling plasma calcium after ingestion of a high calcium meal.

In addition to its well established action on bone, calcitonin has important effects on a number of other tissues. Calcitonin receptors are present in the kidney as well as bone (Marx et al., 1972), and calcitonin has a marked natriuretic, diuretic and calciuric effect in the rat (Keeler et al., 1970) and man (Bijvoet et al., 1971). The calciuric effect may be masked by the induced hypocalcemia. Injection of calcitonin into the lateral ventricle inhibited gastric secretion (Morley and Levine, 1981), and acts on the appetite center in the hypothalamus to cause anorexia (Levine and Morley, 1981). However, the most striking effects of calcitonin are in the central nervous system, where receptors are found in the hypothalamus and nuclei of the limbic system and in the critical periaquaductal grey matter which is the major pain pathway (Henke et al., 1983). Administration of calcitonin into the cerebral ventricles has a very potent analgesic effect (Pecile et al., 1975), which is explained in part by an increase in beta-endorphins, but occurs even when this path is blocked by naloxone (Braga et al., 1978). This is shown in Figure 3. Clementi et al. (1985) have linked this to the serotoninergic system, while Rohner amd Planche (1985) present evidence for a morphine-like and cortisone-like effect. It is also significant that calcitonin suppresses prostaglandin production in bone and has an anti-inflammatory effect (Cesarani et al., 1979).

Human CGRP has been demonstrated in the brain and in the thyroid and circulates at a level five times that of calcitonin (Girgis et al., 1985). Tippins et al. (1984) demonstrated a log-dose related stimulation of contraction of strips of guinea pig ileum, and a positive inotropic and chronotropic effect on strips of rat atria. However, the most interesting effect is vasodilation (Brain et al., 1985). Gennari and Fischer (1985) gave human subjects a single dose of 25.3 nM of hCGRP i.v. and observed a decrease of 26 mm Hg in systolic pressure and 20 mm Hg in diastolic pressure, along with an increase in heart rate of 41 beats per minute. The same dose (25.3 nM) of human calcitonin had no effect. Struthers et al. (1986) obtained similar results. They consider it the most potent vasodilator known, and since it circulates in plasma at levels of 25 pM/L., they feel it may have an important role in cardiovascular regulation. Indeed, the combination of vasodilation and a positive inotropic effect on the heart suggests that CGRP may have a useful role in the treatment of hypertension.

CALCITRIOL (1,25 dihydroxycholecalciferol)

There is an excellent recent review on role of the vitamin D endocrine system in health and disease (Reichel et al. 1989) and also one by A.W. Norman in this volume. The prohormone of calcitriol, cholecalciferol (vitamin D3) is formed from 7-dehydrocholesterol in the skin under the action of UV light, and is only a true vitamin in northern climes during the dark winter months. The critical experiments of Kodicek (1974) and DeLuca (1974) showed that cholecalciferol (vitamin D3) was oxidized in the liver to 25-hydroxycholecalciferol and ultimately in the kidney to the most active metabolite, 1,25 dihydroxycholecalciferol (CALCITRIOL), the most active metabolite in terms of increasing the production of calcium transport proteins in gut, kidney and bone. The ultimate proof that this was an important calcium regulating hormone came with the demonstration of negative feedback control of its production, in which a low level of plasma calcium, (with increased production of PTH) activated the 25-hydroxycholecalciferol-1-hydroxylase to produce calcitriol (Boyle et al., 1971) as did a low level of plasma phosphate (Tanaka and DeLuca, 1973). The hormone acts on the cells of gut, kidney and bone to produce a specific calcium binding protein which facilitates calcium transport and is essential for the action of PTH. It is now clear that receptors for calcitriol are present in many tissues other than those involved in calcium regulation, where it may effect the intracellular calcium concentration and affect cellular biology. Of particular interest is the maturing effect on hemopoietic cell which may have a potential for treatment for certain leukemias.

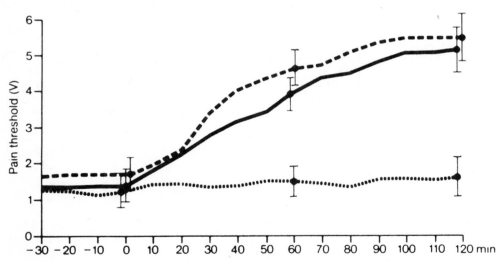

Fig. 3. Analgesic effect of salmon calcitonin as indicated by increased pain threshold in rabbits injected into the cerebral ventricle with calcitonin (12 U/kg; solid line); naloxone injected subcutaneously (1 mg/kg; dotted line) or both treatments (broken line). From Braga et al., (1978), courtesy author and publisher.

B.   OTHER SYSTEMIC HORMONES ACTING ON BONE

Note: These are discussed in the review by Raisz (1988b).

1.   GROWTH HORMONE (pituitary)

The pituitary growth hormone has a stimulating effect on growth of all tissues of the body, including bone, and indeed the early assays for the hormone were based on its stimulation of growth at the epiphyseal plate in growing rats. Because of its anabolic effect, it has been used in treating pituitary dwarfism.

2.   THYROID HORMONES T3 and T4 (thyroid)

These hormones are involved in the metabolic activity and maturation of all tissues, including bone and the first evidence of thyroid deficiency may be a delay in eruption of teeth and appearance of ossification centers.

3.   GLUCOCORTICOIDS (adrenal cortex)

These hormones, so frequently used in the management of allergic and rheumatic disease, inhibit protein synthesis and cell growth and are antiosteogenic. This is clearly evident in the reduction of osteocalcin levels in patients on cortisol therapy, and creates a real problem of osteopenia in patients on prolonged cortisol therapy .

4.   GONADAL STEROIDS (ovary and testis)

The role of the gonadal steroids in the morphometric development of the skeleton have long been recognized, but they also have an important function in maintaining the integrity of bone. Removal of the gonads by castration (Foresta et al., 1985) or ovariectomy (Gordan and Vaughan, 1980) is associated with a loss of bone mass, which is associated with decreasing levels of calcitonin. Indeed, the most important cause of osteoporosis is the loss of gonadal hormones after the menopause. Even the temporary loss of ovarian function in some athletes and in patients with anorexia nervosa is associated with serious loss of bone mineral (Brotman and Stern, 1985).

C.   LOCAL FACTORS

In recent years, over 30 local factors have been discovered which regulate bone at the cellular level (Raisz, 1989A, 1989B). These include prostaglandins, cytokines such as OAF (Osteoclast Activating Factor) and interleukins and interferon, as well as local growth factors and colony stimulating factors. None are currently used therapeutically, but they do have a potential in the treatment of local lesions such as fracture healing. One of the most promising is osteogenin, a specific polypeptide which has been isolated by Sampath et al. (1987), and is discussed in detail by Reddi in this volume. Because it is a potent stimulator of osteogenesis, it should have a potential in human therapy.

INORGANIC FACTORS (Calcium and Phosphate)

It has long been known that the level of Ca and phosphate in the plasma has an important effect on bone mineralization, so that a CaxP product of less than 40 led to impaired mineralization and rickets (in the young) or osteomalacia (in adults). The homeostatic mechanisms described above to keep these levels within the normal range are so efficient that there is no significant drop in plasma calcium even when the calcium intake is deficient. However, a severe deficiency of phosphate in young rats produces a rapid loss of mineral from the skeleton to provide for the phosphate needs of the soft tissues (Day and McCollum, 1939), while the hypophosphatemia produced by such a regimen was associated with a marked reduction in the response to both PTH and calcitonin (Copp, 1971).

CURRENT TRENDS IN USE OF BONE REGULATORY FACTORS AS THERAPEUTIC AGENTS

With increased understanding of the bone regulatory factors, there has been increased use of these agents in treating bone diseases. Of these, the most important has been postmenopausal osteoporosis – the accelerated bone loss which occurs in women after the menopause, which leads to fractures of spine, wrist and hip. This condition affects one in four women over age 65 and is estimated to cost the health care system in North America over $8 billion per year. Two hundred years ago, this was not a problem, since few women lived past the menopause. It is a tribute to our health care system that women may expect to spend a third of their lives beyond the period of reproductive activity. Postmenopausal bone loss is a consequence of this achievement, and a challenge to physicians who wish to make these years comfortable and productive. Prophylaxis for this condition consists primarily by building up the bone mass during adolescence and early adulthood by assuring adequate exercise and a high calcium intake, particularly during pregnancy and lactation. Once menopause has occurred, it is now generally agreed that in addition to the above, there should be replacement of the ovarian hormones no longer secreted by the ovary (Osteoporosis Consensus Conference, 1985). There appears to be a strong racial factor in this disease. Alhava and Puittinen (1973) have shown that the incidence of hip fractures in women in Sweden, Israel, Hong Kong and Finland increased rapidly after the menopause in women. The sole exceptions were the bantu women in Johannesburg. This occurred in spite of a very poor diet (low in calcium and other nutrients). An explanation may be the relatively high levels of calcitonin observed in black men and women compared to caucasians (Stevenson et al., 1984). This may reflect an adaptation to the high solar incidence and resulting high level of production of calcitriol in blacks. Nonetheless, it is important to recognize that, in general, blacks do not develop osteoporosis.

The disease, which affects primarily postmenopausal caucasian and oriental women, results from the lower bone mass and plasma calcitonin levels compared to men (Parthemore and Deftos, 1978; Hillyard et al., 1978) and the accelerated bone loss which occurs after the menopause, with the sudden reduction in estrogens and fall in plasma calcitonin (Milhaud et al., 1978). The current recommendation for prevention and control of this condition (Osteoporosis Consensus Conference, 1985) is an adequate calcium intake, appropriate exercise, and a low dose and cycled estrogen/progestin replacement therapy (Gordan and Vaughan, 1980; Maresca, 1985). There is considerable evidence that estrogens stimulate endogenous calcitonin secretion (Stevenson and Evans, 1982) and that this may, in fact, be an important factor in the response. Fears concerning possible increases in ovarian and uterine cancer have now been largely dispelled, and there is the additional benefit of reduced incidence of heart disease.

However, there is still the problem of those who, for a number of reasons cannot tolerate estrogen therapy, or those in which osteoporosis is far advanced and symptomatic (e.g. fractures) and more specific therapy may be indicated. This is still an area of major controversy, particularly since assessment of the efficacy of treatment requires long and precise measurement of changes in bone density (using the most accurate and reproducible procedures such as dual photon X-ray absorption densitometry (DPX). It is an expensive and time consuming investigation. These problems will be considered in evaluating the current trends in the use of bone regulatory factors in human therapy.

It is significant that the same risks occur for hypogonadal men in whom low levels of testosterone and calcitonin are associated with osteoporosis, while administration of testosterone restored the calcitonin levels (Foresta et al., 1985) and presumably had the same beneficial effects as estrogens had in women. Calcitonin has also been effective in the treatment of established osteoporosis, where it prevents further bone loss and may increase skeletal mass, at the same time reducing pain and increasing mobility (Aloia, 1985; Francheschini et al., 1984; Gennari et al., 1985; Mazzuoli, 1986). Indeed, the analgesic effect of calcitonin may prove to be of major importance.

Parathyroid Hormone

While not officially approved for general use in treatment of osteoporosis, in clinical trials, the 1-34 fragment of bovine PTH has been shown to increase (Slovik et al., 1986). It may have a useful role in ADFR (Activate, Depress, Free, Repeat) therapy, through activation of osteogenesis.

Calcitriol

Calcitriol is well established as a therapeutic agent, either by itself, or as its immediate precursor, 1-alpha-hydroxycholecalciferol which is converted to calcitriol in the kidney. In Japan, the 1-alpha-cholecalciferol is used extensively in the treatment of osteoporosis (70%); there are also reports of its efficacy in treatment of osteoporosis (Canniggia, et al., 1988). The rational is based on the assumption that the dietary calcium intake and absorption from the gut is reduced with age, along with a reduced synthesis of calctriol, so that the loss of bone is really due to calcium deficiency. Although this is certainly a rational approach, and assurance of an adequate dietary and vitamin D intake is important in the management of osteoporosis, use of calcitriol should be considered only when there is a positive indication.

However, in addition to the use of calcitriol in osteoporosis, it should be recognized that it has an important place in the treatment of renal osteodystrophy (when loss of renal cells interferes with the normal synthesis of calcitriol). It is also the treatment of choice in certain types of rickets. Recently, there has been special interest in its action to cause maturation of hemopoietic cells (Abe et al., 1981) with a potential for the treatment of leukemia if a derivative can be obtained with this effect but without stimulating osteolysis.

CALCITONIN

Calcitonin is by far the most extensively used of the bone regulatory factors in human therapy. World sales in 1988 exceeded $500 million US and approached those of insulin. It has been used primarily in treatment of osteoporosis (80%), Paget's disease (10%) and relief of pain (10%), although it also appears to have a role in controlling pain and in the management of acute pancreatitis.

Tumor marker: The radioimmunoassay for human calcitonin has proven to be particularly useful in detecting patients with medullary carcinoma of the thyroid--an inherited tumor of the C cells which is associated with high levels of calcitonin in the plasma (Goltzman et al., 1974). It has been used to screen families at risk and to determine the effectiveness of surgical removal of the tumor. It also appears to be useful diagnostically in patients with bronchogenic cancer (Silva et al., 1979).

Therapeutic Use: This has been reviewed by Stevenson and Evans (1982) and Austin and Heath (1981). It is based primarily on its established anti-osteolytic action (Rico, 1985), although recent studies suggest that it may also have a useful role as an analgesic agent (Szanto et al., 1986). Calcitonin has been used to treat the intractable pain in patients with terminal cancer (Allen, 1983). The early experiments which indicated a homeostatic role in controlling hypercalcemia clearly indicate a potential therapeutic use in this condition in patients with active osteolytic bone disease (Silva and Becker, 1973) such as hyperparathyroidism (Au, 1975) and multiple myeloma (Behn and West, 1977). It has also been used to treat the hypercalcemia resulting from prolonged immobilization (Carey and Raisz, 1985), a matter of some importance to astronauts. It is the preferred treatment of Paget's disease of bone (Avramides, 1977; Martin, 1981)--a disease affecting 2-4% of the population over age 60, which is characterized by high bone turn-over, fractures, pain and immobilization. De Rose et al. (1974) reported effective treatment of this condition with porcine and salmon calcitonin over a 3 year period, in spite of the development of neutralizing antibodies in 30% of the patients receiving salmon calcitonin and 60% of those receiving the porcine hormone. The availability of synthetic human calcitonin may reduce this problem (Singer, 1977).

However, the greatest potential use of calcitonin is in the treatment of osteoporosis (Rico, 1985; Maresca, 1985)--a condition in which the bone mass is reduced to the point at which fractures of spine, wrist and hip occur spontaneously or with minimal trauma. Major problems in the widespread use of calcitonin, particularly as a prophylactic approach to osteoporosis, are the high cost (which may be solved by recombinant DNA technology) and the parenteral route of administration. Many patients accept the latter, as do diabetics, because of the relief of pain. However, a number of approaches have been investigated, including an intranasal spray, orally administered liospheres containing calcitonin, and rectal administration. The intranasal spray is the only one to be widely used, and appears to be effective in Paget's disease (Reginster et al., 1985).

OTHER FACTORS

In recent years, a number of factors have been used therapeutically which are not true bone regulatory factors but which do have an important effect on bone metabolism. While they are not in the purview of this paper, they should be mentioned. Foremost are the diphosphonates, which block bone resorption and are widely used in the management of osteoporosis. The early diphosphonates also produced a kind of osteomalacia (not seen with the second generation of these compounds). There is also wide spread use of fluoride as an osteogenic agent, based in part on the observation that osteoporosis is rare in women living in areas of high natural fluoride, and the well documented fact that F administration increases bone mass. However, in a retrospective study of 416 osteoporotics treated with F for more than 1000 patient years, Riggs et al. (1987) found no significant effect on the incidence of hip fractures.

CONCLUSIONS

The growing multiplicity of bone regulatory factors has provided major opportunities for their use in the management of bone disease. It is important that this be based on solid physiological grounds. Currently, the major problem is the management of postmenopausal osteoporosis, and the most promising approach is diet (calcium, vitamins and proteins), exercise and ovarian hormone replacement (or testicular hormones for the male) and calcitonin and diphosphonates when the loss of bone mineral is producing fractures. Calcitonin may also have an important role as a very potent and safe analgesic.

REFERENCES

Abe, E., Miyaura, C., Sakagami, H.,Takeda,M., Konno, K., Yamazaki, T., Yoshiki, S., and Suda, S. (1981). Differentiation of mouse myeloid leukemia cells induced by 1-alpha-dihydroxyvitamin D_3. Proc. Nat. Acad.Sci.USA 78: 4990-4994.

Alhava, E.M., and Puittinnen, J. (1973). Fractures of the upper end of the femur as an index of senile osteoporosis in Finland. Ann. Clin. Res. 5, 398-403.

Allen, E. (1983). Calcitonin in the treatment of intractable pain from advanced malignancy. Pharmatherapeutica 3, 482-486.

Aloia, J.F. (1985). Calcitonin and osteoporosis. Geriatric Medicine Today 4, 20-28.

Amara, S.G., Jonas, V., Rosenfeld, M.G., Ong, E.S., and Evan, R.M. (1982). Alternative RNA processing of calcitonin gene expression generates mRNAs encoding different polypeptide products. Nature 298, 240-244.

Au, W.Y.N. (1975). Calcitonin treatment of hypercalcaemia due to parathyroid carcinoma. Arch. Intern. Med. 135, 1594-1597.

Austin, L.A., and Heath, H. (1981). Calcitonin: Physiology and Pathophysiology. New Engl. J. Med. 304, 269-278.

Avramides, A. (1977). Salmon and porcine calcitonin treatment of Paget's disease of bone. Clin. Orthopaed. 127, 78-85.

Azria, M. (1989). "The Calcitonins--Physiology and Pharmacology". S.Karger, Basel. 152 pages.

Behn, A.R., and West, T.E.T. (1977). Emergency treatment with calcitonin of hypercalcemia associated with multiple myeloma. Br. Med. J. 1, 755-766.

Bijvoet, A.L.M., van der Sluys Veer, J.V.D., De Vries, H.R., and van Koppen, A.T.J. (1971). Natriuretic effect of calcitonin in man. New Engl. J. Med. 284, 681-688.

Boyle, I.T., Gray, R.W., and DeLuca, H.F. (1971). Regulation by calcium of in vitro synthesis of 1,25 dihydroxycholecalciferol and 21,25 dihydroxycholecalciferol. Proc. Natl. Acad. Sci. USA 68, 2131-2134.

Braga, P., Ferri, S., Santagostino, A., Olgiati, V.R., and Pecile, A. (1978). Lack of opiate receptor involvement in centrally induced calcitonin induced analgesia. Life Sciences 22: 971-978.

Brain, S.D., and Williams, T.J. (1985). Calcitonin gene-related peptide is a potent vasodilator. Nature 313, 54-56.

Brain, S.D., MacIntyre, I., and Williams, T.J. (1986). A second form of human calcitonin gene-related peptide which is a potent vasodilator. Eur. J. Pharmacol. 124, 349-352.

Brotman, A.W., and Stern, T.A. (1985). Osteoporosis and pathological fractures in anorexia nervosa. Am.J.Psychiatr. 142: 495-496.

Cannigia, A., Nuti, R., Lore, F., Martini, G., Righi, G., and Turchetti, V. (1988). Long-term calcitriol treatment in postmenopausal osteoporosis: Follow up of two hundred patients. In: Vitamin D Molecular, Cellular and Clinical Endocrinology. Proc. 7th Workshop on Vitamin D., April, 1988. Eds. A.W. Norman, K. Schaefer, H.-G. Grigoleit, and D. v. Herrath. Walter de Gruyter, Berlin. pp. 807-816.

Care, A.D., Bates, R.F.L., Swaminathan, R., Scanes, C.G., Peacock, M., Mawer, E.B., Taylor, C.M., DeLuca, H.F., Tomlinson, S., and O'Riordan, J.L.H. (1975). The control of parathyroid hormone and calcitonin secretion and interaction with other endocrine systems. In: "Calcium Regulating Hormones", eds. R.V.Talmage, M.Owen, and J.A.Parsons, Excerpta Medica, Amsterdam, ICS 346, pp. 100-110.

Carey, D.E., and Raisz, L.G. (1985). Calcitonin therapy in prolonged immobilization hypercalcemia. Arch. Phys. Med. Rehabil. 66, 640-644.

Cesarani, R., Colombo, M., Olgiati, V.R., and Pecile, A. (1979). Calcitonin and prostaglandin system. Life Sciences 25: 1851-1856.

Clementi, G., Amico-Roxas, M., Rapisardi, E., Caruso, A., Prato, A., Trombadore, S., Priolo, G., and Scapagnini, U. (1985). The analgesic action of calcitonin and the control of the serotoninergic system. Eur. J.Pharmacol. 108, 71-75.

Collip. J.B. (1925). The extraction of a parathyroid hormone which will prevent or control parathyroid tetany and which regulates the level of blood calcium. J.Biol.Chem. 63: 395-438.

Copp, D.H. (1967). Hormonal control of hypercalcemia. Historic development of the calcitonin concept. Am. J. Med. 43, 648-655.

Copp, D.H. (1969). Endocrine control of calcium homeostasis. J. Endocrinol. 43, 137-161.

Copp, H. (1971). Effets d'un regime pauvre en phosphore sur l'homeostasie du calcium et de l'ion phosphate chez le rat jeune. In: "Phosphate et Metabolisme Phosphocalcique." Ed. D.J. Hioco. Sandoz Laboratories, L'Expansion Scientifique Francaise, Paris pp. 111-116.

Copp, D.H., and Shim, S.S. (1965). Extraction ratio of Sr^{85} as a measure of effective bone blood flow. Circulation Res. 16: 461-467.

Copp, D.H., and Davidson, A.G.F. (1961). Direct humoral control of parathyroid function in the dog. Proc. Soc. Exp. Biol. Med. 107, 342-344.

Copp, D.H., Davidson, A.G.F., and Cheney, B.A. (1961). Evidence for a new parathyroid hormone which lowers blood calcium. Proc. Can. Fed. Biol. Soc. 4, 17.

Copp, D.H., Cameron, E.C., Cheney, B., Davidson, A.G.F., and Henze, K. (1962). Evidence for calcitonin--a new hormone from the parathyroid that lowers blood calcium. Endocrinology 70, 638-649.

Copp, D.H., Cockcroft, D.W., and Kueh, Y. (1967). Calcitonin from ultimobranchial glands from dogfish and chickens. Science 158, 924-925.

Day, H.G., and McCollum, E.V. (1939). Mineral metabolism, growth and symptomatology of rats on a diet extremely deficient in phosphorus. J.Biol.Chem. 130: 269-283.

DeLuca, H.F. (1974). Vitamin D : the vitamin and the hormone. Federation Proc. 33: 2211-2219.

DeRose, J., Singer, F., Avramides, A., Flores, A., Dziadiw, R., Baker, R.K., and Wallach, S. (1974). Response of Paget's disease to porcine and salmon calcitonins. Am. J. Med. 56, 858-866.

Foresta, C., Zanata, G.P., Busnardo, B., Scanelli, G., and Scandellari, C. (1985). Testosterone and calcitonin plasma levels in hypogonadal osteoporotic young men. J. Endocrinol. Invest. 8, 377-379.

Francheschini, R., Bottaro, P., Panapoulos, C., and Messina, V. (1984). Long term treatment with salmon calcitonin in postmenopausal osteoporosis. Current Therapeut. Res. 34, 795-800.

Friedman, J., and Raisz, L.G. (1965). Thyrocalcitonin: inhibitor of bone resorption in tissue culture. Science 150: 1465-1467.

Gennari, C., and Fischer, J.A. (1985). Cardiovascular action of calcitonin gene-related peptide in humans. Calcif. Tiss. Intern. 37, 581-584.

Gennari, C., Chierichetti, S.M., Bigazzi, S., Fusi, L., Gonneli, S., Ferrara, R., and Zacchei, F. (1985). Comparative effects on bone mineral content of calcium and calcium plus salmon calcitonin given in two different regimens in postmenopausal osteoporosis. Current Therapeut. Res. 38, 455-464.

Gibson, S.J., Polak, J.M., Bloom, S.R., Sabate, I.M., Mulderry, P.M., Chatel, M.A., McGregor, G.P., Morrison, J.F.B., Kelly, J.S., Evans, R.M., and Rosenfeld, M.G. (1984). Calcitonin gene-related peptide immunoreactivity in the spinal cord of man and eight other species. J. Neurosciences 4, 2101-2111.

Girgis, S.I., Stevenson, J.C., Lynch, C., Self, C.H., MacDonald, D.W.R. Bevis, P.J.R., Wimalawansa, S., Morris, H.R., and MacIntyre, I. (1985). Calcitonin gene-related peptide: potent vasodilator and major product of the calcitonin gene. The Lancet ii,14-16.

Goltzman, D., Potts, J.T., Ridgway, E.C., and Maloof, F. (1974). Calcitonin as a tumor marker--use of the radioimmunoassay for calcitonin in the post-operative evaluation of patients with medullary carcinoma. New Eng. J. Med. 290, 1035-1039.

Gordan, G.S., and Vaughan, C. (1980). Use of sex steroids in the clinical management of osteoporosis. In "Clinical Use of Sex Steroids" (Givens, J.R., ed.), pp. 69-94, Yearbook Medical Publishers, Chicago.

Gray, T.K., and Munson, P.L. (1969). Thyrocalcitonin--evidence for a physiological function. Science 166, 1512-1513.

Guttmann, S. (1981). Chemistry and structure-activity relationships of natural and synthetic calcitonins. In: Calcitonin 1980, Proc. Int. Symposium in Milan. Ed. A.Pecile. Excerpta Medica Int. Congr.Ser. 51: 11-24. Amsterdam.

Guttman, S., Pless, J., Huguenin, R.L., Sandrin, E., Bossert, H., and Zehnder, K. (1969). Synthese von Salm-Calcitonin, einem hochaktiven hypocalcamischen Hormon. Helv. Chim. Acta 52, 1789-1795.

Henke, H., Tobler, P.H., and Fischer, J.A. (1983). Localization of salmon calcitonin binding sites in rat brain by autoradiography. Brain Res. 272, 371-377.

Hillyard, C.J., Stevenson, J.C., and MacIntyre, I. (1978). Relative deficiency of plasma-calcitonin in normal women. The Lancet i, 961-962.

Hirsch, P.F., Voelkel, E.F., and Munson, P.L. (1964). Thyrocalcitonin: hypocalcemic hypophosphatemic principle of the thyroid gland. Science 146, 412-413.

Hock,J.M., Hummert,J.R., Boyce, R. Fonseca, J., and Raisz, L.G. (1985) Resorption is not essential for the stimulation of bone growth by bPTH (1-34) in rats in vivo. J.Bone & Mineral Res. 4, 449-458.

Kallio, D.M., Garant, P.R., and Minkin, C. (1972). Ultrastructural effects of calcitonin on osteoclasts in tissue culture. J. Ultrastruct. Res. 39, 205-216.

Keeler, R., Walker, V., and Copp, D.H. (1970). Natriuretic and diuretic effects of salmon calcitonin in rats. Can. J. Physiol. Pharmacol. 48, 838-841.

Kittur, S.D., Hoppener, J.W.M., Antonarakis, S.E., Daniels, J.D.J., Meyers, D.A., Maestri, N.E., Jansen, M., Korneluk, R.G., Nelkin, B.D., and Kazazian, H.H. (1985). Linkage map of the short arm of human chromosome 11: location of the genes for catalase, calcitonin and insulin-like growth factor II. Proc. Natl. Acad. Sci. (USA) 82, 5064-5067.

Klein, D.C., and Talmage, R.V. (1968). Thyrocalcitonin suppression of hydroxyproline release from bone. Proc. Soc. Exp. Biol. Med. 127, 95-99.

Kodicek, E. (1974). The story of vitamin D, from vitamin to hormone. The Lancet i, 325- 329.

Le Douarin, N., and Le Lievre, C. (1970). Demonstration de l'origine neurales des cellules a calcitonine du corps ultimobranchial chez l'embryon poulet. C.R.Acad.Sci. Paris 270, 2857-2860.

Lee, Y., Takami, K., Kawai, Y., Girgis, S.I., Hillyard, C.J., MacIntyre, I., Emson, P.C., and Toyama, M. (1985). Distribution of calcitonin gene-related peptide in the rat peripheral nervous system with reference to its coexistence with substance P. Neuroscience 15, 1227-1237.

Levine, A.S., and Morley, J.E. (1981). Reduction of feeding in rats by calcitonin. Brain Res. 222, 187-191.

Lewis, P., Rafferty, B., Shelley, M., and Robinson, C.J. (1970). A suggested physiological role for calcitonin: the protection of the skeleton during pregnancy and lactation. J. Endocrinol. 49, ix-x.

MacCallum, W.G., Voegtlin, C. (1909). On the relation of tetany to the parathyroid glands and to calcium metabolism. J.Exp.Med. 11: 118-151.

MacDonald, B.R., Gallagher, J.A., and Russell, R.G.G. (1986). Parathyroid hormone stimulates the proliferation of cells derived from human bone. Endocrinology 118: 2445-2449.

MacIntyre, I. (1984). Katacalcin: discovery of a new hormone with implications for our general concepts of treatment in bone disease. Acta Med. Austriaca (Suppl). 30, 17-18.

MacIntyre, I., and Craig, R.K. (1981). Molecular evolution of the calcitonins. In: "Neuropeptides--Basic and Clinical Aspects." (Proc. 11th Pfizer Internat. Symposium) pp. 254-258. Churchill Livingston, Edinburgh.

MacIntyre, I., Hillyard, C.J., Murphy, RP.K., Reynolds, J.J., Das, R.E.G., and Craig, R.K. (1982). A second plasma calcium-lowering peptide from the human calcitonin precursor. Nature 300, 460-462.

McLean, F.C. (1957). The parathyroids and bone. Clin.Orthopaed. 9, 46-60.

Marcus, R., and Aurbach, G.D. (1969). Bioassay of parathyroid hormone in vitro with a stable preparation of adenyl-cyclase from rat kidney. Endocrinology 85, 801-810.

Maresca, V. (1985). Human calcitonin in the management of osteoporosis: a multicentre study. J. Int. Med. Res. 13, 311-361.

Martin, T.J. (1981). Treatment of Paget's disease with calcitonin. Aust. N. Z. J. Med. 9, 36-43.

Marx, S.J., Woodward, C.J., and Aurbach, G.D. (1972). Calcitonin receptors of kidney and bone. Science 178, 999-1000.

Mazzuoli, G.F., Passeri, M., Gennari, C., Minisola, S., Antonelli, R., Valorta, C., Palunneri, E., Cervellin, G.F., Gonnelli, S., and Francini, G. (1986). Effects of salmon calcitonin in postmenopausal osteoporosis: a controlled double-blind study. Calcif. Tissue. Internat. 38, 3-8.

Milhaud, G., Benezech-Lefevre, M, and Moukhtar, M.S. (1978). Deficiency of calcitonin in age related osteoporoses. Biomedicine 29, 272-276.

Morikawa, T., Munekata, E., Sakakibara, S., Noda, T., and Otani, M. (1976). Synthesis of eel calcitonin and (Asu 1,7)-eel-calcitonin: Contribution of the disulfide bond to the hormonal activity. Experientia 32, 1104-1106.

Morley, J.E., and Levine, A.S. (1981). Intraventricular calcitonin inhibits gastric acid secretion. Science 214, 671-673.

Moseley, J.M., Kubota, M., Diefenbach-Jagger, H., Wettenhall, R.H., Suva, L.J., Rodda, C.P., Ebeling, P.R., Hudson, P.J., Zajac, J.D., and Martin, T.J. (1987). Parathyroid hormone-related protein purified from a lung cancer. Proc. Nat. Acad. Sci. USA 4, 5048-5053.

Neher, R., Riniker, B., Rittel, W., and Zuber, H. (1986). Menschliches calcitonin. III. Struktur von calcitonin M. und D. Helv. Chim. Acta 51, 1900-1905.

Niall, J.T., Keutmann, H.T., Copp, D.H., and Potts, J.T. (1969). Amino acid sequence of salmon ultimobranchial calcitonin. Proc. Natl. Acad. Sci USA 63, 771-778.

Niall, H.D., Keutmann, H.T., Sauer, R., Hogan, M., Dawson, B.F., Aurbach, G.D., and Potts, Jr., J.T. (1970). The amino-acid sequence of bovine parathyroid hormone. Hoppe-Seylers Z. Physiol. Chem. 351, 1586-1588.

O'Dor, R.K., Parkes, C.O., and Copp, D.H (1969). Amino acid composition of salmon calcitonin. Can. J. Biochem. 47, 823-825.

Osteoporosis - Consensus Conference. (1986). J. A. M. A. 252, 799-802.

Osteoporosis - Consensus Conference. (1986). J.Am.Med.Assoc. 252, 799-802.

Otani, M., Noda, T., Yamauchi, H., Watanabe, S., Matsuda, T., Orimo, H. and Narita, K. (1975). Isolation, chemical structure and biological properties of ultimobranchial calcitonin of the eel. In: "Calcium Regulating Hormones", eds. R.V.Talmage, M.Owen and J.A.Parsons, Excerpta Medica, Amsterdam, ICS   pp. 111-115.

Parsons, J.A., and Reynolds, J.J. (1968). Species discrimination between calcitonins. The Lancet i, 1067-1070.

Parthemore, J.C., and Deftos, L.J. (1978). Calcitonin secretion in normal human subjects. J.Clin.Endocrinol. & Metab. 47, 184-188.

Pearse, A.G.E. (1966). The cytochemistry of the thyroid C cells and their relationship to calcitonin. Proc. Roy. Soc. London (Ser. B) 164, 478-487.

Pearse, A.G.E., and Carvalheira, A.F. (1967). Cytochemical evidence for an ultimobranchial origin of rodent thyroid C cells. Nature 214, 929-930.

Pecile, A., Ferri, S., Braga, P.C., and Olgiati, V.R. (1975). Effects of intracerebroventricular calcitonin in the conscious rabbit. Experientia 31, 332-333.

Potts, J.T., Niall, H.D., Keutmann, H.T., Brewer, H.B., and Deftos, L.J. (1968). The amino acid sequence of porcine thyrocalcitonin. Proc. Natl. Acad. Sci. USA 59, 1321-1328.

Raisz, L.G. (1988a). Bone metabolism and its regulation: an update. Triangle 27, 5-10.

Raisz, L.G. (1988b). Local and systemic factors in the pathogenesis of osteoporosis. New Engl. J. Med. 318, 818-828.

Reichel, H., Koefler, H.P., and Norman, A.W. (1989). The role of the vitamin D endocrine system in health and disease. New Engl. J. Med. 320, 980-991.

Reginster, J.Y., Albert, A., and Franchimont, P. (1985). Salmon-calcitonin nasal spray in Paget's disease of bone: preliminary results in five patients. Calcif. Tiss. Internat. 37, 577-580.

Reynolds, J.J. (1968). Inhibition by calcitonin of bone resorption induced in vitro by vitamin A. Proc. Roy. Soc. London (Ser. B) 170, 61-69.

Rico, H. (1985). Calcitonin and treatment of osteoporosis. J. Med. 16, 493-495.

Riggs, B.L., Baylink, D.J., Kleerekoper, M., Lane, J.M., Melton, L.J., and Meunier, P.J. (1987). Incidence of hip fractures in osteoporotic women treated with sodium fluoride. J.Bone and Mineral Res. 2, 123-126.

Rohner, A., and Planche, D. (1985). Mechanism of the analgesic effect of calcitonin. Evidence for a two-fold effect: morphine-like and cortisone-like. Clin. Rheumatol. 4, 218-219.

Sampath, T.K., Muthukumaran, N., and Reddi, H.(1987). Isolation of osteogenin, an extracellular matrix associated bone-inductive protein by heparin affinity chromatography. Proc. Nat. Acad. Sci. USA, 84, 7109-7113.

Silva, O.L., and Becker, K.K. (1973). Salmon calcitonin in the treatment of hypercalcaemia. Arch. Int. Med. 132. 337-339.

Silva, O.L., Broder, L.E., Dippman, J.L., Snider, R.H., Moore, C.F., Cohen, M.H., and Becker, K. (1979). Calcitonin as a marker for bronchogenic cancer. Cancer 44, 680-684.

Singer, F.R. (1977). Human calcitonin treatment of Paget's disease of bone. Clin. Orthopaed. 127, 86-93.

Slovik, D.M., Rosenthal, D.I., Doppelt, S.H., Potts, J.T., Daly, M.A. Campbell, J.A., and Neer, R.M. (1986). Restoration of spinal bone in osteoporotic men by treatment with human parathyroid hormone (1-34) amd 1,25-dihydroxyvitamin D. J. Bone Mineral Res. 1, 37-381.

Stevenson, J.C., and Evans, I.M.A. (1982). Oestrogens, calcitonin and parathyroid hormone secretion. Maturitas 4, 1-7.

Stevenson, J.C., Myers, C.H., and Ajdukiewics, (1984). Racial differences in calcitonin and katacalcin. Calcif. Tiss. Int. 36, 725-728.

Struthers, A.D., Brown, M.J., Macdonald, D.W.R., Beacham, J.L., Stevenson, J.C., Morris, H.R., and MacIntyre, I. (1986). Human calcitonin gene-related peptide: a potent endogenous vasodilator in man. Clin. Sci. 70, 389-393.

Szanto, J., Jozsef, S., Rado, J., Juhos, E., Hindy, I., and Eckhardt, S. (1986). Pain killing with calcitonin in patients with malignant tumors. Oncology 43, 69-72.

Tanaka, Y., and DeLuca, H.F. (1973). The control of 25-hydroxyvitamin D metabolism by inorganic phosphate. Arch. Biochem. Biophys. 154, 566-571.

Tauber, S.D. (1967). The ultimobranchial origin of thyrocalcitonin. Proc. Nat. Acad. Sci.USA, 58, 1684-1687.

Tippins, J.R., Morris, H.R., Panico, M., Etienne, T., Bevis, P., Girgis, S., MacIntyre, I., Azria, M., and Attinger, M. (1984). The myotrophic and plasma-calcium modulating effects of calcitonin gene-related peptide (CGRP). Neuropeptides 4, 425-434.

Wolfe, H.J. (1982). Calcitonin: perspectives and current concepts. J. Endocrinol. Invest. 5, 423-432.

Zaidi, M., Bevis, P.J.R., Abeyasekera, G., Girgis, S.I., Wimalawansa, S.J., Morris, H.R. and MacIntyre, I. (1986). The origin of circulating calcitonin gene-related peptide in the rat. J. Endocrinol. 110, 185-190.

AUTHOR INDEX

SUBJECT INDEX